QUACK MEDICINE

**Recent Titles in
Healing Society: Disease, Medicine, and History**
John Parascandola, Series Editor

From Snake Oil to Medicine: Pioneering Public Health
R. Alton Lee

A History of Multiple Sclerosis
Colin Talley

Sex, Sin, and Science: A History of Syphilis in America
John Parascandola

A History of Infectious Diseases and the Microbial World
Lois N. Magner

A History of the Birth Control Movement in America
Peter C. Engelman

QUACK MEDICINE

A History of Combating Health Fraud in Twentieth-Century America

ERIC W. BOYLE

Healing Society: Disease, Medicine, and History
John Parascandola, Series Editor

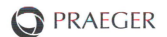 PRAEGER

AN IMPRINT OF ABC-CLIO, LLC
Santa Barbara, California • Denver, Colorado • Oxford, England

Copyright 2013 by Eric W. Boyle

All rights reserved. No part of this publication may be reproduced, stored in a retrieval system, or transmitted, in any form or by any means, electronic, mechanical, photocopying, recording, or otherwise, except for the inclusion of brief quotations in a review, without prior permission in writing from the publisher.

Library of Congress Cataloging-in-Publication Data

Boyle, Eric W.
    Quack medicine : a history of combating health fraud in twentieth-century America / Eric W. Boyle.
        p. cm. — (Healing society: disease, medicine, and history)
    Includes bibliographical references and index.
    ISBN 978–0–313–38567–4 (hardcopy : alk. paper) — ISBN 978–0–313–38568–1 (e-book) 1. Quacks and quackery—United States—History. I. Title.
    R730.B69   2013
    615.8′56—dc23   2012028059

ISBN: 978–0–313–38567–4
EISBN: 978–0–313–38568–1

17 16 15 14   2 3 4 5

This book is also available on the World Wide Web as an eBook.
Visit www.abc-clio.com for details.

Praeger
An Imprint of ABC-CLIO, LLC

ABC-CLIO, LLC
130 Cremona Drive, P.O. Box 1911
Santa Barbara, California 93116-1911

This book is printed on acid-free paper ∞

Manufactured in the United States of America

This book is dedicated to my mother, Gail Marie

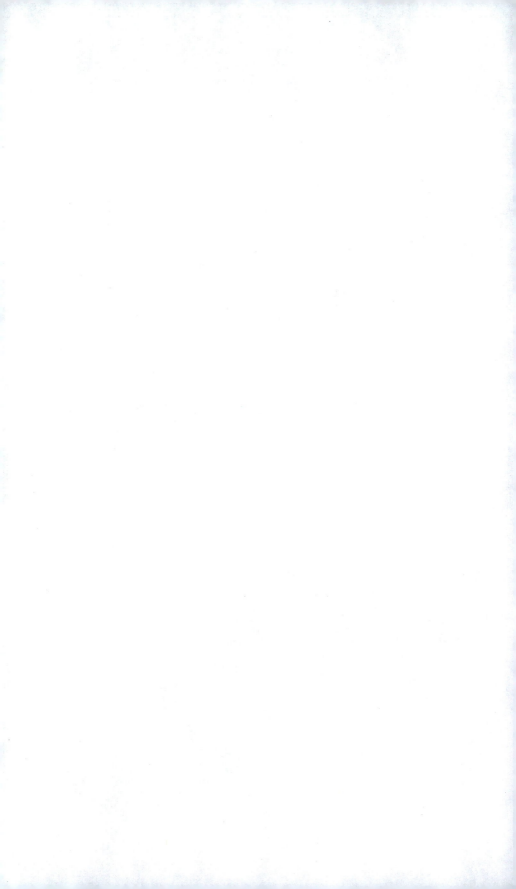

CONTENTS

Contents

SERIES FOREWORD

The Praeger series *Healing Society: Disease, Medicine, and History* features individual volumes that explore the social impact of particular illnesses or medically related conditions or topics for a broad audience. The object is to publish books that offer reliable overviews of particular aspects of medical and social history while incorporating the most up-to-date scholarly interpretations. The books in the series are designed to engage readers and educate them about important but often neglected aspects of the social history of medicine. Disease and disability have significantly influenced the course of human history, and the books in this series will examine various aspects of that influence.

Quack Medicine: A History of Combating Health Fraud in Twentieth-Century America is about an important and fascinating aspect of the history of medicine that is the efforts of reformers to curb the charlatans who prey on the unfortunate victims of disease. Quackery is as old as medicine and will undoubtedly remain with us in some form as long as there are sick people and unscrupulous charlatans willing to take advantage of them. Eric Boyle traces the history of the antiquackery crusade in the United States from its beginnings in the nineteenth century up through the present day.

Boyle places the history of medical quackery in America within a broader social and cultural context. He examines the roles of the various players involved in combating health fraud in the United States, from organized medicine to muckraking journalists to consumer advocates to government agencies. He traces the development of legislation and regulatory requirements aimed at controlling the sale of questionable medicines and medical services. Boyle also explores the reasons for the persistent appeal of medical quackery, which has resisted the efforts of reformers to eliminate it, concluding that by the end of the twentieth century quackery was better controlled, "but arguably still as popular as ever."

The book expands on previous work on the history of quackery and efforts to combat it, and will be of considerable interest to scholars of medical history, health professionals, and government regulators. Given the continued significance of health fraud in today's world, it should also appeal to members of the general public who wish to learn more about the subject.

—John Parascandola

ACKNOWLEDGMENTS

Many people have made this book possible. First, I owe thanks to my colleagues and advisers. From my time in graduate school at the University of California–Santa Barbara (UCSB) to my postdoctoral work at the Office of History at the National Institutes of Health, many people have offered kind encouragement, sharp critiques, and thoughtful advice. Many helpful comments and suggestions have come from audience members at various conference presentations as well. I apologize for not being able to acknowledge by name all the people who have generously offered their help along the way. I would also like to express my gratitude to countless librarians, archivists, historians, and staff members who have helped me acquire, engage, and understand the materials necessary for completing my research. I want to specifically thank the generous people who helped me navigate the following collections on which this book is based: the College of Physicians of Philadelphia Library, the American Medical Association Archives, the American Institute of the History of Pharmacy, the American Philosophical Society Library, the National Library of Medicine, the Francis A. Countway Library of Medicine, the Library of Congress, the Social Welfare History Archives at the University of Minnesota, the Carnegie Institution Archives, and the New York Academy of Medicine Library.

My research has been funded by several generous sources, including the UCSB Graduate Division; the UCSB History Department; the UCSB History Associates;

the UCSB New Visions of Nature, Science and Religion Program; the UCSB Interdisciplinary Humanities Center; the UCSB Affiliates; the University of California Humanities Research Institute's Andrew and Florence White Scholarship; the American Institute of the History of Pharmacy; the University of Minnesota; the Bakken Library and Museum; the New England Regional Fellowship Consortium; the American Philosophical Society; the Rockefeller Archives Center; the National Science Foundation; and the Chemical Heritage Foundation.

To my friends and family, I owe more than I could possibly express. My father and sister have been there at every step. My second family at Cashion's generously provided love and laughter throughout. Specifically, I'd also like to thank Sarah, whose love and encouragement made it possible for me to finish this book.

ABBREVIATIONS

Organizations, Journals, Legislation, and Concepts

AMA	American Medical Association
CAM	Complementary and alternative medicine
DSHEA	Dietary Supplement Health and Education Act
FDA	Food and Drug Administration
FDCLJ	*Food, Drug and Cosmetic Law Journal*
FDCLQ	*Food, Drug and Cosmetic Law Quarterly*
FFDCA	Federal Food, Drug and Cosmetic Act
FTC	Federal Trade Commission
JAMA	*Journal of the American Medical Association*
NCAHF	National Council Against Health Fraud
NCCAM	National Center for Complementary and Alternative Medicine
NEJM	*New England Journal of Medicine*

Archives

AIHP   American Institute for the History of Pharmacy

APS   American Philosophical Society

CPP   College of Physicians of Philadelphia Library

HHF   Historical Health Fraud Collection (American Medical Association)

NA   National Archives

NLM   National Library of Medicine

SWHA   Social Welfare History Archives (University of Minnesota)

INTRODUCTION

Voltaire's dictum, that the charlatan was born when the first knave met the first fool, was but a half-truth. Quackery is rampant in many fields—in religion, in politics, in literature, in economics, and in medicine. As Voltaire had the medical field in mind when he visioned his epigram, he must stand corrected, for it is not the juxtaposition of knavery and foolishness that gives birth to the quack but that of knavery and ignorance. Credulity is bred less by a lack of brains than by a dearth of knowledge. We are all credulous when we wander in fields that are strange to us. Knowledge, rather than intelligence, is the best antidote for credulity.

—Dr. Arthur J. Cramp (1936)[1]

Dr. Arthur J. Cramp did more than perhaps anyone to combat quackery in the twentieth century. As the first director of the Bureau of Investigation of the American Medical Association (AMA), he helped establish an antiquackery surveillance network that investigated, exposed, and attempted to regulate allegedly fraudulent therapeutic approaches to health and healing under the banner of consumer protection and a commitment to medical science. These efforts to combat medical quackery shaped debates about the place of drugs in the realm of health care among medical professionals, scientists, legislators, drug makers, and consumers for much of the twentieth century. By the standards Cramp and other members of the antiquackery network set, these efforts nevertheless failed.

At the beginning of the twentieth century, reformers intent on launching a crusade against the forces of quackery faced a number of challenges that limited the impact of their work. The success of education as a primary tool for reform depended on the validity of the assumption that people made poor choices due to a lack of knowledge. As it turned out, people chose a wide range of alleged forms of quackery for a variety of other reasons. While efforts to establish, enlarge, and police the boundaries of therapeutic acceptability ultimately helped instill confidence in the authority of physicians, the standard historical narrative exaggerates the extent to which professional authority determined the therapeutic choices made by the public and physicians alike. Therapeutic reformers could measure their success in the proliferation of new regulations, new institutions, and innovative therapies, but alleged quack alternatives maintained their positions in the marketplace.[2]

Reformers also struggled with the basic task of defining the terms "quack" and "quackery." In his files, Dr. Cramp kept a folder in which he had typed out the following standard dictionary definition of a quack: "(noun): a boastful pretender to medical skill; (adjective): pertaining to, or characterized by, boasting and pretension; as, a quack medicine; a quack doctor; (verb transitive): to make extravagant claims or to advertise boastingly; to treat or to manage as a quack would." For Cramp, quackery simply consisted of the acts, arts, or pretensions of a quack. A quack boasted or bragged inordinately of his or her ability. But this did not necessarily imply either the lack of legal qualifications to practice medicine or even the complete lack of skill. In fact, Cramp admitted that many quacks were, doubtless, highly skillful, and a very large number of quacks were legally licensed to practice medicine. The quack claimed to cure diseases he simply could not. He lied about the contents of the remedy he promoted. He made promises that could not be kept. Accusing someone of being a quack, or dismissing a remedy as quackery, remained an easy task. Proving it was entirely more difficult.[3]

Aside from moral outrage and a genuine desire to protect hapless victims, reformers embraced various reasons and techniques for combating quackery. Chapter 1 begins by identifying the professional, economic, and cultural origins of the antiquackery crusade in the nineteenth century. Cognizant of a growing variety of practitioners and an expanding national drug trade, medical professionals led the crusade against quackery in the early to mid-nineteenth century by developing a two-pronged strategy: (1) educational and legal reforms from within the profession and (2) public education. Despite these efforts, a flood of self-treatment options, in the form of brand-name patent medicines, coincided with the rise of unorthodox medical systems such as Thomsonianism, homeopathy, hydropathy, chiropractic, and osteopathy. While on the eve of the Civil War the proprietary medicine industry raked in $3.5 million annually, by the turn of the twentieth century that sum had multiplied by more than 20 times. Drug promoters took advantage of promising prospects in the medical field, as well as persistent therapeutic weaknesses, in pioneering new advertising techniques that included planting articles in medical periodicals and reporting exciting therapeutic advances that had yet to be confirmed in the laboratory. Marketers of secret remedies such as Radam's Microbe Killer and Cureforhedake Brane-Fude mimicked the vocabulary and concepts of medical science, just as scientific advances were used by medical professionals to promise a therapeutic revolution that would ultimately rid the nation of the quackery menace. Yet, in the waning years of the nineteenth century, orthodox physicians continued to prescribe proprietary drugs in large numbers, while unorthodox schools of medicine grew in popularity.[4]

At the dawn of the twentieth century, major organizational and educational reforms within the medical profession coincided with the first successful efforts to regulate an increasingly crowded medical marketplace. Chapter 2 illustrates how the AMA took the lead in the effort to define the difference between acceptable and fraudulent medicines by introducing a framework for evaluating and standardizing drugs. At the same time, a broad coalition of reformers—from drug manufacturers and chemists to muckraking journalists and women's clubs—played important roles in securing legislative reform. The institutionalization of these reforms established mechanisms for communicating new medical knowledge to the public and profession. During this period, a network of professional quackery adversaries joined forces to exchange information and coordinate regulatory efforts.

In addition to securing the landmark Pure Food and Drugs Act of 1906, reformers pushed to eliminate the advertising of questionable drugs and medical services. Chapter 3 illustrates how these efforts had some of the desired effects on restricting the most egregious offenders, but drug manufacturers continued to employ ingenious marketing measures and encouraged doctors to use their products despite regulatory restrictions and professional condemnation. An analysis of advertising materials aimed at doctors illustrates how drug promoters successfully marketed their products by using advertising techniques that undermined the reform measures discussed in Chapter 2. Collectively, these marketing strategies undercut the effect of efforts to eliminate the advertisements of questionable quack remedies from the popular and medical press, and allowed drug manufacturers and distributors to capitalize on new standards and regulatory requirements. Disclosing ingredients, guaranteeing chemical purity, and claiming adherence to high scientific standards became one way to reassure doctors about a drug's safety and effectiveness. Recounting historical experience or employing the latest, modern, progressive methods also undoubtedly helped convince doctors and consumers that treatments actually worked. Anecdotal evidence brought together each of these themes by using the satisfied customer and the authority of physicians, institutions, and scholarly journals to legitimize therapies that had been deemed quackery by reformers. As a result, while the work of a growing antiquackery network, the restrictions of the Pure Food and Drugs Act, and advertising reformers helped eliminate much of the secrecy of patent medicines and led to the prosecution of thousands of allegedly fraudulent medicine makers, these efforts ultimately did not definitively establish the boundary lines between quackery and nonquackery. Meanwhile, the manufacturers and distributors of countless questionable remedies still continued to turn massive profits.

Chapter 4 examines how the AMA accelerated its antiquackery activities as part of a broader effort to define the boundaries of scientific medicine and therapeutic acceptability. The AMA's Propaganda Department, officially established in 1914 to gather and disseminate information concerning health fraud and medical quackery, revealed a complex of economic, philosophical, and professional motivations involved in this work. The Propaganda Department helped remove some medicines from the market and helped legitimize the AMA as a professional organization of expert scientists and practitioners committed to protecting the public. The AMA also played a pivotal role in establishing a national network of antiquackery surveillance at this time, with its close work with municipal, state, and federal government organizations. The association collaborated with businesses, other allied health professionals, and private voluntary health organizations to establish a correspondence network with doctors, scientists, educational organizations, editors of magazines and newspapers, and a growing number of people searching for an authoritative voice in a highly contested medical marketplace. The Propaganda Department also used the antinostrum crusade as a mandate to expose other approaches to therapeutics deemed quackery and "pseudomedicine," including homeopathy, naturopathy, osteopathy, and chiropractic.

Despite the best efforts of the antiquackery network, Chapter 5 illustrates how these and other targets of the crusade continued to have widespread appeal into the 1930s. The popularity of secret nostrums and unorthodox systems of medicine left many reformers perplexed. Disappointed with the results of the antiquackery crusade, some blamed the inadequacy of the 1906 Pure Food and Drugs Act. Amidst widely publicized reports that dangerous and deadly drugs were still being sold to millions of unsuspecting consumers, reformers initiated a long campaign to revise and extend regulatory restrictions. A protracted struggle ensued as members of an otherwise united campaign disagreed on the best path to reform. Reports of the tragic deaths of more than a hundred people from a new drug in 1938 ultimately helped tip the scales. Consequently, the Federal Food, Drug and Cosmetics Act of 1938 represented both a major breakthrough and a compromise among stakeholders. The 1938 law ultimately required manufacturers to demonstrate the safety of drugs under the conditions recommended in packaging and advertising, but the new law said nothing about the government's right to control the way drugs were used. The newly empowered U.S. Food and Drug Administration (FDA) only had the power to regulate what manufacturers said about a drug. Enforcement officials soon found that while rank fraud and known poisons were easy to identify, a more difficult problem was posed by newly developed drugs whose potency was not in doubt but whose benefit depended on the supervision of a doctor and the precautions taken in their use.

Chapter 6 explores how a flood of new drugs in the 1940s, part of what has been called a chemotherapeutic revolution, created a double pressure for many of the targets of the antiquackery network. As the drug revolution surged on, many proprietary formulas became outmoded by new prescription medications because little research had been published in the medical literature regarding their efficacy while the proprietary industry failed to keep pace with conducting its own innovative research. Meanwhile, pharmaceutical manufacturers began to enter the self-medication field, and the earlier distinction between ethical drugs and secret proprietaries on the one hand, and between prescription drugs and self-medication on the other, began to break down as firms diversified, and pharmaceutical and proprietary companies merged into large firms that made and marketed drug products of all types. During this period, the prescription drug industry became increasingly entangled with the booming commercial economy, and consolidation of businesses not only blurred previously established lines between ethical drug companies and proprietary firms but also heralded a revolution in medical economics as well as therapeutics. Nostrum sellers adapted. They employed alternative means of collateral advertising in the form of pamphlets, newspaper spreads, placards, roadside signs, and travelling pitchmen. They embraced parallel changes in the kinds of therapeutic promises made in the wake of legislative reform. They moved into the gray areas where medical science offered little therapeutic benefit or where scientific opinion had not yet reached consensus on effective treatment. Regulatory institutions could not keep pace with the expansion in the drug market.

By the mid-1950s, members of the antiquackery network admitted that quackery was alive and well, just as the age of wonder drugs peaked. Chapter 7 discusses a new wave of muckraking journalists who reported that the total cost of "pseudo-medical deception" to the American public had come to $1 billion a year in 1960. Quackery's most knowledgeable enemies were forced to reassess its significance. Many of the prominent individuals who had been branded as quacks in the 1930s and 1940s had responded to regulatory attacks by banding together. In joining forces with the National Health Federation, formed by leading medical gadget and food fad promoters, they waved the banner of "medical freedom" in an appeal to Americans who felt disenchanted with American health care. They gained ready converts who were willing to believe that the real problem was not with "medical irregulars" but was instead with an evil conspiracy among bureaucrats, doctors, and the makers of drugs. At the same time, the hazards of allegedly fraudulent medicine became a theme widely treated in printed and broadcast journalism. The antiquackery network capitalized on renewed interest. The government created educational films that warned Americans about the dangers of quackery and taught vulnerable citizens how to spot a quack. Agencies reinvigorated their educational and regulatory campaigns. The new secretary of health, education, and welfare, Arthur Fleming, made headlines by holding press conferences pointing out the dangers of quackery in the nutrition and weight-reducing fields. Professional and voluntary organizations expanded their own educational campaigns and attempted to persuade newspapers, magazines, radio, and television to raise their advertising standards.

As the 1950s gave way to the 1960s, Americans witnessed a more persistent and varied barrage of criticism aimed at medical quackery than ever before. Under the joint sponsorship of the AMA and FDA, these efforts culminated with the first National Congress on Medical Quackery in 1961, when 700 representatives from public and private agencies and organizations around the country met to discuss the problem. In addition to sharing information, these representatives launched critiques against physicians, regulators, and the media (each deemed responsible for part of the problem) and proposed plans for confronting the enemy through more vigorous law enforcement, more ample funding, self-regulation by the media with respect to advertising, and above all else an all-out campaign of public education. At the same time, disagreements among members of the antiquackery network ignited over the issue of regulatory reform. The 1962 Kefauver-Harris Amendment to the Federal Food, Drug and Cosmetics Act, which came partly in response to the thalidomide drug tragedy, required drug manufacturers to provide proof of safety and effectiveness before their products were approved for use, which granted the FDA unprecedented power and authority. Although the new law had been primarily aimed at abuses associated with prescription drugs, new weapons against quackery resulted in a series of pioneering cases that broadened the scope of the FDA's control over the medical market. Nevertheless, at the meeting of the Third National Congress on Medical Quackery in 1966, prosecutor John W. Miner of California reported that the financial toll of medical quackery had topped $2 billion, despite the revival of the antiquackery crusade in the preceding decade.

Chapter 8 begins with an examination of new studies in the 1970s that were designed to explain the persistent appeal of quackery. Despite the qualified optimism of reformers, regulatory control of quackery receded in the 1970s. A 1976 amendment to the Federal, Food, Drug, and Cosmetics Act of 1938, for example, prevented the FDA from limiting the potency of vitamins and minerals in daily supplements as well as classifying vitamins and minerals as drugs. This marked the first retrogressive step in federal legislation with regard to self-treatment wares since the initial Food and Drugs Act became law in 1906. Advertisers subsequently resorted to tried and true techniques in the absence of regulatory oversight. They also developed new, more sophisticated methods by involving M.D.s and Ph.D.s in copywriting and tapping into new electronic networks. Meanwhile, the AMA, which had played a dominant role in the antiquackery crusade since early in the century, abolished its quackery committee and closed down its Department of Investigation in 1975. The most controversial episode involving antiquackery crusaders came with the case launched against the cancer drug Laetrile, which provoked what one observer called "one of the most politicized medical disputes in American history." The Laetrile controversy highlighted weaknesses in the antiquackery network but also inspired a new generation of antiquackery professionals.

While this new band of self-proclaimed"quackbusters" revived interest in the waning antiquackery crusade in the 1980s, the 1990s heralded a fundamental shift in the enduring effort to combat quackery. Whereas federal policies had predominantly been used in the past to support the objectives of antiquackery forces—first with the Pure Food and Drugs Act of 1906; then with the Federal Food, Drug and Cosmetic Act of 1938; and then with the Kefauver-Harris Amendments in 1962—remarkable changes in the 1990s frustrated these efforts. First, with the creation of the Office of Alternative Medicine at the National Institutes of Health, the federal government got directly involved in the study of a number of questionable approaches to medical therapies that had long been relegated to fringe status by the antiquackery network. Second, passage of the Dietary Supplement Health and Education Act (DSHEA) of 1994 signaled a broader push to relax regulatory restrictions on a broader class of therapies often grouped under the banner of complementary and alternative medicine, or CAM. Mixed responses to these developments vividly illustrated a lack of consensus within the antiquackery network, which led the crusade against health fraud for much of the twentieth century.

Throughout the century, the crusade against quackery nevertheless shaped the medical marketplace in profound ways. It helped to secure professional authority for M.D.s, changed the way the government controlled access to drugs, and undoubtedly protected millions from dangerous and deadly medicines. The crusade also effectively denied people access to medical therapies, demonized well-intentioned practitioners, and dramatically restricted therapeutic practices. Still, despite concurrent advances in modern medical science, and the parallel expansion of legislation designed to protect consumers from dangerous or ineffective medical therapies, efforts to establish an exact border between quackery and nonquackery ultimately failed in some cases. This is partly because competing professional, economic, and political priorities often encouraged the drawing of arbitrary or poorly defined boundaries between what some defined as true, orthodox, or good medicine, versus quack medicine. Controversial therapies were dismissed without being tested. Licensed practitioners of alternative systems of medicine were sometimes relegated to the same quack status as rank charlatans. Meanwhile, reformers stubbornly believed that quackery could be largely eliminated by educating the public and enforcing existing laws. This strategy failed to accomplish its goal. Even when opponents of quackery used prevailing scientific standards and methodologies to challenge the effectiveness of questionable medical therapies, consumers continued to use many of them regardless of results.

Part of the credit for the failure of the antiquackery crusade can be given to those pilloried as quacks. Advocates of questionable medicines marketed their wares to consumers by appealing to vanity, instilling fear, creating hope, and promoting the freedom of unfortunate victims of disease. Simultaneously, alleged quacks ingeniously used advertising outlets and media channels to promote their wares while cleverly handling the opposition. Despite grave warnings and earnest appeals for consumers to base their decisions on reasoned, scientific evidence, people continued to use drugs and other drugless approaches to medical therapy that had been judged useless or dangerous by antiquackery professionals and authorities. In the end, quackery—as the quackbusters defined it—was better controlled, but arguably still as popular as ever.

ONE

QUACKERY UNMASKED

Although quackery is everywhere acknowledged to be a crying evil, some appear to think that it should not be opposed. You can do nothing, they say, to suppress or diminish it; it is useless to try. Is this a good philosophy? Do sound statesmen or moralists ever act upon such a principle? Certainly not. The most efficient and moral means are constantly employed against vice. And will any physician who regards the honor and usefulness of his profession, or any intelligent citizen who values the good of society, stand still and look on in culpable apathy whilst the tide of empiricism rolls on, prostrating at the same time the honor of the profession and the best interests of humanity? . . . It is idle to say that nothing can be done.

—Dr. Dan King, M.D. (1858)[1]

In his 1858 book *Quackery Unmasked*, Massachusetts physician Dan King blew the whistle on the various forms of nineteenth-century quackeries he deemed most dangerous to public health. Patent medicine peddlers travelled the country selling their secret nostrums and "snake oils." Uncounted cancer doctors, bonesetters, inoculators, and abortionists operated without professional sanction. Female practitioners, Native American healers, and clergymen offered medical care in the homes of sick patients, despite their lack of formal education and training. Representatives of dangerous new medical sects, including homeopaths, Thomsonian herbal healers, eclectics, and hydropaths offered allegedly natural cures that ran counter to thousands of years of knowledge accumulated by the medical profession.

King asserted that over the course of the first half of the nineteenth century, Americans had become "great lovers of nostrums," devouring whatever was new with insatiable voracity. "Staid Englishmen," meanwhile, "looked on in astonishment. . . . They call us pilleaters and syrup-drinkers, and wonder at our fickleness and easy credulity; so that we have almost become a laughing-stock in the eyes of the world." Medicine mongers continually catered to the public taste. As soon as one dish became stale, the "table was being bountifully reset with new varieties in the greatest profusion." Tennessee physician J. P. Epperson agreed that the time had come to address the problem of quackery in its ever growing number of forms. "Every age and country has been infested by such ignoramuses," Epperson asserted, "but the present age and this country appear to have more than their proportional share of them." Quackery had assumed so many shapes that it had become nearly impossible to identify it in all its forms.[2]

The proliferation of quack critics coincided with a tumultuous first half of the nineteenth century for American physicians. At the beginning of the 1800s, state laws governing licensure had helped define the medical profession and supported a virtual monopoly for "regular" physicians whose diplomas served as evidence of their authority and expertise. Even elite physicians, however, were still actively conscious of their precarious cultural authority. A second tier of practitioners included surgeons, apothecaries, and ethnic practitioners, from Native American healers and slave doctors to smaller groups such as the descendants of New Amsterdam's Zieckenstroosters ("comforters of the sick"), who ministered to their own and to neighbors. Between domestic and professional medicine, lay healers provided much of the primary care for the rest of the population. They operated as a sort of medical counterculture and often adopted positions hostile to the medical profession's therapeutic tenets and its social aspirations. Given the complexity of the medical landscape, the relationship between the profession and society remained peculiarly tense. The Boston Medical Association expressed a contradiction that remained hard to explain, noting that "as a community, physicians are, more than most classes of men, made the butt of ridicule, and not infrequently the subjects of sweeping and unsparing censure, while as individuals, no class of men are more honored and trusted."[3]

By the 1830s, the political forces of Jacksonian democracy had validated the fears of regular physicians and helped create a largely unregulated medical marketplace with the widespread repeal of licensing laws. In the pervasive atmosphere of *caveat emptor* (let the buyer beware!), medical self-help options also expanded dramatically as "irregular" practitioners joined name brand medicine makers in offering an ever increasing range of alternatives to regular doctoring. As the accepted monopoly enjoyed by regular physicians effectively ended, what became known as the medical

sectarian movement emerged as an alternative in the 1820s and 1830s. The proliferation of "sectarianism" reflected a variety of concurrent developments, including a
vacuum of legal control, a desire on the part of dissident groups to assert their claims
against the dominant profession, and the growing public dissatisfaction with the dog-
matic adherence by regulars to their regimen of what was called "heroic medicine,"
which included bloodletting, emetics, poisonous evacuants, and other harsh
therapies.[4]

The genius of medical sectarians was to express their protests against the dominant
order in terms of therapeutic alternatives as well as political, social, and religious ideas.
Accusations of quackery were also launched in retaliation against the regular profession. In response to the fining and imprisonment of an herbal practitioner in 1839,
"for no other cause than curing a man given over to die by the legal doctors," an editorialist conveyed his complaint in verse:

Shall a self-created band
Govern with supreme command
(While their deeds of quackery stand,)
All through the country?

Shall they thus monopolize,
Deceive the people with their lies,
Sink the truth no more to rise
In this happy land?

In the same issue of the *Independent Botanic Advocate*, another article reported that a
"scientific M.D. quack" had recently been prosecuted and fined for bleeding a patient
to death. The editorialist suggested, "Should every regular calomel (mercury chloride)
peddler in the State of New York receive his just desserts for his poisonous and murderous practice, in the same manner that Wallace has, there would not be jails and
prisons enough in the State to contain them."[5]

The first wave of the sectarian assault on orthodox heroic practices by
Thomsonians, homeopaths, eclectics, hydropaths, health reformers, mesmerists, and
other irregular healers denounced regular physicians as "learned quacks" and offered
alternative sources of medical care. Sectarian rhetoric identified learned quackery with
aggressive and depletive "heroic" therapies that depended on an outdated and overly
speculative "rational" approach. In actuality, regular doctors relied on visible and
physiological evidence for therapeutic effectiveness, but their ability to explain and
predict these effects helped establish their authority. Purges purged, emetics caused
vomiting, opium soothed pain, bleeding affected blood pressure or changed the pulse.
As historian John Harley Warner argues, "What was essential was that the physician
be able to act, and to do so in accordance with regular values . . . it was practice that

mattered most to physicians in assessing the orthodoxy of their fellows." This could create problems. As one physician complained, the young practitioner was often compelled "to give medicine when it is not plainly indicated" because "he must cure quickly, or give place to a rival."[6]

Regular practitioners were pejoratively portrayed by their critics as "mineral doctors," "the poison depletive quacks," "mercury dosers," "drug doctors," and "the knights of calomel and the lancet." Their entire system of regular medicine, meanwhile, was styled as "the murderous system," "the calomel and blue pill school of medicine," and "the mineral, humbuggery practice." Bloodletting and large doses of mineral-based drugs had been virtually banished from sectarian practice. Thomsonians and eclectics substituted plant remedies, homeopaths employed only very minute doses of any drug, and hydropaths replaced nearly all treatments with the creative use of water. "The essential difference," one homeopath noted, "between the old and the new school, consists in an entire rejection of the latter, of the materia medica, and therapeutics of the former." "The old school physician lifts his fatal club and strikes at random," wrote one Thomsonian doctor, "the force of which oftener comes on the head of the healing principle that exists in man, termed nature, than on his enemy, disease."[7]

Patent medicine promoters also railed against the dangers of regular medicine and its heroic manifestations, even as they maintained their own secrecy. The term "patent medicines" did not necessarily indicate a patent of any kind. When used in common discourse, the words "patent" or "proprietary" instead referred to the secrecy in which their formulas were held. Manufacturers rarely patented the key medicine in bottles or, in most cases, the composition of the entire formula. They sometimes patented the distinctive shape of the bottle, the box the medicines came in, the type styles and pictures on the labels, and the advertising associated with it all. These strategies, along with the emphasis on secrecy, represented a major break with the past, as doctors and lawmakers had long worked to establish a known, stable list of medicines and their ingredients via pharmacopoeias and national formularies.[8] In "their flaming advertisements," wrote Dr. Epperson, in his pamphlet dedicated to the exposure of quackery, "we have an exhibition of it (secrecy) at once sublime and ridiculous." Advertising campaigns capitalized on fear, in particular, depicting death, suffering, and evil at the hands of regular doctors. Such advertisements in newspapers and magazines were complemented by "pamphlets, calendars, almanacs, books of stories, cookbooks, joke books, and various other publications with advertising interspersed throughout the text like commercials in a television show." Advertisements entertained consumers while they emphasized the value and ease of self-treatment.

Numerous factors broadened the market for vendors of packaged medicines at the time, including rapid growth in population, the spirit of therapeutic laissez-faire in a democratic age, and the constant growth in media for advertising. High-volume patent medicine makers were the first American manufacturers to seek out a national market, the first large-scale producers to go directly to consumers with a message about their product, and the first to employ a multitude of psychological techniques to entice buyers. In addition to playing on fears, advertisements enticed readers with sexual innuendo, appealed to interest in the exotic and mysterious, and played on patriotic sentiments by depicting American heroes and even presidents in their advertisements. Frederick Fact, who was also a Thomsonian sympathizer, was not alone in offering his own patent medicine alternatives in response to "the wishes, prayers, petitions, remonstrances, tears and groans for all those not fattening on the prerogative to poison by rule, or destroying by chartered right." Fact cultivated customers by offering his remedies as answers to consumers' desires.[9]

Irregular practitioners also divorced themselves from regular medicine in their method for obtaining their therapies. They portrayed regulars as tied to old-fashioned stationary dogmas of the past. Homeopaths referred to them pejoratively as "allopaths" who merely treated the symptoms of disease, rather than its root causes. Along with other "sectarians," by contrast, they claimed to derive their therapies from empirical experience. In his book *Quackery Exposed*, a defender of Thomsonianism published a copy of a letter from a disillusioned former lecturer at Cambridge University that summed up the value of empiricism. "I am indeed so disgusted with learned quackery," wrote Dr. Benjamin Waterhouse, "that I take interest in the honest, humane and strong minded empiricism; for it has done more for our art, in all ages and in all countries, than all the universities since the time of Charlamagne." A number of sectarians agreed. As one botanical doctor explained, "I confess my inability to perceive the allopathic practice of medicine as a science, or as being even reasonable; it is based on apparently plausible but really false theories." While learned quackery remained overly rationalistic and relied too much on theory, its critics claimed to trust in experience.[10]

EXPLAINING THE PERSISTENCE OF QUACKERY

Part of the appeal of the empirical approach—which predominantly used the symptoms of the disease as the data upon which to base diagnosis and treatment, and often included a mistrust of anatomy and physiology as sources of medical knowledge—could be found in what it promised that regular medicine could not. When outlining his list of other delusions that helped explain the persistence of quackery, Dr. D.H. Nutting, a Boston physician, argued that the "effrontery and boldness of quackery," the "credulity and perseverance of patients," and "incorrect experience or observations in medicine" deserved the most credit. The "inordinate desire of life" also explained how quacks capitalized on the desperation of the deathly ill. In the case of fatal diseases, where science knew no curative drug, Nutting recounted another common series of events: "The regular physician, finding no room for hope, gives no promise of recovery, and is discarded for one who will. He, failing to cure, is dismissed for one more ignorant still; for each promises more confidently, in proportion to his ignorance, and they feed delusive hope on these promises, although they know them to be 'empty as the wind.'" Alleged quacks offered hope for a cure where regular medicine remained ineffective.[11]

Antiquackery forces also blamed newspapers and magazines for exacerbating the problem. Many earned the bulk of their revenue from advertising nostrums (a common name for questionable medicines with unproven effectiveness and often secret ingredients). According to Dr. Epperson, these advertisements encouraged "the fanciful quest of fountains of rejuvenescence, and the vain hope of discovering one remedy for all diseases, or at least a specific remedy for each disease, although the obvious fact that the same disease presents many points of variation in every different person, and even in the same person at different times, renders the hope totally and plainly absurd." A commitment to freedom of the press nevertheless made it virtually impossible to restrict nostrum advertisers.[12]

Advertisements capitalized on the mystery in which regular doctors often enshrouded the whole subject of medicine. It remained difficult for regular doctors to determine the exact nature of many diseases, and there were many more that no art could cure. In other cases, it was virtually impossible to determine accurately the precise results of treatment, nor did regular doctors have the means of comparing the results of alleged quack treatments with those of the "scientific physician" so that the masses could see the difference. Nutting argued the masses took for granted that there were no fixed principles in medicine, that disease and the action of remedies were all haphazard. "Crafty men were ready to take advantage of this," Nutting reasoned, "and though ignorant as the masses, contrived, by loud-sounding words, to involve them in greater darkness than before, and yet persuade them they knew it all. In consequence, quackery flourished, while the regular physician was neglected." According to Nutting, the physician needed to enlighten the masses on the laws of health, the structure and functions of the body, drawing on the latest study of anatomy and physiology. "It is to this change," he concluded, "that I look with strongest hope for the overthrow of quackery, whether in or out of the regular profession."[13]

In enumerating some of the other causes that contributed to the support of alleged quacks, physicians acknowledged that professional discord and low educational standards were also contributing factors. Lowered standards of medical education in the United States also made the profession relatively easy to access and allowed incompetent individuals to enter its ranks. Physicians who obtained diplomas without more than a smattering of medical knowledge were "easily induced to abandon the profession altogether, or to embrace some variety of quackery," one critic observed. Meanwhile, neighboring physicians were often either open or secret enemies; "they were jealous and envious of each other, too ready to publish each others' faults, and with a fiendish gladness rejoice at each others' misfortune." At least one physician believed that if regular doctors could cure this self-interested "moral disease," dismiss private jealousies and animosities, and cordially unite, "quackery of every name and form and color would soon take wings and fly away." In the long run, increased professional harmony failed to deliver on this promise, but it did have its benefits for physicians[14]

DEFINING BOUNDARIES BETWEEN REGULAR AND IRREGULAR MEDICINE

The expansion of sectarian alternatives and patent medicines encouraged unity among physicians and commanded boundary-setting actions. It heightened regular practitioners' group identity and actually helped define, strengthen, and fortify the concept of orthodoxy as distinct from its heterodox counterparts. From the orthodox perspective, sectarians appealed to credulity and lived on vanity and speculation, while "science, professionalism and ethics demanded a sound thinking faculty, reason, honesty, modesty, and common sense." The crystallizing of these features of orthodox identity in the middle third of the 1800s was expressed most visibly in the proliferation of explicitly orthodox institutions. Along with the multiplication of local and state medical societies, the national American Medical Association (AMA) was formed in 1847 partly to distance regulars from sectarians. Sectarians were barred from the AMA as well as most state and local medical societies and thereby denied access to one source of distinction, knowledge, and business. The regulars also explicitly forbade consultation with sectarians in their codes of ethics, closed the doors of their schools to unorthodox practitioners, revoked diplomas from alumni who took up sectarian practice, and expelled students who associated with sectarians. Orthodox medical journals, meanwhile, also multiplied rapidly and offered a platform for denouncing sectarian ways and consolidating authority. Sectarian practitioners also created their own distinct identity and their own distinct set of institutions. The sectarian challenge subsequently shaped both the structure of the profession and efforts to reform the medical marketplace for years to come.[15]

The largest and arguably most respected group of sectarians, the homeopaths, epitomized the nature of the sectarian challenge. In direct opposition to the excesses of heroic medicine associated with what homeopaths deemed "allopathy"—the term used to describe orthodox medicine's treatment by *opposites*—homeopathy was rooted in the mild therapeutic principles of its founder Samuel Hahnemann, which treated by the principle of similars. Homeopaths were roundly criticized for their approach to therapeutics, most famously by Oliver Wendell Holmes, whose 1842 address "Homeopathy and Its Kindred Delusions" was the most thoroughly explicated attack on homeopathy as a dangerous and deadly error. According to Holmes, homeopathy was a "mingled mass of perverse ingenuity, of tinsel erudition, of imbecile credulity, and of artful misrepresentation." Homeopathy was quackery *par excellence*. Homeopaths, nevertheless, increasingly attracted patients and became the largest irregular group of practitioners by the end of the nineteenth century.[16]

Some historians believe that sectarians collectively compelled regular physicians to change their approach to therapeutics by demonstrating the effectiveness and appeal of milder alternative interventions. However, the sectarian assault on orthodox therapy had two very different effects. On the one hand, it incited patients to resist heroic therapies and obliged some regular physicians to either renounce or moderate their use. On the other hand, medical sectarianism operated as a conservative force on regular medicine by encouraging some regular physicians to proclaim their allegiance to medical tradition and the enduring features of their practice in order to define orthodoxy in opposition to alleged quackery and to secure their own identity as legitimate physicians. Long after the appearance of sectarians, many regular doctors continued to use heroic therapies. A manual on the principles of physiology and medical botany in 1859, for example, asserted: "We affirm that the cure always consists of producing perspiration, restoring vital action, removing obstructions with emetics and evacuants, and equalizing the circulation [with bleeding]." The author celebrated the famous advocate of heroic therapies, Dr. Benjamin Rush, as the model to follow and set out to prove the essential unity of all diseases in relationship to a distinctly "regular" allopathic practice. Sectarianism, in this case, helped make the regular profession think and act like a sect of its own.[17]

While many regular physicians were preoccupied with maintaining the appearance of therapeutic unity, in their fight against quackery and elsewhere, dissention and debates within orthodox circles were also driven by the rise of the experimental medical sciences during the second stage of change in medical therapeutics between 1860 and 1885. From roughly 1820 to 1860, orthodox medical therapeutics had undergone a dramatic transformation, as American doctors reevaluated the usefulness of traditional therapies. By 1891, at the fifteenth anniversary of the Johns Hopkins University, Dr. William Osler argued that medicine had progressed with "extraordinary rapidity" in the preceding generation. He nevertheless attributed its "complete revolution" primarily to advances in disease prevention and a better understanding of microbiology. Osler noted that the past half-century had placed only half a dozen "absolutely indispensable drugs" in the hands of doctors, while changes in diet and nursing had supplanted heroic measures of the past. "We recognize daily the great fact that disease is only a modification of the normal processes of health," Osler admitted, "and that there is a natural tendency to recover. We cannot claim in the medicinal treatment of disease to have made great positive advances; still, to have learned not to do what we did is for the poor patients a great gain."[18]

During the last third of the century, a new orthodoxy rooted in the knowledge generated and validated by experimental science held that universality in treating diseases was not only possible but preferable. An emphasis on objective evidence from anatomy, physiology, and pathological changes encouraged a more universal approach to particular ailments, which served to demarcate the boundaries of orthodoxy because it ran counter to the prevailing current in irregular circles that approached disease as a unique and subjective experience. An earlier generation of antiquack crusaders had argued that it was utterly absurd to think that any one remedy could cure any malady or even be beneficial except by pure accident, given the innumerable variations of disease produced by age, sex, climate, habits, complications, and so on.[19]

The claim of laboratory science to practical relevance in medical therapeutics did much more than challenge the empiricism associated with a growing list of alleged quack medical schemes. Warner shows how "it urged a thoroughgoing rearrangement of the relationships among therapeutic practice, knowledge, and professional identity." What was known with certainty, and rationally explained, was elevated to the "science of therapeutics," and the concurrent spread of scientific ideology transformed orthodox therapeutic approaches by emphasizing knowledge over behavior as the basis for professional identity. This shift from behavior to ideology transformed the doctor-patient relationship because the newly objectified concepts of disease and therapy directed attention away from sick individuals, and their social and physical environment, which increasingly became the domain of public health reformers. An introductory lecture in the medical department of Dartmouth College reflected this shift by defining disease as "an entity, as something distinct from, or added to, a person." No longer considered a disturbance from the natural balance between an individual and his or her environment, disease was described here and elsewhere as a deviation from a normal physiological state, which altered the categories by which clinical thinking organized therapies. For doctors, this was the "fundamental proposition of all pathology or knowledge of disease" and provided evidence that "the positive progress of our science enables us to stand to-day on a firmer platform than our forefathers." New diagnostic technologies, furthermore, facilitated efforts to identify specific targets for therapeutic intervention and discouraged the use of many indiscriminate older therapies.[20]

In the late nineteenth century, the most common objection to grounding therapeutics upon experimental science was simply that the laboratory offered the practitioner nothing of immediate practical therapeutic value. Many of those who rejected the therapeutic claims of experimental science did so because the traditional ideal of clinical empiricism appeared to offer a more solid foundation for therapeutic practice and progress. A medical lecturer at the University of Virginia in the late 1880s, for example, told his class that great progress in physiology did not necessarily imply therapeutic improvement. Therapeutics had already been "groping in the dark two decades by studying the physiological action of drugs on inferior animals," so he urged his students to take as their guide clinical observation, not "the recreations of science."[21]

While a lack of laboratory-generated therapeutic applications allowed room for sectarian alternatives, the advent of pathological anatomy and experimental physiology upset traditional notions of bodily functions in health and disease that had previously been commonly shared by patients and their physicians. This set the stage for backlash and retrenchment. The notion of an increasingly fragmented body composed of discrete organs and systems selectively afflicted by disease offered immense promise in terms of new therapeutic interventions. At the same time, the popularity of alternative medical systems such as homeopathy and hydropathy, with their holistic therapies, appealed to those disillusioned with the growing therapeutic skepticism of mainstream medicine. In some ways, sectarians offered a throwback to the individuality and holism in therapy offered by humoralism, an older bygone form of medical orthodoxy.[22]

A flood of self-care options from the patent medicine trade further complicated efforts to define the boundaries of medical orthodoxy in the late nineteenth century, in no small part because advertisers capitalized on orthodox advances in selling their wares. On the eve of the Civil War, the proprietary medicine industry raked in $3.5 million annually. By the turn of the century, that sum had multiplied by more than 20 times. As historian James Harvey Young argues, the "chameleon-like creatures" of the patent medicine trade continued to expand their market share during the late nineteenth century by taking advantage of orthodox medicine's promising prospects as well as its persisting weaknesses.[23]

Patent medicine promoters employed a wide range of advertising techniques that simulated the methods of medical and pharmaceutical science as well as capitalized on recent discoveries. Patent medicine makers planted articles in medical periodicals, reported alleged therapeutic advances, and encouraged doctors to prescribe products that the consumer could subsequently buy at the local drug store. "Hand in hand with the progress of medical science," one physician warned, "we see an army of pseudo-scientific quacks who trade upon the imperfect knowledge of the masses, and by plausibly written advertisements convince many, even of the educated classes, that their particular method of treatment is based upon the latest scientific discoveries." In the scientific journal *The Bacteriological World*, for example, the Aerated Oxygen Compound Company reported that just as scientists discovered the bacterium that caused tuberculosis, their company used the latest knowledge to begin affecting immediate cures. Companies also exploited similar advances in the physical sciences. With the discovery of radium, for example, came advertisements for "radium-impregnated" cures for cancer. Other similar examples abounded, especially in the fields of electrotherapy—which included cure-all electric belts, finger rings, and an array of microbe killers that promised to rid the blood of pathogenic bacteria.[24]

Thus the marketers of alleged "quack," patent, and secret remedies mimicked the vocabulary and concepts of medical science just as orthodox practitioners used them to promise their own therapeutic revolution. Herein lay a paradox: while patent medicine promoters capitalized on the distinction of science, never before had there been so firm a foundation of medical and pharmaceutical knowledge on which to build a sound critique of the most outlandish forms of patent medicine quackery. As Dr. Osler noted in his anniversary address at the Johns Hopkins University in 1891, at the very time that physicians were beginning to embrace a more rational, scientific approach to the treatment of disease, the public appeared to "delight more and more in patent medicines" and remained "at the hands of advertising quacks."[25]

COMBATING QUACKERY

Dr. Nutting insisted it was the "duty of the regular physicians, as conservators of the public health, not only to cure disease, but to expose the practices of those who would tamper with the public health." Dr. Epperson agreed and admitted "to oppose the empty pretentions of patent medicines by serious argumentation, seems on the one hand ludicrous, but on the other necessary." It was commonplace for advertisers to proclaim the infallibility of nostrums for virtually any disease under the sun, and the "extravagant certificates" and "pompous assertions" of thousands cured appeared to serve as ample evidence of patent medicine makers' excesses. The discoverer of a secret nostrum often informed the public that his medicine alone was valuable, and that all others were "rascally impositions." As Dr. Epperson noted, "This game of mutual crimination goes on till, like the celebrated cats, they eat each other almost totally up. These witnesses, therefore, of equal incredulity, destroy the testimony of the other." Despite the promise to annihilate the "whole tribe of human maladies," Epperson insisted that "every one [of approximately 20,000 nostrums in his estimation], although infallible," had disappeared from the light of trial, "like gaseous meteors from the morning sun, in less than a dozen years from the time of its fabrication." While overly generalized and arbitrarily measured, Epperson's point was commonly expressed by quackery critics: if nostrums cured the diseases they claimed, then the survival of the former would have been jeopardized by the demise of the latter. Nevertheless, the people remained "as ardent in the pursuit of infallible cures as they ever were."[26]

In exposés in popular magazines and newspapers, articles in medical journals, pamphlets, books, and public lectures, critics of patent medicines used what they believed would be the most valuable weapon in the war against "flim-flam": public education. As Dr. Epperson explained, the public failed to understand that medical science was not the experience of one man, or of one age, but rather "the accumulated experience of all physicians, of more than two thousand years." If only the public knew that medical science was "a system which must have been, and has been built, like the coral reef, by the long continued and joint labors of a vast multitude," they would respect it. As it was the common resort of quacks to persuade the masses that they had been initiated into the secrets of medicine, or been given all the skill and power of the regular doctor, it was the duty of the physicians "to claim for themselves the competency to judge of every system and mode of practice." Women were incited to protect their families from unscrupulous advertisers. Clergymen were implored to respect the authority of physicians and their expertise in the laws of medical reasoning and evidence. Publishers were asked to embrace a higher standard by universally rejecting nostrum advertising.[27]

Unfortunately, the public had so long been accustomed to the use of patent medicines and sectarian practices that many considered them indispensable. Furthermore, the sheer volume of patent medicine advertising could not be matched. Perhaps most importantly, in many cases regular doctors had limited alternatives to offer to replace patent medicines, whether they worked or not.

The fight against patent medicines had nevertheless been a primary objective of the American Medical Association since its founding in 1847. Its original *Code of Ethics* categorically stated that it was "derogatory to professional character" for a physician "to dispense a secret nostrum, whether it be the composition of exclusive property of himself or others."

> For if such nostrum be of real efficacy, any concealment regarding it is inconsistent with beneficence and professional liberality; and if mystery alone give it value and importance, such craft implies either disgraceful ignorance or fraudulent avarice. It is also reprehensible for physicians to give certificates attesting the efficacy of patent or secret medicines, or in any way to promote the use of them.

At the preliminary convention of the AMA, a special Committee on Education also recommended adopting a rule that would forbid any physician from patronizing a druggist who dealt in patent or secret remedies. Two years later, the AMA's Committee on Medical Science moved to establish a board to analyze alleged quack remedies and nostrums and to "enlighten the public in regard to the nature and dangerous tendencies of such remedies."[28]

In the decades to come, the AMA approved a series of similar resolutions and proclamations on proprietary medicines, but a lack of finances and effective organization hampered efforts to reform the medical market for the remainder of the nineteenth century. It was easy for most physicians to simply ignore the mandates of the association. Until reforms within the AMA dramatically increased membership in the early twentieth century, many considered it an upstart, regional organization that remained heavily weighted toward academic and hospital physicians. The AMA had relatively little influence outside the northeastern United States. Some members of the AMA, meanwhile, continued to patronize druggists and apothecaries dealing in nostrums, while other physicians continued to promote their own proprietary remedies with little or no consequence. Fifty years after its formation, the AMA still had not established a board to analyze alleged quack remedies.[29]

Meanwhile, the AMA had taken only tentative steps to preclude the advertisement of secret remedies in medical journals. As early as 1850, the House of Delegates adopted a resolution that the AMA "regard it as contrary to its system of ethics for medical journals to advertise nostrums or secret remedies although their composition may have been known to the editor." Thirty years later, the House of Delegates went a bit further, adopting resolutions that recommended that editors of all medical journals "refuse to notice all patent medicines . . . [and] works of unprofessional or unscientific character." Additionally, the AMA threatened to refuse membership for noncompliant journals in the Association of Medical Journal Editors, which had been organized by the AMA for the purpose of casting its influence on the side of improvement in scientific publications. The AMA's own board of trustees, furthermore, mandated that the editor of the *Journal of the American Medical Association* (*JAMA*; est. 1883) must exclude all advertisements of proprietary, trademarked, copyrighted, or patented medicines. Over the first two decades of the *Journal*'s existence, however, it regularly advertised alleged quack remedies. After facing mounting criticism, the Trustees promised to appoint a Special Committee on Advertising in 1894 and admitted that during the entire existence of the *Journal*, no question had presented greater difficulty or afforded the Board more embarrassment than the contents of its advertising pages. The Board asserted that the formula of all secret and proprietary remedies should be submitted to the Committee on Advertising before being advertised in the *Journal* but acknowledged that enforcing this requirement would likely result in a considerable financial loss. Consequently, an official change in *Journal* policy was delayed several years.[30]

While little had been done to effectively limit patent medicine advertising by the end of the nineteenth century, quackery critics helped secure some reforms in the areas of medical education and licensing during the final third of the century, but with limited effect. Mid-century quackery exposés frequently noted that low standards of medical education had made the profession too easy to access, which allowed incompetent individuals to enter its ranks. As Dr. King maintained in *Quackery Unmasked*, "The distinction between men learned and skilled in the profession, and ignorant pretenders, should be made wider and more apparent . . . In this land of boasted liberty, public opinion is opposed to arbitrary rules, and the right of every man to medicate whomsoever he pleases is everywhere conceded." The end result in his mind was clear, "our State governments always appear disposed to allow quackery its largest liberty." Between 1875 and 1890, forty state governments addressed this problem by passing laws that regulated medical practice and licensing, including higher educational standards. A lack of uniformity in legislation and enforcement resulted in limited impacts. Some reformers argued that defective licensing laws actually helped facilitate the practice of medicine by quacks and charlatans. An editorial in *Science* in 1887 argued that "no law has yet been passed which has had the slightest effect in suppressing quackery or protecting the community against imposture." In 1889, Bellevue Hospital's professor of physiology August Flint maintained it was not an exaggeration to say that in the United States, the door to quackery was still left "wide open." "It is time, at last," Flint argued, "for the profession to make a united effort to protect the people against quackery; for the disjointed, spasmodic, and crude attempts that have been made in this direction have resulted in but little good in a few States."[31]

The "Report of the Illinois State Board of Health on Medical Education," released in 1891, provided evidence of improved standards among medical colleges, but also exposed the fatal flaws of state-based regulation. While some states enacted licensing boards and required diplomas from medical colleges "in good standing," several states still had no laws regulating the practice of medicine. Of the 135 medical schools in operation in the United States, 23 had been deemed "fraudulent diploma mills." Some of the worst and most fraudulent colleges, which offered diplomas for a fee with little to no educational requirements, had nevertheless been "legally chartered."[32]

The most innovative period of educational reform between 1880 and 1900 took place primarily at major medical schools such as Harvard, Pennsylvania, Michigan, and Johns Hopkins. Reformers introduced a more rigorous curriculum that incorporated the latest scientific advances from abroad. They added many new subjects such as physiological chemistry, pharmacology, and bacteriology. Clinical teaching expanded its scope to include new courses in specialties like gynecology, dermatology, psychiatry, and pediatrics. In the closing decades of the nineteenth century, a conceptual revolution also changed how medical students were taught. The introduction of hands-on work in laboratories and hospitals made students active participants. Teaching changed from predominantly didactic to practical. A 1901 *JAMA* report on medical education concluded: "Medical education in this country is a different thing from what it was two decades ago."[33]

Medical education, however, was never monolithic and controversies over standards, research priorities, the role of professors, relationships with universities, and admissions requirements continued into the twentieth century. The AMA endorsed reforms as essential to making regular medical practice more scientific, while simultaneously capitalizing on changes in an effort to discredit much of the sectarian competition on the basis of their educational deficiencies.[34]

Nevertheless, by the closing decade of the nineteenth century, the regulars and sectarians still managed to find common cause on some issues. In addition to general advances in a wide range of scientific disciplines and their application to medicine, exciting advances in surgery, preventative medicine, and pharmacology emerged by the 1880s, stemming in part from educational reforms, and the public and sectarians alike responded enthusiastically. Homeopaths and Eclectics began to blend their teachings with orthodoxy, partly in response to patient requests, and many sectarian schools made efforts to incorporate educational reforms begun by regular schools. The growth of specialization also increased interdependence in the profession, as orthodox specialists depended on homeopathic and Eclectic general practitioners for referrals. Conversely, the growth of hospitals made sectarian general practitioners depend on regular hospital administrators for access to the increasingly important facilities that the specialists controlled. The licensing movement of the late nineteenth century also promoted collaboration between regular physicians and their most highly educated sectarian counterparts, in order to win laws that would protect all of them from competition with poorly trained practitioners, who were still graduating in large numbers from proprietary operations that served as diploma mills.[35]

AMA gestures of accommodation toward old adversaries also reflected a more general effort to unify and strengthen the medical profession. In addition to elevating educational standards, the profession's leaders advocated new understandings about the cause of disease, and adopted new methods of treatment. Yet despite these advances, the status, power, and income of most doctors remained low and inadequate according to the profession's spokespersons. Critics attributed the root cause of this lack of respect and authority to the overcrowding and disunity of the profession. In addition to excessive numbers of regular physicians, the *Journal of the American Medical Association* and many leading state journals fumed about the large number of irregular doctors and quacks who further limited the doctors' income and status. A 1901 *JAMA* article on the state of medical education identified "the multiplication of facilities for medical education," motivated not by the needs of the profession but the greed of their founders. The proliferation of these diploma mills "cheapened the profession" by lowering its standards, and the *Journal* suggested that "if we wish to make ourselves respected we must make ourselves respectable" by elevating the profession as a whole.[36]

CONCLUSION

While reformers remained steadfast in their belief that public education could curb the excesses of the most egregious quacks, they still unhappily noted that "the demand for panaceas and for the services of those who claim to cure by extraordinary means" was "not confined to those who are deficient in intelligence or weakened and discouraged by exhausting diseases." Mid-nineteenth century reformers had likewise admitted that they could never expect quackery's complete extermination. "History informs us," Dr. King noted, "that it has always existed in some form or other, and a consideration of the human propensity leads us to conclude that it always will." King nevertheless concluded: "Spread before them the necessary intelligence, and public opinion will, to a great extent, correct errors and reform abuses. Knowledge is the sovereign remedy against error; and although its effects may not be seen immediately, it will eventually succeed." Toward the end of the 1800s, some reformers nevertheless admitted that "the 'quack,' the 'shyster,' and the 'sheep in wolf's clothing'" would always exist.[37]

Such an admission reflected how the therapeutic marketplace had become more crowded with options than it had ever been. Patent medicines proliferated, new sectarian schools of medicine introduced alternative treatments, and orthodox doctors employed a series of new drugs. Collectively, they promised cures for virtually any ill one could conceive. As a result, orthodox reformers faced the challenge of redefining the boundaries of therapeutic orthodoxy in order to clearly distinguish their approaches from their alleged quack competitors.

In this crowded medical marketplace, orthodox physicians in the early twentieth century sought to redefine and reestablish the basis of their professional and cultural authority. Scholars have emphasized the important role played by a number of changes in this period that facilitated the transformation of the medical profession, including the introduction of medical practice acts, the revival of licensing legislation, and reforms in medical education. Each of these developments helped define professional boundaries between orthodox and unorthodox practitioners. However, scholars have undervalued the important role that combating quackery, and redefining the boundaries of therapeutic orthodoxy, played in establishing the modern medical profession as we know it.

TWO

RATIONALIZING AND REGULATING THE THERAPEUTIC MARKETPLACE

And all of them were pernicious, because they fostered the idea that a man—it was usually a woman—could treat his own ailments. They made drugging easy; it should be made hard. I can never speak calmly of those patent medicines that intentionally preyed upon their victims by dosing him with alcohol or dope. A manufacturer who produces a "medicine" like that, knowing that all his victim will get from it will be false stimulation, which when it has fastened upon him will be a far worse disease than the one he started with, deserves to boil for a million years in a cauldron of his own mixture. He is a wretch beneath all human contempt.

—C. H. La Wall[1]

In an address on the progress of medical therapeutics delivered before the Philadelphia County Medical Society in 1900, Dr. Solomon Solis-Cohen lamented "the great flood of proprietary remedies, secret or half-secret, that has been let loose upon the profession and the public." He condemned physicians who remained lazily content to use a drug exploited by some manufacturing firm, rather than use their own brains to find a remedy. Insofar as these remedies were secret nostrums, Solis-Cohen maintained they undermined the openness of scientific inquiry and threatened to destroy all therapeutic science by encouraging ignorance. A physician at the annual meeting of the American Medical Association (AMA) that same year echoed these concerns, suggesting that "the first stupendous error, one which is so vast in its influence that it hangs like a withering blight over the individuality of every man in the profession, is the dictation of the innumerable pharmacal companies, the self-constituted advisers in the treatment of diseases about which they know nothing, to the entire profession." Likeminded doctors worried that drug companies threatened to undermine the authority of physicians to diagnose diseases and prescribe the proper remedies.[2]

Meanwhile, despite the fact that regular and irregular practitioners sometimes found common cause in lambasting individual drug proprietors and larger drug firms as unconscionable quacks and nostrum peddlers, patent medicine companies continued to expand their share of the market. By some estimates, patent medicine makers had become a more formidable financial challenge to regular doctors than their irregular counterparts. By pioneering techniques and strategies used in nationwide advertising, a trickle of patent medicines had quickly become a flood. Proprietary compounds grew to dominate the U.S. drug market, growing from 28 percent of all drugs produced in 1880 to 72 percent in 1900. The patent medicine industry subsequently became a major factor in the growth and development of professional advertising itself, and created unprecedented challenges for both patients and practitioners trying to make sense of marketplace options. In addition to selling drugs, they offered general advice about medical problems, and distributed guides to health and happiness. Some claimed to be doctors themselves when they actually were not. Others operated health institutes and medical colleges, and gained endorsement from eminent physicians. As a result, patent medicine manufacturers and distributors represented a much greater threat than might be presumed—they offered competition beyond the drug they might sell versus a drug that a physician would prescribe.[3]

Despite widespread condemnation of patent medicines, as the bane of the medical marketplace, their place in orthodox therapeutic practice remained ill defined. Some doctors prescribed them to patients. Others packaged and sold their own proprietary medicines. As the market became increasingly flooded with new drugs, it became increasingly difficult for physicians and patients alike to distinguish drugs that had been isolated in laboratories and clinically tested for effectiveness from drugs that capitalized on this research but failed to undergo testing. The patent medicine trade exploited almost every major innovative discovery in medical science, from the synthetic chemicals of the 1880s and 1890s, to the serums and vaccines of the 1890s and 1900s, to the biological therapies such as hormones in the 1920s and 1930s. Innumerable patent medicines claimed to contain these substances but simply did not.[4]

While such patent medicine promoters were roundly denounced as quacks by the profession, they were not the only "drug pushers" guilty of mislabeling and misrepresenting their wares. Medicines prescribed and recommended by regular mainstream medical practitioners as safe and nonaddictive often contained such drugs as opium, heroin, and cocaine. Pills were regularly sold without any restriction. Labeling often gave no hint of the presence of these ingredients and rarely included warnings against misuse.[5]

On numerous occasions in the late 1800s, medical reformers argued that manufacturers should be compelled by law to print the composition of patent medicines on packages, in order to eliminate secrecy and allow consumers to make informed choices. "Such a regulation," argued a 1880 editorial in the *Pharmacist*, "would do more towards abating the swindling operations now practiced in that class of goods in a month than all the harangues and anathemas of the justly indignant medical profession in a century." Despite some inroads at the state level at the close of the nineteenth century, little progress was made on creating a national law.[6]

THERAPEUTIC REFORMERS

Historian Harry Marks has identified what he calls a group of therapeutic reformers at the turn of the century who sought to use science to create a more rational approach to choosing drugs and protecting consumers. The combined excesses of drug advertisers and traveling medicine showmen, along with the exploitation of remedies believed to be dangerous or inert, inspired reformers to establish a program of what they called "rational therapeutics" to direct medical practice. The notion of a rational approach to therapeutics referred to "the use of therapeutic agents whose mechanisms of action were scientifically established prior to their introduction into clinical practice," and restricted clinical practice to the use of drugs with known pharmacological activity and effects. Put simply, drugs would not be used on patients until the effectiveness of their ingredients had been proven in the laboratory or the clinic. The challenge was how best to harvest the riches of the laboratory while protecting medical practice from the incursions and temptations of the market. Reformers wanted to ensure that physicians would use drugs effectively and appropriately, which meant drawing a line between the commercial influences of patent medicine quacks and a new rationally based therapeutic orthodoxy advocated by the profession.[7]

To establish the boundaries of therapeutic orthodoxy and overcome the efforts of drug advertisers to bypass the physician as a source of therapeutic information and authority, advocates of reform promoted both a new system for evaluating drugs and the use of regulatory mechanisms to control the introduction and promotion of new remedies. The remainder of this chapter demonstrates how the AMA took the lead in both of these efforts and became the central player in redefining therapeutic boundaries.

THE AMA AND PROPRIETARY MEDICINES

Prior to 1905, the AMA failed to apply its own *Code of Ethics* when it came to provisions against patent medicines and advertising in its journal. The Pennsylvania State

Medical Society condemned the AMA's Board of Trustees for this very reason in 1895, claiming the *Journal of the American Medical Association* (*JAMA*) had continued to publish unethical advertisements for secret remedies with seemingly miraculous curative powers. AMA Trustees responded by asking the journal to tweak its advertising policy, requiring proprietors to supply a formula with the "official or chemic name and quantity of each composing ingredient to be inserted as part of the advertisement." This had virtually no immediate impact.[8]

Steadily increasing advertising revenue in the nineteenth century might explain why *JAMA* did not lead the crusade against patent medicines until after the turn of the century, but the move for advertising reform should also be understood in terms of the AMA's broader effort to consolidate professional authority. As of 1900, the association had only 9,000 members, while the total membership of all local, state, and national medical societies was approximately 33,000. Another 77,000 physicians belonged to no professional association whatsoever. In an effort to consolidate professional support, the AMA revised its constitution in 1901, and in order to transcend its regional character it became a confederation of state medical societies that in turn drew its membership from the smaller county societies divided into local chapters. Membership skyrocketed. Members rapidly achieved the unity and coherence that had for so long eluded them, and benefits soon came from their newfound political power in the form of support for new licensing restrictions that reduced competition. By 1903, *JAMA* revenue topped $88,000, nearly double the numbers brought in before the AMA's reorganization. By 1909, the *Journal* was earning $150,000 a year for the AMA, having become its major source of income. Increased *JAMA* revenues reflected the dramatic growth of the AMA itself, along with an increase in the number of subscribers. The total number of subscribers in 1900 barely topped 13,000, while that number reached 80,000 by the early 1920s.[9]

In 1900, the AMA's House of Delegates also resolved once again to fulfill the express will of its members by finally excluding from its journal's columns those embarrassing advertisements of nostrums and secret preparations. A series of eight articles appeared in the *Journal* between April 21 and July 14 under the heading "Relations of Pharmacy to the Medical Profession." The articles discussed the problematic nature of proprietary medicines and promised to expose corruption in the patent medicine trade. An address on "Progress in Therapeutics" delivered before the Philadelphia County Medical Society and reprinted in *JAMA* later echoed this sentiment: "In so far as these remedies are secret nostrums, they threaten to destroy all therapeutic science; for ignorance, which is the aim of secrecy, is the very antithesis of science."[10]

Meanwhile, the *Journal* still published advertisements of questionable and allegedly fraudulent remedies, despite the resolution by new editor George H. Simmons to end this practice. Simmons had quickly established a reputation as a maverick, so this appeared to be no empty promise. He actually began his career as a practicing homeopath after graduating from Hahnemann Medical College in 1882. Toward the end of the 1880s, however, he altered his therapeutic views, and he secured a degree from Rush Medical College of Chicago in 1892. He then returned to his native Nebraska, where he served as secretary of the State Medical Society and editor of the *Western Medical Review*, which he had founded, and which also adopted a pronounced antihomeopathic stance. In 1899, when the AMA's Board of Trustees appointed a new secretary and *Journal* editor, they selected Simmons for the post. His dual role as general secretary and general manager of the AMA, from 1899 to 1911, and editor of the *Journal* from 1899 to 1924, gave him considerable influence. Simmons helped reinvent the organization as a representative of average practitioners and helped reinvent its journal as the voice of the profession. His obituary reads: "Unquestionably he was the greatest figure in his generation in the development of the American Medical Association and the profession which it represents."[11]

As early as 1900, Simmons had argued that secret medicines should not be "patronized" by members of the profession. But he also admitted that the advertising pages of the *Journal* contained "announcements that . . . ought not to be there." P. Maxwell Foshay, the editor of the *Cleveland Medical Journal,* explained this apparent contradiction by identifying the financial dilemma created by proprietary medicines. "The greed for advertising patronage," he said, "leads the editor only too often to prostitute his pen or his pages to the advertiser, so long as he can secure the coveted revenue. So our journals are filled with articles and editorials containing covert advertisements of this and that remedy." Foshay observed that given the multiplicity of medical journals, few of them could survive only on their subscription receipts. Drug promoters knew this and often resorted to coercion with journal editors and advertising managers by stipulating in their contracts that in addition to standard advertisements in designated pages of the journal, certain advertising matter must appear among original articles and editorials. Out of the 250 medical journals published at the time, meanwhile, not a dozen made a rigid separation between advertisements and editorial matter. In fact, a large proportion of medical journals had a department devoted to special advertisements under the guise of abstracts, reading notices, commercial news, therapeutic notes, and other apparently valuable summaries of medical progress that seemed to put the editor's stamp of approval on thinly disguised promotional materials.[12]

While the *Journal* was not the most egregious offender in this regard, advertisements for proprietary medicines were common in its pages. A single issue of the *Journal* in 1900 contained the following ads spread over 25 pages: Bethesda Mineral Spring Water, which claimed to have been "proved absolutely and permanently curative" for 14 different diseases, including diabetes and rheumatism; Gardner's Hypophosphate Ammonium, which promised to "instantly relieve laryngitis, pharyngitis, catarrh and all inflammations of the respiratory tract"; Platt's Chlorides, "The True Disinfectant," which would "cool and purify the air by liquid evaporation and chemical absorption" if diluted with water and wafted about the sick room by towel or sheet; Schieffelin and Company's heroin pills indicated in "the so-called functional neuroses, neurasthenia, hysteria, and other general nutritional disturbances of the nervous system"; J. S. Tyree's Antiseptic Powder, which promised to be "absolutely cleansing and curative" for gonorrhea when used as a douche; Pepto-Mangan, a true "blood builder"; Hagee's Cordial of Cod Liver Oil, which would allegedly "restore tone to the nervous system, and is the indicated remedy for the run down in health and for those who want to grow fat"; and Liberty Chemical Co.'s Thermol, an "antiseptic in the blood ... proven by its specific action against typhoid." None of these claims had been substantiated by scientific evidence.[13]

Finally, in 1905, the AMA created its Council on Pharmacy and Chemistry to carry out the Simmons mandate to test and evaluate drugs before they were advertised in *JAMA*. The council would determine which proprietary medicines were therapeutically valuable, worthy of physicians' patronage, and thereby worthy of being granted permission to advertise in the *Journal*. The need for such protection was made evident by a 1906 *Journal* article, which estimated that about 50 percent of prescriptions in large cities were for proprietary remedies lacking independent analysis of either contents or effectiveness. The overall figure for proprietary medicine prescriptions in New York City that year topped 70 percent. Another analysis of prescriptions in Philadelphia in 1905 found that 41 percent called for remedies of unknown composition. Committed to protecting the medical consumer and creating a well-informed medical profession, and determined to redefine the boundaries of therapeutic orthodoxy, the Council on Pharmacy and Chemistry embarked upon its daunting tasks.[14]

THE COUNCIL ON PHARMACY AND CHEMISTRY

The AMA's new council addressed the widespread concern that neither physicians nor laypersons could make sense of a nostrum-corrupted medical marketplace. Its primary objective would be not only to delegitimize useless nostrums but also to ensure that physicians chose effective drugs. To overcome the prevailing therapeutic skepticism of the day, the council would evaluate new drugs based on the combined use of chemical analysis and existing clinical knowledge about the efficacy of drug components. In the process, the council ultimately provided three major benefits to the AMA: (1) it created an opportunity for the association to establish its own set of professional standards for evaluating new drugs for doctors to use in treating their patients, (2) it offered a method for determining which drugs would be allowed to advertise in the *Journal*, and (3) it cemented a crucial relationship with the federal government by providing the analytical work of the AMA's chemical laboratory to the Department of Agriculture, which had begun conducting its own similar investigations.[15]

Throughout 1905, the *Journal* went to great lengths to explain the need for the council, its objectives, the scope of its work, and its potential benefits. An editorial acknowledged the seriousness of the problem and introduced readers to the council by revisiting an important distinction:

> Technically, there is no difference between the proprietary medicines manufactured for physicians' use and the "patent medicines" exploited to the public, both being protected simply through copyright or trade-mark names. Yet the relation of the physician to these preparations is very different; about the latter he has little direct concern, save that he regrets that our laws permit the foisting on a suffering and unsuspecting public of preparations that are usually dangerous and always irrational. In the former he is directly and intensely interested, for they compose a part of the armamentarium which he is expected to use. On them he often has to depend, or at least does depend, consequently on them rest his success and the health, sometimes the lives, of those who place themselves in his care.

The implications of this position for the operation of the council and the future of the AMA and its *Journal* were threefold: (1) the council would not analyze and evaluate patent medicines aimed at the public, at least initially, but instead would concentrate on proprietary medicines; (2) this would help cement a close, dependent relationship between the medical profession and the proprietary medicine trade by establishing a standard for approving drugs and then admitting them for *Journal* advertising; and (3) this would ultimately increase income for the AMA because those proprietaries that disclosed their contents and met with approval were also implicitly granted a new status as safe, effective, and scientifically sound. Proprietary medicine manufacturers often subsequently purchased advertising space not only in the *Journal* but also in the physicians' book of medicines that conformed to the new standard, the AMA's *New and Non-Official Remedies*.[16]

From *Journal* editor Simmons's perspective, the creation of the council and chemical laboratory was also essential because proprietary medicines had been introduced to the profession under very different conditions in the nineteenth century. For the first two-thirds of the 1800s, doctors were provided with pharmaceutical or descriptive names, the drugs were of well-known composition and standard formulae, and they were manufactured by pharmaceutical houses that took pride in their products. In the last third of the nineteenth century, however, more and more preparations had been introduced with nondescriptive names protected by copyright or trademark, and with mysterious and even fictitious formulae. By making extravagant claims and resorting to persistent and exploitative advertising, furthermore, manufacturers labeled their products with therapeutic or disease-sounding names that appealed to doctors because they were "convenient, palatable, and, at least, satisfactory placebos." This saved the doctor the trouble of writing a full prescription. The real problems began, however, when the fancy, catchy names became popular with the public, who in turn found full directions for use and the names of diseases in which these remedies were indicated on their labels. Thus, the physician became "the unpaid peddler of secret nostrums" who "encouraged his patient to prescribe for himself." In the process, the secret nostrum manufacturer became richer and the physician became poorer.[17]

The Council on Pharmacy and Chemistry intended to play the crucial role of restoring order to a chaotic therapeutic marketplace by separating the wheat from the chaff. Could the physician be expected to be a chemist and a pharmacist as well, examining all the products he or she prescribed? Of course not. The number of remedies on the market had become so great that any attempt to separate safe and effective remedies from their quack counterparts was bewildering. The result of it all, Simmons worried, was that the "educated, thinking physician—he who is honest with himself and his patient—refuses to prescribe any proprietary mixture," becoming a therapeutic nihilist. Part of the goal of the council was to provide a system of "rational therapeutics" in contrast to this therapeutic nihilism that patent medicines had helped create.[18]

According to the AMA, the task of separating legitimate chemical and pharmaceutical preparations from those it called secret nostrums had also become virtually impossible for medical journals. By employing the notion of a rational therapeutics, the council would help identify legitimate therapeutic agents whose mechanisms of action had been scientifically established prior to their introduction in clinical practice. The distinguishing characteristics of a rational (as opposed to empirical) remedy included its demonstrability in the laboratory and its action on the cause (as opposed to the symptoms) of the disease. According to Solomon Solis-Cohen, who had led the Philadelphia County Medical Society's earlier critique of *JAMA* advertising policy and helped initiate the broader professional crusade against patent medicines, rational symptomatic treatment was considered acceptable only in the absence of a known cure, but even here there was an expectation to demonstrate and explain the mechanism at work. In terms of rational medical practice, the council's purpose would be to ensure that the profession officially endorsed only specific dosages and uses of demonstrably effective drugs in accordance with existing knowledge about pharmacological activity and effects.[19]

Endorsing a rational approach to therapeutics offered a solution to the advertising dilemma faced by the *Journal* because doing so legitimized its rationale for the inclusion or exclusion of drugs based on scientific evidence. In theory, forcing manufacturers to reveal the contents of their drugs, and requiring evidence for the therapeutic efficacy of those contents, would allow the council to discriminate between drugs of merit and worthless nostrums. All varieties of proprietaries marketed and sold to doctors would be subjected to analysis, including synthetic chemical compounds and pharmaceutical specialties put out under trademarked names.

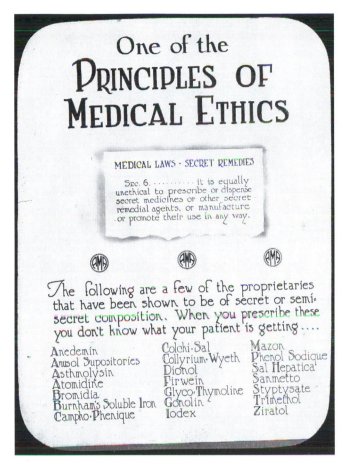

One of the

PRINCIPLES OF
MEDICAL ETHICS

MEDICAL LAWS · SECRET REMEDIES

Sec. 6. ·········· it is equally
unethical to prescribe or dispense
secret medicines or other secret
remedial agents, or manufacture
or promote their use in any way.

The following are a few of the proprietaries
that have been shown to be of secret or semi-
secret composition. When you prescribe these
you don't know what your patient is getting ....

Anedemin	Colchi-Sal	Mazon
Anusol Suppositories	Collyrium-Wyeth	Phenol Sodique
Asthmolysin	Dionol	Sal Hepatica
Atomidine	Firwein	Sanmetto
Bromidia	Glyco-Thymoline	Styptysate
Burnham's Soluble Iron	Gonolin	Trimethol
Campho-Phenique	Iodex	Ziratol

Lantern Slide #834 (ca. 1912).
(© American Medical Association. Courtesy of AMA Archives)

Preparations that conformed to the standards of the council would not only be allowed to advertise in the *Journal* but would also be incorporated in the AMA's new reference book, *New and Non-Official Remedies*. This accessible, authoritative book was designed to serve a pressing need for the busy physician. But its value would be proportional only to its completeness. This meant, therefore, that *New and Non-Official Remedies* proposed to be "as liberal in approving articles for the book as is consistent with justice and equality to the public, to the manufacturing pharmacist and chemist, and to the physicians."[20]

Scholars have underestimated the significance of the liberal standard of the council by emphasizing the value of this quasiregulatory effort primarily in terms of the restrictions it put in place. As a result, the AMA has been widely praised for applying the yardstick of science in excluding secret remedies from its journal. In Paul Starr's analysis, for example, the council's rules established an unprecedented advertising standard that required drug companies to choose their market because if they wished to advertise a drug to doctors in the pages of the association's *Journal*, they could not advertise it to the public or instruct the laity in its use. Starr also notes that the *New and Non-Official Remedies* became widely used—both by medical journals in setting advertising standards and by doctors in prescribing medicines. For the public, meanwhile, James Burrow argues that the council was seen largely as an agency dedicated to consumer health protection and committed to detecting and exposing proprietary frauds. This triumphal narrative, however, neglects a crucial development. The combination of restrictive requirements and liberality governing the acceptance of drugs allowed the AMA simultaneously to attack the greatest financial threat to physicians (secret nostrums advertised directly to the public) while courting the association's biggest financial ally (proprietary drug manufacturers who paid for advertising in the pages of *JAMA*). Advertising revenue was the association's principal source of income. As noted earlier, revenue increased dramatically from $88,000 in 1903 to the post-council sum of $150,000 a year by 1909. This advertising revenue made the expansion of the AMA into professional, political, and public circles possible.[21]

In spite of this apparent commercial incentive for the council's work, the AMA presented these reforms as an attempt to moderate the excesses of capitalism, embodied by the unchecked exploitation of consumers by patent medicine manufacturers. "Honest advertising is a necessary feature of civilization—at least it is not an unmitigated evil," observed one prominent council member, whereas, "fraudulent advertisements are one of the curses of civilization." Simmons argued that the commercial domination of therapeutics through advertising had not only led to the "debauching of our journals" and the "tainting of our textbooks," but had also undermined the scientific basis for a rational therapeutics. For Progressive-Era therapeutic reformers, science operated as a moral as well as an intellectual source of reform.[22]

The liberal nature of the standard that governed the acceptance of drugs by the Council of Pharmacy and Chemistry allowed it to claim the moral high ground. At the same time, it promised to eliminate the most exploitative nostrums and simultaneously offer redemptive possibilities for effective therapeutic elements that had been advertised in a questionable fashion. Liberal standards also allowed the AMA to increase its advertising revenue at the very moment when restricting advertisers could have threatened the financial future of the *Journal* and the AMA itself.

Because the 10 rules governing inclusion in *New and Non-official Remedies* played such an important role, they merit examination. The first three rules mandated disclosure of ingredients and required evidence for their identity, purity, and strength. Collectively, these rules also attempted to establish clear boundaries between orthodox and unorthodox drug therapies by outlining specific duties for manufacturers and physicians regarding each. No compound advertised to the public would be admitted. New drugs were not to be prescribed by doctors unless they met with the council's approval. If proprietary manufacturers fulfilled the duties laid out by these rules, the council would have the power to identify and pass negative judgment on inert proprietary medicines with no active ingredients and alleged miracle cures without a clear identity. All patent medicines marketed and sold directly to the public would bear the mark of noncompliance, and physicians were implored to not use any patent medicines.[23]

Of all the provisions, rule 4 was arguably the most important in the effort to define boundaries between acceptable and unacceptable therapeutic practices because it completely disallowed all therapeutic agents that made claims about efficacy in treating specific diseases. These restrictions did not, however, cover the advertising of therapeutic agents in medical journals or literature distributed solely to physicians. As the *Journal* conceded, the fourth rule appeared "radical" to some because it helped delegitimize the prescribing of medicines that did not make it into the pages of *New and Non-Official Remedies*. Rule 4 also undercut the recommended use of those drugs by manufacturers and pharmacists. Only the physician was deemed qualified to prescribe or recommend any medicine for the treatment of specific diseases, even if some therapeutic reformers admitted privately that the physician's training was likely to be such that he or she could "not distinguish the rank fraud from the efficacious remedy, honestly made and sold." The council believed that the application of rule 4 would force manufacturers to make a choice about what they would rather have: the preference and favor of the medical profession's most authoritative and influential body or the doubtful support of a rapidly disappearing minority of practitioners.[24]

The provisions in the fifth and sixth rules regarding misleading statements allowed the council a considerable amount of leeway in denying questionable remedies and required several manufacturers to change their advertising strategies. No article with "unwarranted, exaggerated, or misleading statements" would be admitted, even if no clear standard for making this judgment existed. Efforts to make this judgment proved particularly difficult with newly developed drugs. These rules, however, did not necessarily disqualify proprietors from advertising in the *Journal* if satisfactory changes were made.[25]

The remainder of the council's rules required additional information from the manufacturer, including full disclosure of dangerous ingredients, composition, registration, and patents. While these strictures eliminated the most egregiously fraudulent nostrums from appearing in any *JAMA* publication, they still allowed some questionable proprietary medicines to claim new status as being accepted by the AMA.

An editorial comment in the *Journal* summarized the new standards of therapeutic orthodoxy established by the council, which merely required that "the composition of the remedy be non-secret, that its uniformity be safeguarded, that no false claims be made regarding its therapeutic properties, and that its use shall be based on at least a probability of therapeutic merit."[26] However, "probability of therapeutic merit" represented a potentially dangerous and malleable provision. Such a subjective standard operated in an uncomfortable tension with the rigid objectivity (and well-established pharmacological tradition) of chemical analysis. When applied liberally, it could allow for the acceptance of dangerous unproven therapeutic agents; when applied restrictively, it could delegitimize promising therapeutic agents.[27]

Harry Marks argues that establishing a rational therapeutic regime meant providing an experimentally grounded chain of evidence linking laboratory knowledge to treatment at the bedside. In the practical work of the council, however, such a link was sometimes impossible because of either a lack of evidence or conflicting opinions about the motives of the manufacturers who were mandated to provide that evidence. Analyzing the chemical constituents in the AMA's new chemical laboratory in Chicago was most often a straightforward process. Drugs whose principal ingredients turned out to be misrepresented or whose active ingredients were not standardized or accurately reported were readily dismissed. Evidence was more often equivocal when it came to therapeutic efficacy due to a lack of unified standards for measuring and evaluating laboratory and clinical data.[28]

The council also lacked the resources to conduct its own clinical experiments and relied on clinical consultants who were generally medical school faculty and experts on either the disease or the type of drug in question. In some of these cases, evidence of the character of the proprietor aided the decision of the consultant. Products from firms that had proved reliable in the past were scrutinized less than habitual offenders. Data from the "high-minded men" and "institutions" of clinical science was considered more trustworthy than data either paid for or produced by proprietors' own laboratories.[29]

Regardless of the origin of the data, the council remained committed to experimental science as a corrective tool in evaluating evidence. The acknowledged leader of the council over the next four decades, Torald Sollman, professor of pharmacology at Western Reserve University, and author of the first American textbook on the new laboratory-based pharmacology, argued that in the preclinical evaluation of drug chemistry and the clinical evaluation of therapeutic efficacy, the council was committed to following "the canons of other scientific experimentation. Otherwise, its usefulness is nil, and even its practical usefulness is, at best, doubtful." Evaluating therapeutic efficacy according to the standards of experimental science, however, was much easier said than done. As Sollman admitted, "Experiments may be framed so loosely, the observation may be so superficial, the analysis of results so careless, the deductions so illogical, that the experiment has no permanent value—it is not an experiment in the precise sense of the word." The council intended to create a "corps of medical consultants" composed of physicians connected to hospitals in various parts of the country to "make physiological and therapeutic tests" of preparations under investigation and produce reliable evidence for a drug's efficacy.[30]

Initially, however, the council relied predominantly on experimental evidence submitted by the drug's manufacturer. This was supplemented by existing research and animal testing, which had its own limitations because some drugs could not be reliably tested on animals. The persistence of clinical skepticism regarding the laboratory also made it difficult for the council to dismiss a drug on the basis of animal studies alone. As a result, Marks has suggested clinical investigations constituted the "weakest link" in the council's work due to ongoing disputes about the value of evidence. Even with the formation of a staff of clinical consultants to advise the council in 1908, "honest differences" of opinion existed among researchers. In cases where reports from these referees doubted the value of a compound but lacked the evidence to prove it worthless, the council had few options besides negotiating with the manufacturer to tone down its therapeutic claims. By 1911, the AMA authorized a Committee on Therapeutics to conduct its own original pharmacologic research in order to address this problem, but limited funding and a small staff meant few disputed questions were resolved. In the absence of reliable evidence, the council's rules were sufficiently vague to allow for the judgment of its members regarding claims for the therapeutic value of drugs under investigation.[31]

RESPONSES TO THE CREATION OF THE COUNCIL AND ITS EARLY WORK

To garner support for the council, the AMA sent out a preliminary announcement to all drug manufacturers, requesting feedback on the creation of this new body. The association also published supportive comments from a wide range of pharmaceutical manufacturers, medical journals, and medical societies in the newly created pharmacology department of the *Journal*. E. B. Squibb & Sons, Merck & Co., Crowell & Co., Fritzsche Brothers, Victor Koechl & Co., Gardner-Barada Chemical Co., White Co., Organic Chemical Mfg. Co., American Ferment Co., and Frederick Stearns & Co. all offered words of support for the "right direction," "safe and honest service," and "pioneer and systematic step" that the council represented. From the perspective of some drug makers, the council was promising to "promote the interests of ethical medicine and pharmacy" as the "bulwark for the protection of the good name of the American manufacturer." Words of praise also came from medical societies, other medical journals, and the primary organs of pharmaceutical and manufacturing houses.[32]

The only major criticism reproduced in the pages of *JAMA* came from the *New York Medical Journal*, which approved of the council's 10 rules and the expertise of its members but worried that "even with the best intention and with the most expert administration, the establishment of such a censorship is likely to prove a source of serious contention, and will undoubtedly involve the association in trouble of a kind that it has been heretofore free from." The *Western Druggist* echoed this sentiment with its prediction that "the 'community of interest' among the manufacturers" would certainly prompt them to "view with suspicion the creation of an official outside authority over their products." Knowing that the council's plan would work only if the most popular preparations used by the profession placed themselves "under the council's censorship," the *Western Druggist* anticipated they would "be slow about entering the seductive little parlor of the council." After all, few manufacturers would willingly make themselves perpetually accountable "to a group of critics who may or may not be governed at all times by infallible intelligence or by recognized principles of mercantile equity."[33]

Outside the pages of the association's *Journal*, criticism from observers in the medical field was easier to find. The *Medical Council*, for example, a journal that claimed a circulation of over 25,000 practitioners, sympathized with the reform program of the AMA but was not blind to the fact that there were some "defects in the details of both plan and findings." While many readers of the *Medical Council* supported the AMA's reform program and wholeheartedly endorsed the effort to "raise the standard of American medicine," others were more critical. Answering a call by the journal to evaluate the reform program of the AMA, many doctors questioned the value of some AMA council reports due to their lack of evidence for the therapeutic value of new drugs as based on clinical observations and evidence. As one doctor in Mississippi surmised, "It is interesting to know how a certain drug acts on a guinea pig, but far more important to know how it acts on a sick man." Another doubter, from Indiana, rhetorically asked whether the AMA laboratory scientists and the editorial staff were actually engaged in the active practice of medicine, suggesting that if they were not, they had little to offer on therapeutic advice. After all, according to a physician from Colorado, laboratory findings were important, but not the last word by any means. Another practitioner from Illinois agreed: "I am a laboratory man but trust that I am broad enough to regard all laboratory findings as *aids*—aids to the man who must interpret them at the bedside; aids to him who receives the ultimate benefit, the sick man." The last word on the subject came from Chicago: "The time is past when a man can sit in his laboratory and dictate to the physician his diagnosis, or his treatment, or his prognosis. The real man is the one who has the responsibility, and that is the physician in charge." Many practicing physicians remained unconvinced that therapeutic progress would originate in the laboratory.[34]

Many of these critiques reflected the fact that the council, as a creation of the AMA's Board of Trustees, represented the views of the professions' national leadership, and was heavily weighted toward specialists and medical educators rather than local practitioners. Of 10 initial council members, seven were professors of pharmacology, pharmacy, or chemistry, while two worked in government laboratories responsible for the evaluation of vaccines and drugs. Simmons, *JAMA*'s editor, was the tenth. In this era, influence in the medical community was still measured first by local and then by national reputation, so the council's composition also placed it at a disadvantage. Although six of the 10 held medical degrees, none was regarded as engaged in the *practice* of medicine, and only Simmons was widely known in the profession.[35]

Another common critique of the council focused on the perception that since it represented professional interests, it could not be considered a neutral body. The strongest view in this regard came from a doctor in Wisconsin: "I have no faith at all in the work of the Pharmacy Board, or any of the work of the A.M.A, or the U.S. Association of Surgeons, being done 'for the good of the public.' I am not a pessimist, but that claim has been advanced too often in getting legislatures to pass stringent medical and pharmacy laws . . . to secure a monopoly." A physician from New York agreed: "Bossism in medicine is quite similar to that in politics. We should have none of it." While this reflected a common criticism of the AMA more broadly during the Progressive Era, more measured responses also reflected a certain amount of discomfort in placing trust in any single authoritative body. A doctor from Connecticut, for example, suggested, "No one set of investigators can give the only exact findings, nor should their findings be accepted as final until after they have been proven by other laboratory and clinical experiences." These critiques reflected concerns about unmitigated authority.[36]

Even critics were willing to concede, however, that standardization and governmental supervision of drug manufacturers was in the best interest of physicians and consumers. But in these early years of regulatory efforts, there was still reason to doubt whether a sufficiently objective and effective system could be worked out. The AMA repeatedly insisted its work was being done in the "interests of public health." It did not "recommend" any products, nor did it create a "blacklist" of products. It merely published the facts and left it up to physicians to draw their own conclusions about whether they wished to use such products. Not everyone was convinced.[37]

According to an editorial in the *Medical Standard*, a journal devoted to the interests of proprietary manufacturers, the AMA had established its Council on Pharmacy in an effort to ostracize virtually all of the proprietary preparations on the market. Proprietary manufacturers had been offered a choice: provide certain specific information as to the ingredients of their products or be practically blacklisted. This unquestionably had the effect of "weeding out many of the notorious frauds which [had] been thriving under a false conception of their character," but it had also demonstrated that there was little difference "in the estimation of the medical man, between a meritorious preparation which is proprietary and one that is non-proprietary." From the perspective of the *Medical Standard*, reports issued by the "competent medical authorities" of the council illustrated how impure and fraudulent drugs and medicines in the open preparations of the market represented a vastly more dangerous threat than those bearing the mark of proprietorship by a manufacturer who "must protect the stability and integrity of his preparations from debasement and substitution."[38]

The bulk of medicines recommended and prescribed by physicians and prepared by pharmacists, meanwhile, remained notoriously guilty of belying all standards as "trashy and worthless" preparations. As a result, the *Medical Standard* recommended the council "expend a little less of its effort in directions which are already hedged about with natural, economic and legal safeguards, and where possible harm is exceedingly small, and give a little more attention to the supervision of these unprotected channels of fraud and adulteration." A 1916 reprint from *Standard Remedies* titled "How Physicians Regard the Open Formula Requirement as Applied to Their Own Medicines" suggested doctors unfairly targeted secret proprietaries given their own proclivities for secrecy in their own prescriptions. This apparent contradiction was corroborated by a 1915 article from the *American Journal of Clinical Medicine*, which asked doctors whether they felt they should be compelled to inform patients about the ingredients of medicines dispensed. Replies from both orthodox and unorthodox practitioners as well as editors of several medical journals adamantly opposed any such measure. One doctor argued "it is always best that people do not know that they are taking" drugs with powerful or potentially dangerous ingredients, while others worried that "such a practice might lead to self-drugging."[39]

A parallel critique painted the work of the council as a power grab. A reprint of an article in the *National Druggist* claimed the council's rules constituted a threat to boycott all noncompliant manufacturers. The article claimed that many drug makers were unwilling to take the council "into their confidence and to entrust to its keeping the valuable trade secrets upon which the prosperity of their business is based" and predicted decreased advertising revenues for *JAMA*. According to the *National Druggist*, the AMA was "inspired with the hope that it would destroy the proprietary medicine business, and thus confer on themselves and their guild the valuable monopoly of furnishing medicines to the sick."[40]

This critique reflected the commercial interests of proprietary manufacturers and indicated that even without AMA approval, proprietors could still market their medicines directly to doctors through circulars, pamphlets, and trade cards, which will be discussed in Chapter 3. It remained true, however, that many of the most frequently used drugs, prepared by doctors and pharmacists, were not subject to investigations by the AMA's council. The *National Druggist* explained the AMA's subsequent campaign for legislative reform through its committee on legislation as an attack on noncompliant manufacturers. In 1906, the committee had resolved "to bring the influence of the entire medical profession to bear in securing the enactment" of legislation mandating both that all patent or proprietary medicines carry an exact formula of their contents printed on the package and that advertising copy be restricted to the same. As the *National Druggist* saw it, the medical profession's campaign for the passage of the Pure Food and Drugs Act of 1906 appeared to be motivated not by a national call for reform but rather by "the clique of political doctors who, for the time being, are in control of the great American Medical Association."[41]

PURE FOOD AND DRUGS ACT OF 1906

Gullible America will spend this year some $75 million in the purchase of patent medicines. In consideration of this sum it will swallow huge quantities of alcohol, an appalling amount of opiates and narcotics, a wide assortment of varied drugs ranging from powerful and dangerous heart depressants to insidious liver stimulants; and, far in excess of all other ingredients, undiluted fraud. For fraud exploited by the skillfulest of advertising bunco men, is the basis of the trade. Should the newspapers, the magazines and the medical journal refuse their pages to this class of advertisements, the patent medicine business in five years would be scandously historic as the South Sea Bubble, and the nation would be richer not only in lives and money, but in drunkards and drug fiends saved.

—Samuel Hopkins Adams[42]

In promoting its work toward a system of "rational therapeutics," the AMA also capitalized on increased public demands for reform following the muckraking work led by the writer-editor team of Samuel Hopkins Adams and Norman Hapgood. The push for federal legislation to protect the public from the dangers of nostrums also facilitated the movement for a rational therapeutics. Harvey Wiley, the crusading chief of the federal government's Bureau of Chemistry, and the man responsible for administering the Pure Food and Drugs Act, and John Anderson and George McCoy, responsible for testing vaccines and serums for the federal government, held seats on the AMA's Council on Pharmacy and Chemistry and worked closely with it. The federal government also used the AMA's chemical laboratory to conduct some of its early tests for the purity of drugs and food.[43]

The success of the pure food and drug reform movement was also due, however, to the wide range of activists involved in supporting the legislative campaign. This informal coalition of individuals can partly be explained by the dual emphasis on establishing protective measures for consumers in food *and* drug consumption, but new partnerships were also forged out of previously antagonistic relationships. Regular and irregular doctors, for example, found common cause in opposing the nostrum crusade, and a wide range of professional groups, academic institutions and allied organizations, trade associations, individual businesses, consumer groups, magazines and journals, and prominent individuals played important roles in the broadening coalition. Despite their competing objectives and conflicting agendas, all could agree that the patent medicine trade threatened public health. The efforts of the AMA in eliminating the patent medicine menace were bolstered by the support of this informal coalition and the widespread public calls for reform following the graphic documentation of the dangers of nostrums in the popular press. The Council on Pharmacy and Chemistry succeeded partly because the AMA could afford to devote sufficient resources to its work, but this effort was conducted in tandem with expanded governmental organizations devoted to the same cause. The close relationship between the AMA and the broad coalition of pure food and drug reformers, forged by work toward a common end, helped lay the groundwork for a long-term relationship in which the AMA extended and institutionalized the mandate of the Pure Food and Drugs Act.[44]

The architects of the Pure Food and Drugs Act of 1906, however, had a different objective than the Council of Pharmacy and Chemistry. While the council initially focused on protecting consumers by reforming the therapeutic practice of physicians, the Pure Food and Drugs Act had been designed to protect consumers more directly from deceptive advertising practices and secrecy by prohibiting false and misleading labeling and packaging. The act included two main provisions: first, that the presence and amount of 11 different habit-forming drugs should be definitely listed on the label of the bottle or package; and second, that no false or misleading statement whatsoever should appear on the label or package. With the passage of the act, the muckraking Adams suggested patent medicine manufacturers and advertisers had four main options: first, they could go out of business rather than expose the real nature of the concoctions with which they had been so long "doping" the public; second, they could change their formulas, leaving out those dangerous ingredients that now must be specified on the label; third, they could remove from their labels the fraudulent claims and print the percentages or proportions of such ingredients as required; or fourth, they could simply ignore the law. In the immediate wake of the act, it seemed that the "Great American Fraud," identified by Adams, had "foregone its attitude of defiance" as manufacturers made efforts to conform to the new regulations. Still, Adams forewarned that every possible subterfuge might be used to obey the letter of the law by changing the patent medicine label while evading and violating its spirit through its advertising methods.[45]

While the AMA acknowledged similar challenges to the limits of the new federal law, a week after President Theodore Roosevelt signed the Pure Food and Drugs bill, *JAMA* nevertheless referred to its passage as "too good to be true." The next issue of the *Journal* acknowledged that "the law is far better than its most ardent supporters

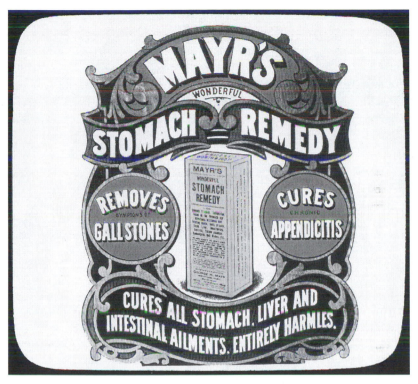

Typical advertisement targeted by the AMA and other advertising reformers (ca. 1912). (Courtesy of American Medical Association Archives)

could reasonably have expected . . . and when we think of the wealth of expert testimony which has been advanced against it, we must confess to a feeling of grateful surprise that the measure is as strong as it is." The act had successfully preserved, for example, the broad definition of a drug as "any substance or mixture of substances intended to be used for the cure, mitigation, or prevention of disease of either man or other animals." This was much to the dismay of the Proprietary Association, the primary professional organ of proprietary drug manufacturers and distributors, which had fought for fewer restrictions on what it deemed the "free market" of the drug trade.[46]

Subsequently, the AMA identified several problems with the act in terms of its limited reach, malleable interpretation, and weak enforcement. Heated arguments over the constitutionality of the law, for example, had limited its reach to the sale of drugs in interstate commerce. An editorial in the *Journal* suggested this meant patent medicines could still "humbug the temperate people" of the states in which they were manufactured, as long as the drugs did not cross state lines. Additionally, while the new law gave people some measure of protection against medicines containing

habit-forming or poisonous drugs, the act offered no protection against other potentially dangerous or useless substances. The AMA saw the need not only for strengthening the legislation and the agencies charged with enforcement, but for confronting
the manufacturing and processing fraternity that might use subtle evasion, lax
enforcement, and favorable judicial interpretations to render the law innocuous.[47]

While the Council of Pharmacy had at least provided a list of drugs that had met
its standards, published in regular *JAMA* articles and compiled in *New and Non-
Official Remedies*, there was no system in place for keeping the public informed about
questionable products investigated under the Pure Food and Drugs Act. A number of
medicines were discontinued or their ingredients were changed to comply with the
new federal law, but many violators simply pled guilty if and when they were charged.
They often paid a small fine and modified or moved their practice. Meanwhile, many
other manufacturers changed their practices to comply with the council's rules.[48]

Enforcement problems were accentuated in 1911, when a federal court judge
ruled in a case involving an alleged cancer cure that the Pure Food and Drugs Act's
restrictions against "false or misleading" advertising did not apply to curative claims.
If the ingredients were correct and only the claims for its ability to cure were false,
no prosecution could go forward. The government appealed to the Supreme Court,
where a majority, led by Oliver Wendell Holmes, agreed that curative claims should
not be settled in a court of law. While the claims for the cancer cure compound were
admittedly misleading if not completely false, Holmes further asserted that Congress
should not get involved in long-running debates about what cured and what did not.[49]

An editorial in *JAMA* quickly charged that the interests benefiting from this decision
were "as cruel a gang of swindlers as ever operated under the protection of the law," and
warned the cancer fakers "who have been driven out of business under the law as previously interpreted, will now be free to resume their damnable trade unmolested." Less than
a month after the Supreme Court's decision, the Los Angeles meeting of the AMA registered its protest and adopted a resolution petitioning Congress to amend the act to outlaw
any false statements regarding therapeutic effectiveness. The secretary of the association
also promptly sent a telegraph of the resolution to the president, the vice president, and
the Speaker of the House. He also sent printed copies to all members of Congress.[50]

A little over a month later, Congress passed an amendment designed to correct the
perceived mistake of the Supreme Court, but the Sherley Amendment, as it became
known, created additional problems. While the amendment stated that it was illegal for
any medicine label to include "false and fraudulent" claims to cure any disease, actually
proving fraudulent intent by a medicine maker was virtually impossible. After all, the
defense could simply claim the patent medicine peddler *believed* that the medicine in
question *did* work. It would be nearly three decades before this loophole in the law could
be closed. Additionally, even when the measure was successfully enforced, the Pure Food
and Drugs Act still had little effect on the advertising of questionable remedies.[51]

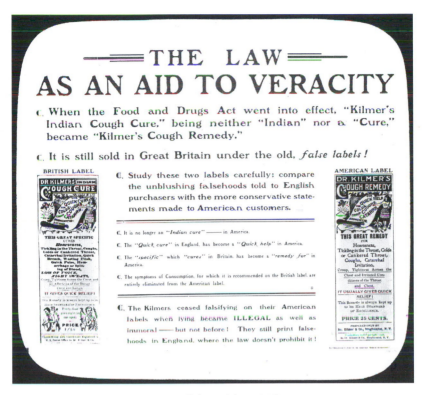

Lantern Slide #14 (ca. 1912).
(Courtesy of American Medical Association Archives)

The success of the Pure Food and Drugs Act rested not only on the strength of a broader coalition for consumer protection, and tightened enforcement measures, but also on the assumption that the public could differentiate between legitimate, legal, or acceptable medicines and their quack counterparts if provided with truthful information about potentially dangerous or addictive contents. This contradicted the Council on Pharmacy and Chemistry's position that even full disclosure was not enough. Acknowledging the chaotic state of the therapeutic marketplace, the council had initially restricted its focus to reforming the practice of physicians. If physicians could not be expected to pass judgment on the secret remedies in the marketplace, certainly the average consumer could not differentiate between nostrums, as the Pure Food and Drugs Act expected. By forcing manufacturers to reveal the contents of their drugs to win AMA approval, the council would theoretically enable physicians to discard redundant or impotent drugs. It could not do the same for drugs advertised directly to consumers no matter how effective the legislation.[52]

CONCLUSION

While it is difficult to quantify the effects of the council on the practice of physi-cians, the *New and Non-Official Remedies* publication nevertheless provided the first reference of its kind for doctors interested in making informed therapeutic decisions. The list of drugs approved for advertisement in *JAMA* adhered to unprecedented standards of full disclosure and experimental evidence. As the first major effort to pass judgment on therapies based on scientific evaluation, the council's rules also provided a model for future regulatory efforts by the federal government. The work to redefine the boundaries of therapeutic orthodoxy, according to standards for purity, safety, and efficacy, nevertheless relied on an ambiguous standard of evidence and placed the decision-making power in the hands of a select group of academic elites. For many new drugs, there was little laboratory or clinical evidence besides that offered to the council by manufacturers. As a result, many drugs were granted experimental status until more conclusive evidence could be acquired. The AMA's chemical laboratory could test for the validity of a drug's chemical constituents but it was not equipped to conduct clinical evaluations for the efficacy of all the drugs it received from manufacturers. Additionally, in some cases where sufficient studies had not been conducted outside manufacturers' laboratories, drugs were disapproved. For consumers, the AMA's refusal to evaluate any patent medicine for the purpose of inclusion in the *New and Nonofficial Remedies* book also left an entire class of drugs initially unconsidered. As a result, many medicine makers protested the judgments of the council while doctors continued to rely on experiential evidence regardless of the AMA's proclamations.

Ideology and circumstances also constrained the regulatory efforts to change the nature of therapeutic practice. As Marks notes, "few physicians shared in the full strength of reformers' convictions that the future of therapeutic progress lay in the lab-oratory." Noncompliant physicians could be changed only by persuasion.[53] But just as the council sought to determine the direction of therapeutic practice, so did drug mak-ers remain committed to the same goal. The Pure Food and Drugs Act successfully prosecuted thousands of manufacturers because they lied about contents, tried to pass off poisonous substances, or falsely labeled their constituent components. But the 1906 law did little to address the issue of whether many drugs marketed to the public were safe and worked as they claimed. The following chapter examines how the limited restrictions of the Pure Food and Drugs Act, combined with exemptions on advertising directly to doctors, played right into the hands of skilled advertisers. Patent medicine manufacturers and advertisers capitalized on the liberal standards of the Council on Pharmacy and Chemistry as well as the limited regulatory reach of the Pure Food and Drugs Act by employing a series of rhetorical strategies designed to successfully promote their drugs to doctors in much the same way they had been doing for decades but without technically breaking the law or violating the standards set by the AMA.

THREE

MARKETING MEDICINES IN AN AGE OF REFORM

A large proportion of medical journals have a department devoted to advertisements under the guise of reading notices, commercial news, therapeutic notes, etc. No pretense is made that these are genuine scientific articles, and it is tacitly understood that these columns are under the control of the advertisers and that the articles are disguised as advertisements . . . As a result, the editor and his contributors exhibit themselves as the willing slave of their proprietary master, having been bought and paid for. The write-up and the apologetic material exhibit the lowest stage of journalistic depravity. An estimate of the extent of this evil can be gained from the statement of a recent writer that the [medical] journals subsidized by the proprietary interests comprise one half of those published in the United States.
—JAMA (1906)[1]

The American Medical Association's (AMA's) Council on Pharmacy and Chemistry helped doctors identify questionable medical therapies by defining some of the characteristics of allegedly quack remedies. To receive the AMA's stamp of approval, the composition of a drug could not be secret, its uniformity had to be safeguarded, and no false claims could be made regarding its therapeutic properties and its use. Drug manufacturers and advertisers also had to provide evidence of at least a probability of therapeutic merit, as demonstrated by laboratory and clinical evidence.

Nevertheless, proprietary firms continued to market drugs to the public and to doctors without the council's approval.

In 1907, the AMA adopted a resolution designed to encourage other medical journals to follow its lead in refusing advertising space to preparations not approved by the AMA's Council on Pharmacy and Chemistry. The resolution requested all other "medical journals to refuse to aid in promoting the sale of preparations which have not been approved by the Council on Pharmacy and Chemistry by refusing advertising space to such preparations" and recommended that AMA members provide moral and financial support to those journals committed to promoting medical science and disregarding commercial interests. Believing that "the press held almost life and death power over the nostrum industry," the association attacked publications that, by advertising nostrums, became "accomplices in deception."[2]

Five years later, in 1912, the AMA denounced the entire business of patent medicine advertising and promised to lead the way in finally eliminating nostrums from the lay and medical press. The *Journal of the American Medical Association* (*JAMA*) declared that all patent medicine advertisements were objectionable, and as a result there could be "no effective censorship of nostrum advertising." In leading an effort to eliminate patent medicine advertising in all medical journals, the association ultimately came up short of its goal.[3]

The AMA nevertheless played a vital role in pushing for the elimination of nostrums from all media. However, an analysis of pamphlets, handbills, trade cards, catalogs, and form letters from the period before and after the advent of regulatory reforms shows that drug manufacturers and distributors employed a wide range of strategies to successfully market their products in spite of regulatory restrictions and the new standards of the Council on Pharmacy and Chemistry. Even when advertisements were banned from medical journals, they still made their way to doctors through the mail. Consequently, the new legislative regime, as well as new institutions designed to protect and inform the public and practitioners, ultimately failed to fully accomplish their goals at least in part because of this loophole.

PATENT MEDICINES AND THE PRESS

To secure advertising reform, the AMA established collaborative relationships with editors and advertising managers from medical and lay journals, magazines, and newspapers. Sympathetic advertising reformers frequently requested information from the AMA's investigatory files, and the association in turn disseminated vast amounts of evidence gathered from a constantly growing number of sources. The managers of the Topeka, Kansas, *Daily Capital*, for example, wrote to the AMA in 1914 in order to provide a copy of its new AMA-inspired advertising policy and to request information about advertisements that had been included in a recent edition of their paper.

The five-page reply from the AMA identified seven different patent medicines, and one patent medicine peddler, and offered evidence against each, collected from the North Dakota Agricultural Experiment Station, the Food and Drugs Act's Notices of Judgment, the Massachusetts Board of Health, articles by Samuel Hopkins Adams, the New Hampshire State Board of Health, the *Chicago Tribune*, and various AMA publications. Another inquiry seeking the AMA's opinion on the advertising content of the *Tuscola County Courier* in Saginaw, Michigan, sympathized with the magnitude of the problem and the difficulties involved in changing the situation. The response from the AMA expressed gratitude for the copy of the *Courier* but informed the paper's advertising manager: "I am sorry to say I cannot agree with your characterization of it as a 'fairly clean county paper as to patents.'" In the single issue submitted for AMA review, advertisements for 27 nostrums filled its pages.[4]

Beginning in 1914, the *Journal* made a point of commending a revised attitude toward the advertising ethics of the mainstream press by publishing words of praise for cooperative newspapers across the country. *JAMA* articles acknowledged the financial risk that the average newspaper faced when contemplating the elimination of allegedly fraudulent advertising but also warned that public opinion shaped itself so rapidly that soon newspapers would find they could not afford to carry such advertisements for "quack" remedies. According to the *Journal*, it had repeatedly been shown that where publications had thrown out these frauds, their pages had gained not only in self-respect but also in the respect of readers.[5]

The *Journal* overtly praised daily and weekly newspapers around the country for committing to the elimination of patent medicine advertising from their pages. In quoting a Canton, Ohio, *Daily News* editorial that admitted, "it is hard to know where to draw the line," the *Journal* reassured its readers that at least the *Daily News* understood that the work of the Council on Pharmacy and Chemistry offered the means to "intelligently, fairly and scientifically censor" the advertisement of proprietary medicines. The editors of the Phoenix, Arizona, *Republican* informed their readers that a much broader movement for reform was already underway and had already spread throughout the country: "A large number of the better known newspapers are now throwing out patent medicine and other offensive advertising, but it is a matter of pride to the *Republican* that it is making a more thorough clean-up than any other secular newspaper of which we have any knowledge." The *Republican* had found additional benefits beside the approval of its own conscience. In addition to an increased volume of "decent" advertising once the frauds were eliminated, an editor explained how the approval of the people of Phoenix had increased subscriptions as well. The *Republican* predicted, "The time, we believe, is near when a patent medicine advertisement will be found in no newspaper which prefers to claim to decency."[6]

One day's "pickings," [Sunday, Jan. 12], from two papers—one in Minneapolis; one in St. Paul. Advertising of this character is barred from THE MINNEAPOLIS JOURNAL.

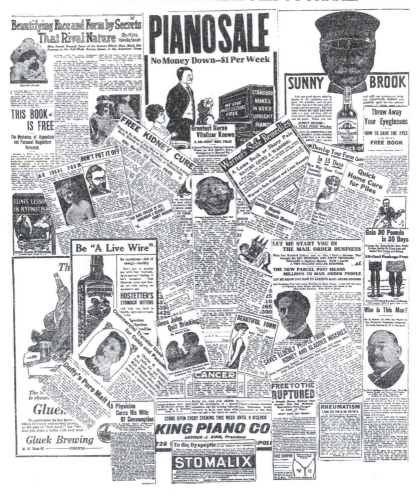

Poster sampling the advertisements banned from the *Minneapolis Journal* newspaper (ca. 1912). (Courtesy of American Medical Association Archives)

The AMA conducted investigations and worked closely with a growing list of advertising reformers both inside and outside the medical profession. Capitalizing on a wave of state laws that regulated advertising on the basis of misbranding and decency, the AMA remained in close contact with newly created protective bureaus and groups such as the Vigilance Committee of the Associated Advertising Clubs of the World. Information was exchanged in both directions. When an agency needed proof of fraudulent claims, misbranding, or expert testimony in court cases, they called on the AMA, which meticulously collected and collated material from a number of private and public sources. When the AMA received complaints from lay observers demanding action, they called on enforcement committees. As a result of this combined effort, the AMA's principal success at purging the secular press from patent-medicine advertisements came from helping to secure the enactment and enforcement of state and federal legislation that prohibited false or misleading advertising. A few states even passed laws making it illegal for newspapers to publish any advertisements for medical practice. By 1919, the U.S. Public Health Service reported that 19,000 out of 20,000 periodicals included in its survey refused to carry any ads for doctors.[7]

The AMA also took direct action in expanding the reform movement among sympathetic members of the medical press. Dozens of state medical society publications almost immediately followed the AMA's lead in eliminating nostrum advertisements from their pages. In 1907, the Kentucky State Medical Association even created its own Committee on Pharmacology, which promised to work closely with the AMA's council. The *Kentucky Medical Journal* implored readers to look through the pages of every medical journal they subscribed to, whether it belonged to a state or national organization, or was supported by the National Proprietary Association, the main organ of proprietary druggists referred to as "the patent medicine vendors' collusive family." If readers found any of the "nauseating advertisements of the blatant frauds already exposed by the Council on Pharmacy and Chemistry," they were urged to write a personal letter to the editor, the publisher, and any other collaborator, calling their attention to such deceptions. Readers were ordered, "Do not talk about it! Write, and write today, and help to save our honorable profession from the vampires who exploit it, to its own shame and dishonor."[8]

The AMA also mercilessly exposed medical journals that refused to eliminate patent medicine advertisements from their pages, despite *JAMA*'s earlier position among the transgressors. In editorials, the *Journal* reported that the *Charlotte Medical Journal*, the *Illinois Medical Register*, the *Atlanta Journal of Medicine*, and the *International Journal of Surgery* were particularly offensive. It described the advertising pages of the latter as "the gallery of nostrums." In 1914, the *Journal* also identified the "Big Six"—the "modest name" assumed by the Associated Medical Publishers in describing their half-dozen medical journals that comprised their organization—as some of the most egregious journals. The Big Six claimed to reach 100,000 physicians every month and promised potential advertisers that since they were the "most aggressive, far-reaching publications of their class," patronizing the Big Six would gain advertisers the "good will, patronage and cooperation of the medical profession of the country." *JAMA* suggested it was more accurate to describe the Big Six as "Six Reasons for the

Perpetuation of the Proprietary Evil." Despite their claims to represent the best in medical science, theory, and practice, in January of 1914, the journals collectively advertised 171 drugs not included in the AMA's *New and Non-Official Remedies*. The *Journal* suggested, "until a majority of the '100,000 of the country's foremost physicians,' who are said to be subscribers to these journals, will devote themselves to the best that is in their profession, we have little or no right to expect that the public at large will believe us to be less gullible than the most unsophisticated layman."[9]

JAMA's relationship with one of the Big Six journals, *Medical Council*, illustrated both the influence of the AMA's Council on Pharmacy and Chemistry and the limits of the reform movement in advertising. In 1914, the June issue of *Medical Council* included an article under the heading, "This Is an Honest Market-Place," which presented the journal as a reliable, scientifically grounded publication useful to the busy medical professional. AMA leadership expressed serious doubts about whether the journal in question represented "an honest marketplace." In the same June 1914 issue of *Medical Council*, the AMA identified 34 medicinal preparations it judged as either "silly," "fakish," "unscientific," or in some instances, "positively harmful." Practically all of these preparations, furthermore, had been criticized specifically in earlier issues of *JAMA*. *Journal* editor George H. Simmons concluded: "It is not creditable—in fact, it is positively brazen—for a medical journal, supposedly published in the interest of the medical profession, to place such advertisements before its readers." *Medical Council* claimed to have 25,000 subscribers, leaving the AMA to lament: "Is it possible that there are this number of physicians who will accept such silly rot through the mails? Truly, were it not pathetic, it would be most humorous."[10]

By the 1920s, the AMA had helped to largely drive the nostrum trade from dozens of medical journals and had at the very least helped raise the standard of medical advertising in the lay press. Improvements could be measured in the less extravagant claims that proprietary manufacturers made for their products, the growing number of states that had enacted some form of new advertising laws, and the thousands of letters the AMA received in recognition of the association's service. In 1927, the Medical Society of the County of New York reported in the *New York Medical Weekly* that most medical journals of standing had by then refused to "accept the advertisements of any product that is not included in *New and Non-Official Remedies*." Many physicians, meanwhile, refused to consider using medicinal preparations unless they had been sanctioned by the Council on Pharmacy and Chemistry. This led the journal to conclude: "The impetus this gives to reliable, high grade medicaments is self-evident." As further evidence of the council's successful work, similar councils had been created elsewhere. This was the path recommended by the American Dental Association to address the problem with proprietary drugs used in dentistry. An article in the *Journal of the American Dental Association* claimed, "It may be succinctly stated that not only has the medical profession of America thrown off the yoke of commercial domination of therapeutics, but also it has gained in self-respect and prestige by having purged itself of much of the baser evils of irrational drug propaganda and therapeutics."[11]

DIRECT MARKETING OF MEDICINES TO DOCTORS

While many reformers considered the effort to purge patent medicines from the medical press a success, the advertising reform movement did nothing to address the direct marketing of questionable remedies to doctors. Literature distributed solely to physicians had been exempted from the rules of the Council on Pharmacy and Chemistry, despite the *Journal's* admission that some physicians could "not distinguish between the preparations that are worthy and those that are unworthy." In public forums, physicians invariably suggested they were sufficiently enlightened and well-educated to separate the wheat from the chaff. As an indication of the faith held by public institutions in this expertise, when the opportunity had arisen to protect physicians from misleading and fraudulent advertising, the Federal Trade Commission (FTC) had exempted advertisements to doctors. So, while state advertising laws banished many nostrums from medical journals and purged them from the lay press, nostrums were still abundantly advertised to physicians via a wide range of direct-marketing techniques.[12]

In the marketing of medicines directly to doctors, the boundaries between patent medicines and the "ethical proprietaries" endorsed by the AMA's council were not always as clearly defined as reformers suggested. Furthermore, despite repeated condemnations by the AMA, direct advertising revealed that many well-respected doctors developed their own patent medicines, and many more provided testimonial support for questionable remedies. Ultimately, the legislation and new standards designed to protect and inform the public and the profession failed to accomplish their goals at least partly because the law could not change the way drug makers sold their wares to physicians. Clever marketers could either bypass regulatory reforms or even co-opt them, which blurred the boundaries between legitimate, safe, and effective drugs and their alleged quack counterparts. If advertisements to doctors provide any indication, many practicing members of the medical profession could still not make this distinction either.

FAITH IN MEDICAL SCIENCE

Medicine manufacturers and distributors had used appeals to scientific evidence to sell drugs long before the reform movements of the early twentieth century, but in the atmosphere of growing fears about patent or quack medicines, advertisements aimed at doctors increasingly emphasized the purity of their products and their "scientific" development. In 1903, for example, the Denver Chemical Manufacturing

Company's pamphlet, "A Study of the Scientific Action and Therapeutic Value of Antiphlogistine," assured doctors that their product had been exclusively "composed of chemically pure" ingredients proven effective by laboratory investigations. Over three decades later, another pamphlet entitled *Infective Wound Therapy* insisted that scientific laboratories had published "experimental evidence confirming our clinical knowledge of the virtues" of the widely advertised ointment Antiphlogistine. The AMA vehemently disagreed. In 1932, the AMA responded to an inquiry regarding Antiphlogistine by asserting, "The unscientific claims made for 'Antiphlogistine' have been commented on in the *Journal*" at various times for decades. Although the Council on Pharmacy and Chemistry never issued an official report, the *Journal* had stated that it was doubtful there was "any real scientific basis for the official product." The claims that had been made for Antiphlogistine also went far beyond the facts and were considered "absolutely unwarranted" and "rather typical of the 'patent medicine' class." These points had been made by the AMA for over 30 years in a series of publications, and they were subsequently corroborated by an article on Antiphlogistine in the *Journal of the American Dental Association* in 1929. The article concluded that "the statements of the wonderful effects of the hygroscopic powers of Antiphlogistine are so manifestly absurd as to be unworthy of further refutation." Nevertheless, no federal action was brought against Antiphlogistine under the Pure Food and Drugs Act. In 1950, the FTC finally filed a complaint under the charges of misrepresentation in the sale of a medicinal preparation for fraudulent and deceptive advertising. Meanwhile, the Denver Chemical Manufacturing Company mailed thousands of advertisements directly to physicians proclaiming the product's scientifically proven, curative powers.[13]

After 1906, many drug manufacturers combined scientific arguments with assurances of legislative or institutional approval. A 1912 ad for the Vanadium Chemical Company, for example, assured doctors that its products were guaranteed by the company "under the Foods and Drug Act, June 30, 1906." Relying on "distinct scientific derivatives," the "newly discovered element vanadium" reportedly "marked an epoch in the history of therapeutics." Following a protracted debate and lengthy correspondence between Vanadium general manager Francis M. Turner, the AMA, and curious doctors, the company submitted five products to the Council on Pharmacy and Chemistry for inclusion in *New and Non-official Remedies* in 1908.[14]

Although the Vanadium Chemical Company included statements and literature regarding the composition of its products and their therapeutic value based on past laboratory and clinical research, the council reported that the evidence was insufficient to warrant the acceptance of the articles. In the first *Journal* report on Vanadium's products in 1908, the council concluded that "the claims made for vanadium have not led to its wide use and until they are confirmed by reliable clinicians

HYGROSCOPIC
ANTISEPTIC   **APPLY**   EXOSMOTIC
ENDOSMOTIC

ANTIPHLOGISTINE

WARM AND THICK

EXPECT IMMEDIATE, DECIDED AND DEFINITE RESULTS

For when within $\frac{1}{64}$ of an inch or less of the circulating blood, it maintains a uniform degree of temperature for from 12 to 24 hours or more; provokes an abundant flushing of the capillaries; apparently through exosmosis a profuse serous transudation, thus depleting the parts, and through endosmosis a stimulating, local, alterative, soothing and tonic effect upon the affected lymphatics and other tissues.

With such processes continuously at work, Inflammation of any kind and Congestions must be and always are promptly benefitted. **Antiphlogistine** is the most effective and deservedly the most popular treatment for

Pneumonia	Chronic Ulcers	Poisoned Wounds
Bronchitis	Orchitis	Dysmenorrhoea
Pleurisy	Buboes	Felons
Pelvic Inflammation	Tonsilitis	Sprains
Osteitis	Piles (external)	Burns
Inflamed Breasts	Boils	Synovitis
Tumors	Erysipelas	Sunburn
Peritonitis	Periostitis	Frost-bites
Rheumatism	Tubercular Pleurisy	Stings

AND FOR ALL CASES WHERE INFLAMMATION OR CONGESTION IS PRESENT AND A LOCAL MEDICINE IS INDICATED

That physicians may know that the medicine has not been exposed and made less capable by absorbing moisture from the atmosphere, they are requested to prescribe in each instance a full package.

Small (actual weight 10½ oz.) ......Price 50 cts.
Medium (actual weight 17½ oz.) ....Price 75 cts.
Large (actual weight 34½ oz.) .....Price $1.25

ANTIPHLOGISTINE is carried in stock by wholesale druggists everywhere. You ought to be able to obtain it promptly in the regular way failing to do so, we will express it to you, prepaid, upon receipt of price.

The Denver Chemical Mfg. Co.

(INCORPORATED 1893)

451-453 WASHINGTON STREET

(Home Office, DENVER)   **NEW YORK**

"Antiphlogistine" (Denver Chemical Co. Pamphlet, 1912).
(Courtesy of the National Library of Medicine)

the remedy must be regarded as in the experimental stage."[15] The council asked Vanadium to provide additional pharmacological evidence for the therapeutic claims in the accompanying advertising literature. Meanwhile, mass mailings of Vanadium literature to doctors continued.

By 1912, a review of the advertising literature directed at doctors revealed a wide range of remarkable claims, including the suggestion that Vanadium could be used as an antiseptic and antitoxin in combating tuberculosis. A special summary pamphlet on Vanadium preparations reported that the council had concluded that "the company has not, and never has had, any reliable evidence on which to base the therapeutic claims it has presented to the medical profession." From the AMA's perspective, it also probably did not help Vanadium's case that a favorable review of vanadium in treating tuberculosis appeared in the *Journal of the American Institute of Homeopathy* in 1912.[16] Meanwhile, the *Journal* also reported in 1912 that it had learned that the general manager of Vanadium was connected to a fraudulent obesity cure firm and was not authorized to use the title M.D. as he did in its advertising literature.[17]

In a January issue of the *Journal* in 1913, the AMA attempted to put the issue to rest by clarifying that the Council on Pharmacy's report on certain proprietary preparations of the Vanadium Company was not a judgment on vanadium itself as a potentially valuable therapeutic agent. The article conceded there was evidence of vanadium's value, but the only way it would be proved was by the "careful and painstaking use of preparations put on the market honestly and free from the bias that is inseparable from proprietaries that are sold under grossly exaggerated claims."[18]

Advertisers moved quickly to equate AMA approval with scientific validity, even when contradictory evidence about the safety or effectiveness of certain drugs persisted. A 1920 pamphlet for the drug Luminal, entitled "A Dramatic Event in the History of a Distressful Disease," emphasized the drug's acceptance by the AMA's Council on Pharmacy and Chemistry in 1913. Luminal had initially been approved for use as a sedative and a hypnotic, but the same year it had been described in *New and Non-Official Remedies*, other medical journals warned practitioners about the dangers of using phenobarbital (the scientific name for the proprietary Luminal). Some of the clinical reports in subsequent years warned of its toxic effects and uncertain results, but other researchers promoted its use, as long as it was under the supervision of a physician.[19]

The controversy peaked in the early 1920s, following reports of the successful use of Luminal in treating epilepsy. That same year, a letter to the editor of *JAMA* warned that until there was a better understanding of the "exact pharmacologic action" of the drug, not to mention a better understanding of epilepsy itself ("if one were to ask a hundred practitioners probably as many definitions would be received," the letter suggested), use of Luminal was too dangerous. By the end of the decade, these warnings had been illustrated by reports of overdoses and Luminal addiction. The AMA became involved in the discussion only when Luminal became the ingredient of choice in a rash of epilepsy patent-medicine cures that merited the publication of a special pamphlet on the issue and gained the attention of the investigative unit at the new federal Food, Drug, and Insecticide Administration. The Department of Agriculture wanted to push for the elimination of Luminal-bearing epilepsy products from the mails, but the AMA worried that if phenobarbital cures were wiped out, quacks would simply go back to its predecessor, the bromides, which had been deemed even more dangerous and addictive.[20]

Advertisers of the "ethical proprietaries" appealed to this judgment and also tried to bolster the scientific basis of their products by making distinctions between indispensable scientific remedies marketed exclusively to doctors and the illegitimate patent-medicine counterparts advertised directly to the public. Liberty Chemical Company, for example, guaranteed doctors that their "scientific chemical" had been manufactured "for the exclusive use of the medical profession." To distinguish itself from its competitors, Liberty even removed all dosage recommendations and mention of therapeutic uses from the labels of its bottles. This practice quickly became widespread.[21]

Several drug companies also inundated physicians with scientific and educational material designed to simultaneously bring practitioners up to speed on the latest scientific developments and sell their products. The Palisade Manufacturing Company, for example, makers of the antiseptic Borolyptol, sent doctors advertisements for their drugs along with a handbook entitled *Syllabus of Bacteriology: A Compact Treatise Designed to Aid the Physician in the Scientific Diagnosis of Disease*. Pease Laboratories also employed the common strategy of sending supplemental scientific reports such as their *Report in the Matter of the Chemical, Bacteriological, and Biological Investigation of Zonite to Determine Its Value as a Germicide and Local Antiseptic*. Neither Borolyptol nor Zonite ever received the approval of the Council on Pharmacy and Chemistry, in large part because of the typically outrageous claims made by antiseptic pushers. The makers of Borolyptol, for example, argued that if more physicians practiced "Borolyptology," a science closely related to, yet opposed to, bacteriology, "all microbic life would be annihilated, and the bacteriologist, like Othello, would find his occupation gone."[22]

On a visual level, advertisers also used the imagery of science to appeal to doctors and consumers. By the 1920s, advertisements increasingly included various scientific images, charts, and graphs to measure and illustrate the physiological effect of drugs, while both cellular and X-ray photography were used to depict before-and-after images. The pamphlet "An Outline of some of the Uses and Advantages of Petrolagar," for example, by Deshell Laboratories, Inc., illustrated the dissemination of Petrolagar in aqueous solutions in photographs of beakers, diagrams of the effects of emulsification, photographs of the microscopic action of the emulsifier, and X-ray photographs revealing images of an impacted bowel prior to and after the Petrolagar regimen. In an era dominated by patent-medicine cures for constipation, Petrolagar tried to set itself apart from competitors through the use of scientific imagery. The Organic Chemical Manufacturing Company, meanwhile, utilized another common technique by commissioning artists to depict the laboratory origins of its various products replete with elaborate instrumentation and scientific iconography.[23]

Patent medicine makers and ethical drug manufacturers were not alone in appealing to the public's faith in science—"sectarian" forms of medical therapies also used the language and imagery of science to legitimize their products. Advocates of homeopathic therapies frequently emphasized their adherence to the natural laws of healing and scientifically proven principles as well. Boericke & Tafel's guide to treating common ailments, for example, proudly announced on its cover that its "medicines and pharmaceutical preparations were awarded prize medals for purity, accuracy and general excellence at the Centennial Exposition, the Cotton Exposition, and the Columbian Exposition, while no other homeopathic pharmacy received an award." The firm's catalog also provided a list of scientific authorities who endorsed their products, while guaranteeing their laboratory preparation and quality. Three decades later, however, the AMA still reported that these same products were "not considered scientific by the Council on Pharmacy and Chemistry," which precluded conducting any tests. While sympathetic to the fact that a great many homeopaths by that time had become members of the AMA, the "original homeopathic doctrines" supported by Boericke & Tafel were officially considered "contrary to established medical fact" and "practically useless."[24]

Anticipating opposition from the orthodox profession, some sectarian groups such as the Pennsylvania Orthopaedic Institute and School of Mechano-Therapy took the novel approach of promoting their therapies as "subsidiary to the medical profession," as an "aid to the regular practice of medicine." This position, combined with superintendent Max Walter's condemnation of the "danger of charlatanism and quackery," helped assure doctors and consumers alike that their treatments were based on a "universally recognized scientific standpoint."[25]

Collectively, the marketing of the therapies mentioned previously undercut the effort to eliminate allegedly fraudulent advertising, as drug firms blurred the boundaries between "scientific" and "unscientific" by adapting terms to their objectives. To borrow a phrase from Christopher Toumey, drug manufacturers and advertisers "conjured science" with rhetorical techniques, imagery, laboratory reports, clinical studies, and institutional approval. Toumey argues that "to invoke the symbols of science is to make policies sound, commodities desirable, and behavior legitimate."[26] In the case of medical therapies, appeals to science sometimes blurred rather than clarified the boundaries between approved conventional medical therapies and their alleged quack counterparts. At the same time, the cases of Vanadium, Luminal, and Antiphlogistine demonstrate that the proclaimed scientific status of a drug could be

PHYSICIANS'

Price List and Therapeutic Hand Book

Homœopathic Medicines and Books

And All Articles Required by Physicians and Pharmacists

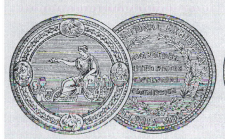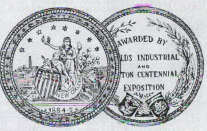

Boericke & Tafel received THE ONLY Medals awarded for Homœopathic
Medicines at the Centennial Exposition in Philadelphia
at the Cotton Exposition in New Orleans and at
the Columbian Exposition in Chicago

BOERICKE & TAFEL

Homœopathic Pharmaceutists, Importers and Publishers

PHILADELPHIA   NEW YORK   CHICAGO
PITTSBURGH   CINCINNATI

"Physicians' Price List and Therapeutic Hand Book" (1922).
(Courtesy of the National Library of Medicine)

highly negotiable. Just because a drug had successfully passed the standards set for evaluation and approval did not necessarily mean that it could be deemed safe and/ or effective. Neither did disapproval necessarily mean that a therapy did not work. Consequently, rhetoric played a crucial role.

HISTORY AND MODERNITY

Another popular rhetorical strategy in advertising therapies to practitioners emphasized either the historical evidence for effective treatments or the modern and progressive nature of new treatments. These strategies proved particularly effective in the marketing of unorthodox remedies deemed quackery by the mainstream medical profession. The historical argument offered by the homeopathic *Humphreys' Specific Manual for the Administration of Medicine and Cure of Disease*, for example, included a scathing critique of the historically excessive treatments used by regular doctors. Humphreys boldly proclaimed the effectiveness of homeopathic treatment, noting that "forty years of experience, of sharp criticism, of professional and popular ridicule and opprobrium" had established "its truth by the stern logic of fact." The AMA Council on Pharmacy and Chemistry never analyzed Humphreys' products, but a reply to an inquiry from the Department of Public Health of Rhode Island decades later typified the AMA's response. The letter asserted, "It is, of course, wholly unwise and not in the interest of public health for such booklets as the Humphreys' Homeopathic Medicine Company distributes to be sent out. We doubt, however, whether the Post Office Department would rule against" the distribution of these particular "nostrum circulars." In a more conciliatory nod, the AMA also suggested more progressive homeopaths were no longer indebted to the outdated therapeutic principles of homeopathy's founder.[27]

Other unorthodox practitioners, meanwhile, argued their therapies could be equated with more progressive orthodox medical practice. A mass mailing advertisement by a physiomedical instrument firm to doctors, for example, included a reproduction of a one-page editorial written by E. L. Shope, M.D., in which the doctor testified to the value of a vibratory massage apparatus, electric light bath cabinet, and hot air treatments. Shope promised readers that adopting such physical or mechanical therapies could be equated with "practicing modern therapeutics." Of course, it was an added bonus for the practitioners that patients would be given the very best advantages in treatments while the doctor also earned a higher income.[28]

In contrast to this modernist argument, advertisers also combined the historical argument with a critique of modern science and its tendency to overlook simple remedies. The Aquatone Lithia Sparkling Water Company of Ambler, Pennsylvania, for example, suggested its spring water could be used to treat rheumatism, despite the fact that the earnest physician, "with his head full of science, busily seeking the latest bacteriological bacillian development, looks far away beyond the medical horizon for a new discovery when the wealth of remedy—simple, safe and certain—lies flowing at his feet." However hyperbolic, the implicit suggestion here—that not man but nature cured—increasingly became a central theme in a series of pamphlets and almanacs produced by both patent-medicine makers and ethical proprietors alike.[29]

In *Nature Cures: The History of Alternative Medicine in America*, historian James Whorton suggests that claims to nature also served as a distinguishing characteristic of alternative medical systems in the early twentieth century. Identifying a shift in the focus of orthodox medical attention in the second half of the eighteenth century toward pathological changes that manifest disease in specific organs, Whorton suggests that alternative practitioners responded to an emphasis on illness as a pathological condition by returning to a more holistic understanding inherited from the Hippocratic tradition. The healing power of nature was a highly controversial and malleable concept for physicians in the late nineteenth century, and was deemed a "heresy" by many orthodox practitioners who roundly criticized their sympathetic colleagues. But for sectarian and proprietor alike, the nature-cure approach represented a more historical *and* a more holistic method in opposition to the modern, mechanistic, reductionistic orientation of mainstream medicine.[30]

While the Kickapoo Indian Medicine Company engaged almost exclusively in marketing directly to consumers, the company distinguished its therapies from those offered by other patent medicine promoters by reassuring readers that "medicines composed of roots, barks, twigs, leaves, seeds, and berries are the most beneficial, because they assist Nature in the right way to make her own cure." Furthermore, the company claimed that as a result of printing all of the ingredients of its medicines on their packages, Kickapoo remedies should no longer be regarded as "patent medicines." As one ornate catalog proclaimed, "One of the most beneficial laws ever enacted in the United States is the Pure Food and Drugs Act of June 30, 1906. That has put out of business more fake 'patent medicines' and so-called 'remedies' containing dangerous drugs than anything else that was ever done in this country." While the AMA's council never conducted tests on Kickapoo Remedies, Kickapoo Cough Cure was declared misbranded under the Pure Food and Drugs Act in 1911 for three reasons: first, because it contained a percentage of alcohol that the bottle's label failed to state; second, it was labeled a "cough cure" when in fact no evidence existed for its curative effects; and third, while it claimed to possess properties recognized by the profession as necessary to the proper treatment of diseases of the lung, it did not possess such properties. The Kickapoo Medicine Company continued to sell several of its nature cures for years to come.[31]

A number of advertisers tried to overcome any rumblings of therapeutic nihilism in their appeal to nature by combining historical and modernist arguments in their appeals to practitioners. The Biogen Company, manufacturers of the "portable oxygen products" Biogen and Dermogen, confirmed the validity of their products by citing the combined historical-modernist argument found in the pages of the *International Journal of Surgery*. The journal article argued that Biogen had remarkably fulfilled the centuries old "ambition of Chemistry to utilize the elements of Nature for the benefit of humanity," which must be of "interest to the progressive physician." As a result, pamphlets suggested Biogen would be the perfect drug for doctors who have "afforded abundant evidence of a disposition to profit in the past by the achievements of chemistry." Biogen never made it into *New and Non-Official Remedies* and was disparaged in the pages of *JAMA* in an article that condemned the "fancy names" of well-known chemical compounds.[32]

Rather than promoting the achievements of science, advertisements employing historical rhetoric often stressed the limitations of a scientific approach. Literature from the bacteriological laboratories of drug manufacturer Dr. George Henry Sherman, for example, argued that all too often years of clinical observations had been dismissed because "the bacteriological pathologists allow their theoretic contentions to outweigh these clinical deductions and continue to keep their objections to the forefront." Jones & Co., meanwhile, similarly marketed their Niagara Folding Hot Vapor Bath Cabinet "for the people's good," suggesting that the effectiveness of the vapor bath cabinet was made self-evident by years of experience. After all, the pamphlet proclaimed, historical experience and "common sense appeals readily to people of intellect."[33]

Collectively, these historical and modernist arguments could either undercut the authority of science or capitalize on its promise. They could lend credence to marginalized therapies by condemning or skirting the judgments of regulatory institutions and encouraging doctors to reconsider their approach to therapeutic practice. Whether these strategies worked is difficult to measure, but they demonstrate the power of rhetoric in marketing efforts designed to encourage doctors to make their own judgments about the medical therapies they employed in their practice, irrespective of conventional admonitions.

ANECDOTAL EVIDENCE

Advocates of unorthodox therapeutic systems, patent medicine makers, and major ethical drug companies also shared a third rhetorical advertising strategy—the use of anecdotal evidence to successfully market their products in spite of regulatory restrictions. In one variation of this strategy, they cited the approval of physicians, medical institutions, and professional journals to capitalize on professional authority. Although this strategy had been used throughout the history of drug advertising, in the wake of the Pure Food and Drugs Act and the creation of the AMA's Council on Pharmacy and Chemistry, the use of anecdotal evidence proved particularly powerful as consumers increasingly relied on the voice of authority to distinguish between effective and ineffective medicines on the market. In another variation of this rhetorical strategy, marketers employed the testimony of satisfied customers as evidence for the efficacy of their products. In the process, anecdotal evidence played a crucial role in legitimizing various types of medical treatment while simultaneously obscuring the border between quackery and nonquackery.

Proprietary drug manufacturers often employed physicians to write reports on the therapeutic effectiveness of their drugs. Dios Chemical Company, for example, reassured physicians about the safety of their sedative product Neurosine by contrasting its qualities with a list of the dangers and disadvantages of other commonly prescribed sedatives. A bibliography listed eight "authoritative works on pharmacology and therapeutics" directly quoted in the brochure, implying the approval of the identified authors. This type of approval mimicked the price list catalogs for ethical proprietary firms like Bayer Pharmaceutical Products, which also frequently included a "select bibliography" of authoritative works on the safe therapeutic action of their drugs, along with the successful experience of quoted physicians. Professor Hans Leo, from the University of Bonn, cited under the heading "Clinical Evidence," confirmed that he had successfully used Bayer's Acidol Pepsin both in personal trials and with hundreds of patients, including very young children. Dios Chemical Company adopted strategies similar to Bayer's by providing detailed case histories testifying to the safety and efficacy of their products. In one pamphlet, 24 references from scientific authorities were used to testify indirectly to the safety of Neurosine.[34]

Of course, none of this advertising material revealed the fact that the AMA considered Neurosine a patent medicine. Neurosine was dealt with critically by the AMA and its journal for decades after it had been introduced. The Council on Pharmacy and Chemistry first published an unfavorable report on this "shot gun nostrum" in 1915. Another unfavorable report followed in 1916. Subsequently, the *Journal* provided a negative review of the product again in 1918 in an article titled "Neurosine and the Original Package Evil," and again in 1925 Neurosine was briefly mentioned for the dangers it presented. In 1931, the *Journal* reported a case of Neurosine poisoning. Anyone writing to the AMA regarding Neurosine received reference to this information in reply. After 1937, AMA responses included references to government bulletins published in May and June of that year, which reported on two cases in which the Neurosine manufacturer had been prosecuted for violating the Pure Food and Drugs Act for adulterating and falsely labeling its product. The principle active ingredients, which included a large proportion of bromides, were not disclosed on the label. Four other potentially poisonous ingredients were also not identified. Without consulting the AMA and its journal, however, doctors relying on advertising literature from Neurosine had plenty of anecdotal evidence to confirm its safety and promote its use.[35]

In contrast to rather tame and measured uses of anecdotal evidence, some companies used anecdotal evidence to confirm the validity of treatments that had been even more widely marginalized or delegitimized by the mainstream medical profession. The Stafford Mineral Springs and Hotel Company of Vossburg, Mississippi, for example, proclaimed in its advertisements to doctors and consumers that their product was "the only Mineral Spring Water in the world, or any other remedy, after

THE SAFETY *of* SEDATIVES
A COMPARATIVE STUDY

By

FREDERIC DAMRAU, M.D.

―――

Since sedatives and hypnotics are among the most widely prescribed of all drugs, their safety is of prime importance. Yet statistics show an alarming increase in deaths and poisoning due to barbital and barbituric acid preparations, and more and more of such products are being offered to the medical profession.

Numerous reports received from physicians by the manufacturers of Neurosine* have emphasized its unparalleled safety even when administered in very large dosage for long periods. These findings contrasted sharply with the known toxicity of many commonly employed hypnotics and sedatives, some of which have a comparatively small margin of safety between the therapeutic and harmful doses. In fact, with susceptible individuals, the therapeutic and toxic doses of barbital and its congeners may partially overlap.

Cases are recorded in which melancholiacs, with suicidal intent, swallowed as much as 6 ounces (24 times the average dose) or more of Neurosine, but suffered no ill effects other than prolonged sleep. The physicians observing these cases found no evidences of depression except drowsiness and stupor, from which the patients eventually awoke refreshed as after a long slumber.

―――

*Neurosine is absolutely free from chloral hydrate, paraldehyde and barbital or its derivatives.

Pamphlet by Frederic Damrau, M.D., "The Safety of Sedatives: A Comparative Study" (New York: Dios Chemical Co., 1935). (Courtesy of the National Library of Medicine)

many thorough tests, pronounced by eminent physicians of New York, New Orleans, Brooklyn and elsewhere, as a cure for Bright's Disease, Diabetes, Cystitis, Dyspepsia, and other diseases of the Kidney, Bladder and Stomach." Stafford even resorted to printing a copy of a letter from the executive mansion, allegedly written by President Grover Cleveland, which asked, "In what larger packages can the 'Stafford Water' be purchased and at what price?" Maximizing the power of anecdotal evidence, Stafford also printed "an unparalleled list" of leading physicians who "have tested" and "are almost daily prescribing it in their practice," offering a free book of their testimonials that promised to "astound and convince the most skeptical."[36]

Testimonials operated as valuable tools for advocates of unorthodox systems of medicine too. Their use helped legitimize unorthodox medical therapies while providing apparent evidence of their efficacy. Boericke & Tafel's catalog of "New Remedies," for example, paired over 130 diseases and conditions with homeopathic remedies, and over 30 different physicians offered testimonials on their behalf. Dr. Coburn, for example, reported that in 10-drop doses and a topical application of *chimaphila umbellata*, a cancerous tumor of the breast had been completely cured. The Pennsylvania Orthopaedic Institute and School of Mechano-Therapy also relied heavily on this type of testimonial, capitalizing on the authority of prominent medical professors and physicians to guarantee the efficacy of treatments including electrotherapy, thermotherapy, hydrotherapy, and corrective gymnastics, all available in their "progressive clinics."[37]

Tyrrell's Hygienic Institute, based in New York City, could reasonably be considered the king of the testimonial, using the words of satisfied customers to promote the J. B. L. Cascade Treatment of "internal baths," also known as self-administered enemas or colonics. In a circular mailed out en masse, Tyrrell's reassured doctors that "thousands of testimonials" were on file in their offices. Tyrrell's Hygienic Institute raised the ante, however, in their 1917 pamphlet that offered a list of "distinguished people and institutions who use the Cascade Treatment," including admirals, colonels, judges, senators, hospitals, sanitariums, and various other institutes. An additional list of "prominent physicians who both use and prescribe it," included M.D.s, D.O.s, and dentists from all over the country. Tyrrell's also employed the common strategy of reprinting commissioned scholarly articles that supported the use of advertised therapies. A pamphlet on internal baths, for example, prominently featured an article from Dr. Frank Crane of the *New York Globe* in the foreword, which was supplemented by the opinions of additional "eminent scientists." Employing another tactic commonly utilized in newspapers and journals, Tyrrell's created advertisements that appeared to be standard journalistic articles, a particularly "insidious piece of quackery" according to one critic.[38]

The president of Tyrrell's Hygienic Institute, Charles A. Tyrrell, operated under the watchful eye of the AMA for years before they came in direct contact. In 1913, when the advertising department of the *American Review of Reviews* contacted the AMA because it was considering dropping Tyrrell's as an advertiser due to complaints from readers, the AMA supplied a special pamphlet they had created on the institute. Here, the *Journal* presented its case against the J. B. L. Cascade Treatment: (1) Tyrrell claimed to be the inventor of the Cascade, while the patent office records showed otherwise; (2) Tyrrell claimed that the Cascade was "the only thing of the kind ever

You're Not Healthy Unless You're Clean Inside

And the one way to real internal cleanliness—by which you are protected against ninety per cent. of all human ailments—is through **proper** internal bathing, with plain warm water.

There is nothing unusual about this treatment—no drugs, no dieting—nothing but the correct application of Nature's own cleanser. But only since the invention of the J. B. L. Cascade has a means for **proper** internal bathing existed.

Only one treatment is known for actually **cleansing** the colon without the aid of elaborate surgical apparatus. This is The Internal Bath by means of the J. B. L. Cascade.

Prof. Metchnikoff, Europe's leading authority on intestinal conditions, is quoted as saying that, if the colon and its poisonous contents were removal, people would live in good health to twice the present average of human life.

Dr. A. Wilford Hall, Ph.D., LL.D., and W. E. Forest, B. D., M. D., two world-famous authorities on internal bathing, are among the thousands of physicians who have given their hearty and active endorsement and support to the J. B. L. Cascade treatment.

Fully half a million men and women and children now use this real boon to humanity—most of them **in accordance with their doctor's orders.**

LET DR. TYRRELL ADVISE YOU

Dr. Tyrrell is always very glad of an opportunity to consult freely with any one who writes him—and **at no expense or obligation whatever.** Describe your case to him and he gives you his promise that you will learn facts about yourself which you will realize are of **vital importance.** You will also receive his book, "The What, the Why, the Way," which is a most interesting treatise on internal bathing. **Consultation with Dr. Tyrrell involves no obligation.**

CHARLES A. TYRRELL, M. D.,
134 West 65th Street, New York.

From Charles A. Tyrrell, *The Royal Road to Health* (New York: Charles A. Tyrrell, 1913). (Courtesy of the National Library of Medicine)

specially designed," which was absurd; (3) Tyrrell claimed that apoplexy, consumption, Bright's disease, syphilis, cancer, and "goodness knows what" all had "their origins in the colon," which "no one but a charlatan and a fool—or both—would claim"; (4) Tyrrell claimed that typhoid fever and appendicitis "may be positively cured" by the use of his apparatus, a statement that was "not only false but vicious"; and (5) Tyrrell fraudulently exploited another device "sold on the strength of faked and fraudulent testimonials and 'analytic reports.'" The AMA distributed this pamphlet to thousands of curious consumers and included excerpts in its journal.[39]

Tyrrell directly challenged the accusations that his advertisements included flamboyant and extravagant claims in the form of testimonials. He insisted no testimonial had appeared in his pamphlets at any time that had ever been solicited in any manner, shape, or form. They all came voluntarily; and when letters of a flattering nature presented themselves, he had invariably asked the writer for permission to use them. Tyrrell believed publishing these testimonials was his duty to the public and emphasized that the people themselves stated they had been cured. He believed in the veracity of the statements because the writers had no object at all in deceiving him. While Tyrrell admitted he was not practicing disinterested philanthropy by any means, he contended that the AMA had gone out of its way to distort the facts. From Tyrrell's perspective, his only offense seemed to be that he was unethical by going outside the "stereotyped lines which govern the medical profession in making the fact of this treatment known to the public at large." If this was his only sin, he confessed with pride that he took glory in it. He concluded: "Every medical man recognizes the fact that there is not finality in medicine; that we have not yet arrived at the point where we can say that this or that is positively accomplished, and therefore it is fully open to discussion, as to what the merits of any particular mode of treatment may be and its effect upon the patient." For the AMA, the case on Tyrrell's Hygienic Institute had already been closed.[40]

Since Samuel Hopkins Adams had uncovered the scheme whereby businesses advertised for, bought, and secured testimonials for drug firms, the AMA had consistently doubted the veracity of such claims and made exposing fraudulent testimonials a top priority. The AMA followed up reports and complaints with its own investigations, which involved tracking down testimonial givers. It found and publicized several cases in which testimonials for an alleged tuberculosis cure were apparently honestly delivered, but then the testimonial givers had subsequently died of tuberculosis. The photos of the tuberculosis victims were widely circulated as part of the AMA's campaign to convince consumers that testimonials were, in fact, worthless.[41]

Despite efforts to undercut the authority of testimonials used by Tyrrell and others, this type of anecdotal evidence had a significant impact in shaping therapeutic choices. For therapies judged inert and either barred or dismissed from the orthodox therapeutic armamentarium due to a lack of scientific evidence for their efficacy, testimonials offered contrary evidence based on experience. While anecdotal evidence could also be used to convey approval from authoritative textbooks, respected medical journals, and highly educated experts, a survey of the marketing material sent to physicians suggests that doctors did not always make therapeutic choices based on experimental laboratory-based evidence. Instead, sometimes experience could be equally compelling.

CONCLUSION

Collectively, these marketing strategies undercut the effect of efforts to eliminate advertisements of questionable remedies from the press and allowed drug manufacturers and distributors to capitalize on new standards and regulatory requirements. Disclosing ingredients, guaranteeing chemical purity, and claiming adherence to high scientific standards became one way to reassure doctors about a drug's safety and efficacy. Recounting historical experience or employing the latest, modern, progressive methods also undoubtedly helped convince doctors and consumers that treatments actually worked. Anecdotal evidence brought together each of these themes by using the satisfied customer and the authority of physicians, institutions, and scholarly journals to legitimize therapies. As a result, while the work of the Council on Pharmacy and Chemistry, the restrictions of the Pure Food and Drugs Act, and advertising reformers helped eliminate the secrecy of patent medicines and led to the prosecution of thousands of fraudulent medicine makers, this ultimately did not definitively establish the boundary lines between quackery and nonquackery. Meanwhile, the manufacturers and distributors of countless questionable remedies continued to turn massive profits.

Having analyzed the conflicting efforts of reformers to regulate the marketplace and drug manufacturers to successfully market their products, the following chapter examines another important tool used by the AMA to fight quackery: the Propaganda Department. The Propaganda Department facilitated efforts to combat patent medicine advertising and established a broadly conceived, multifaceted strategy for leading a wider crusade against all forms of medical quackery.

FOUR

PROPAGANDA FOR REFORM

Is it not naturally the work of the local medical society to educate the people of the neighborhood to a proper appreciation of a profession that concerns them so intimately as does that of medicine, not only individually, but through newspapers and by other printed matter? If it be objected to this that we should be imitating the quacks, I can only answer that as long ago as churches decided that the devil should not have the best music, so now it is surely time that the monopoly by quacks of the best means of disseminating information should cease. "Truth is mighty and must prevail" in a fair field. But if the truth is bottled up and not allowed to get into the open, it is not surprising that falsehood scores a triumph.

—JAMA (1907)[1]

The limited scope of the Pure Food and Drugs Act created an opportunity for the American Medical Association (AMA) to shape the fight against quackery. Drug manufacturers continued to successfully market medicines judged to be quackery. Problems persisted with limited resources for investigating and prosecuting offenders. These shortcomings convinced the federal government that an alliance with the AMA was a necessity. At the same time, the AMA became convinced that it could not rely solely on the work of its own Council of Pharmacy and Chemistry along with the enforcement of federal laws to eliminate the "nostrum menace" through advertising reform. New alliances and a new strategy for reform enabled the AMA to broaden the scope of its effort through the work of its Propaganda Department. This new unit disseminated information not only on the work of the Council of Pharmacy and Chemistry and the Pure Food and Drugs Act but also on all forms of alleged fraud and quackery in the field of medicine more broadly.

The work of the Propaganda Department benefited the association in four significant ways. First, it allowed the AMA to establish itself as the preeminent clearinghouse for information on alleged quack therapies, practitioners, and institutions. The AMA also thereby became the primary arbiter in disputes over the legitimacy of medical therapies. Second, it provided an opportunity to eliminate some of the competition in the medical marketplace by exposing the dangers and deceptions associated with "patent medicine" peddlers and other advocates of what the AMA defined much more broadly as quackery and "pseudomedicine." Third, this broadened campaign against quackery and pseudomedicine became part of an effort to legitimize the AMA as a professional organization of expert scientists and practitioners uniquely qualified for and committed to protecting the public from a very real threat that had been documented extensively by muckraking journalists. Fourth, the AMA's campaign helped create a close working relationship with the government, which facilitated the AMA's move from a position of relative political obscurity at the beginning of the twentieth century to serious political contender in a few short decades. As physicians, the general public, and both private and public organizations became increasingly reliant on the AMA for information, the association attempted to increase the authority of the medical profession by publically proclaiming responsibility for defining the boundaries between safe and effective remedies and their counterparts. Through this work, the AMA became the de facto leader of an informal national network of antiquackery surveillance.[2]

THE PROPAGANDA DEPARTMENT

The AMA's Propaganda for Reform campaign began in the pages of the *Journal of the American Medical Association (JAMA)* in 1907, with a series of articles on questionable drugs. The Propaganda Department advanced the crusade against quackery by investigating and exposing all forms of unorthodox medical practices, including allegedly fraudulent practitioners, questionable medical schools, and unconventional medical organizations, many of which happened to be the AMA's most vocal critics. The campaign established the fight against quackery as one of the most important phases of the AMA's work.

Through the Propaganda Department, the AMA accelerated its drive against the nostrum threat by creating an expansive network of quackery surveillance. While the collection and dissemination of information remained its primary objective, the department also conducted original investigations, collected data received from governmental sources, organized material published in domestic and foreign journals, and filed reports on special commissions. Curious consumers and doctors could receive information about specific drugs, medical practitioners, and therapeutic practices by writing directly to the AMA offices. Educators could inquire about the latest information on medical quackery. Government officials received detailed reports on alleged quacks and quack medicine that were under investigation.[3]

The department divided its work into five main areas that corresponded to different aspects of a constantly growing network of surveillance: (1) publications designed to inform and involve the public in a concerted fight against all forms of health fraud; (2) the creation of educational materials designed to keep physicians, health educators, and the public informed about the latest research and most mendacious quackeries; (3) close work with municipal, state, and federal governmental organizations in fights against quackery on legal fronts; (4) collaboration with business, professional, and other voluntary private organizations in an effort to create a database of questionable practitioners and quasimedical institutions; and (5) correspondence with doctors as well as editors of magazines and newspapers, a growing number of laypersons searching for an authoritative voice in a highly contested medical marketplace, and professional, scientific, and educational organizations. Through this work, the AMA helped establish a network of antiquackery volunteers and professionals that would lead the assault on allegedly fraudulent practitioners and practices for much of the rest of the century.

ARTHUR J. CRAMP: ARCH FOE OF THE QUACKS

The first director of the Propaganda Department, Dr. Arthur J. Cramp, understood the importance of publicity in reform efforts and earned a reputation as a prolific author and the arch foe of the quacks. Colleagues remembered that the diligence in his work reflected his vested personal interest in the fight. Cramp had joined the AMA staff as an editorial assistant with a clear purpose in mind in 1906, the same year he earned his M.D. from the Wisconsin College of Physicians, and the same year Congress passed the Pure Food and Drugs Act. Born in England in 1872, he had come to the United States at the age of 19. Following a move to Milwaukee, he worked as a science teacher at a local high school. When his only daughter fell ill, Cramp called on a local doctor for her care. While it remains unclear what happened with this doctor, Cramp blamed the subsequent death of his daughter on inadequate and inept medical treatment. He was thus inspired to study medicine by a sense of personal mission: an implacable hatred of quacks and the desire to train

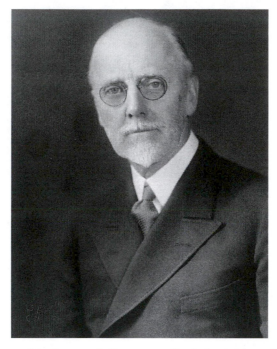

First director of the Propaganda Department, Dr. Arthur J. Cramp (ca. 1920).
(© American Medical Association. Courtesy of AMA Archives)

himself to distinguish between true and false in the realm of medical care. The offer to
join the editorial staff of the *Journal* provided Cramp with the opportunity to devote
his entire career to fighting medical quackery.[4]

Writing reports on AMA investigations of proprietary medicines initially became
his primary task. His early articles from 1906 to 1910 were published in *JAMA*,
and principally dealt with allegedly fraudulent "ethical proprietaries" marketed and
sold exclusively to physicians and druggists. Cramp later recalled that as the physicians of the country "slowly woke up to the fact that they had been deceived and
humbugged by so-called scientific concerns in the field of prescription products, they
began taking an interest in those cruder proprietaries" sold directly to the public.
With virtually no information available at the *JAMA* headquarters for answering
inquiries from physicians about these patent medicines, journal editor George
Simmons turned over all such requests to Cramp. Dissatisfied with informing inquiring physicians that the AMA knew virtually nothing on the subject, Cramp vora-
ciously collected material from all available sources. *JAMA* editor Simmons
suggested the results of this work should be printed in the *Journal* under the title
"Propaganda for Reform in Proprietary Medicines." Given the volume of work

available to Cramp, the AMA then established the Propaganda Department to oversee the project. The creation of the Propaganda Department signaled the growing aggressiveness of the association along with the expansion of its work in taking on the patent medicine menace as marketed directly to the public. The expanded effort was also partly inspired by the conviction that the government had simply not done enough to inform and protect consumers.[5]

FRAMING THE QUACK MENACE

As part of its expanded reform strategy, the AMA had already capitalized on the popularity of muckraking exposés that had played a key role in the passage of the 1906 Pure Food and Drugs Act. The investigatory work of the Council on Pharmacy and Chemistry had hardly begun when the association secured permission to print and circulate a compilation of Samuel Hopkins Adams's articles attacking quackery and nostrums. Within five years of the original publication in *Collier's*, the AMA had printed 150,000 copies of *The Great American Fraud*. By 1913, a fourth edition of the 146-page book, containing 65 illustrations, had been exhausted, and a fifth was in press. The AMA continued to mail out requested copies of *The Great American Fraud*, for less than cost, to libraries and individuals until the 1960s.[6]

To expose quacks as efficiently as possible, the Propaganda Department also issued an ever-growing list of its own best-selling books and pamphlets on the subject. While Adams had offered a relatively general treatment of many alleged fakeries, in 1911 Cramp compiled dozens of detailed case history reports on investigations in book form, which appeared as the 500-page volume *Nostrums and Quackery*. Believing that medical charlatans could survive only behind a "veil of mystery," Cramp's exposés effectively captured the public's attention, offering a glimpse "into the innermost recesses—the holy holies of quackery." Within a year, the printing was sold out, and a second edition was issued, larger by 200 pages than the first. A second volume, described by Cramp as "a veritable Who's Who in Quackdom" was assembled in 1921 and had grown to over 800 closely printed pages.[7]

In *Nostrums and Quackery*, Cramp identified the difficulties involved in classifying the fraud, greed, and dangers involved in patent medicine exploitation specifically, and quackery more broadly. The first section of the book, *Nostrums*, included sections on advertising specialists; alleged cures for cancer, tuberculosis, and female weakness; along with mail order schemes, mechanical contraptions, and fraudulent medical institutes. A second section, *Quackery*, dealt with information on alleged cures for asthma, diabetes, headaches, obesity, rheumatism, seasickness, and kidney problems. This section also included information on "baby killers" (drugs that induced abortions), cure-alls, cough medicines, misbranded drugs, prescription fakes, and other

The Great American Fraud

By Samuel Hopkins Adams

This is a series of articles which contains a full explanation and exposure of the methods of the "patent medicine" men and quacks, and the harm done to the public by these industries, founded mainly on fraud and poison. The object of the series is to make the situation so familiar and thoroughly understood that there will be a speedy end to the worst aspects of the evil. Fully illustrated. Reprinted from *Collier's*. Three series under one cover.

Among the subjects discussed are: Preying on the Incurables, Miracle Workers, Sure Cure, the Specialist Humbug, the "Patent Medicine" Conspiracy Against the Freedom of the Press, Strictly Confidential, the Treatment Accorded Private Letters by the Nostrum Manufacturers, Patent Medicines Under the "Pure Food Law," Peruna, Swamp Root, etc., etc.

The analyses of many patent medicines are given in non-technical language so that their fraudulent composition will be easily understood and indelibly fixed in the mind.

Contents

THE NOSTRUM EVIL
I. Introduction.
II. Peruna and the Bracers.
III. Liquozone.
IV. The Subtle Poisons
V. Preying on Incurables
VI. The Fundamental Fakes

QUACKS AND QUACKERY
I. The Sure-Cure School
II. The Miracle-Workers
III. The Specialist Humbug
IV. The Scavengers

PATENT MEDICINES, THE LAW AND THE PUBLIC
I. The Fraud Medicines Own Up
II. The Fraud Above the Law—"Swamp Root"

[FIFTH ENLARGED EDITION]

Price
Paper cover...15 cents
Cloth cover...50 cents

Stamps are acceptable for amounts up to 50 cents.
Prices on quantities sent on application.

AMERICAN MEDICAL ASSOCIATION
535 NORTH DEARBORN STREET, CHICAGO

From the pamphlet "Obesity Cure Fakes" (1914).
(© American Medical Association. Courtesy of the AMA Archives)

miscellaneous drugs. A third section included supplementary material on confidence schemes crafted by quacks, food preservatives, the manipulation of the press in advertising cures, and the use of testimonials to vouch for the effectiveness of medicines.

Cramp admitted the difficulty in defining clear lines between "quacks" and "nostrum promoters." While some preparations classed as nostrums could be bought at the local drug store, in other cases manufacturers sold them to the "exploited" directly. On the other hand, while the AMA had classed under quackery those drug companies which professed to diagnose and treat disease, some of these manufacturers also produced AMA-approved medicines sold through wholesale and retail drug firms. This left the divisions "purely arbitrary." Cramp admitted there could be "no strict line of demarcation" between various types of nostrums just as there was no "clear-cut division between those members of the profession who belong in the twilight zone of professionalism and the common advertising quack." Cramp's own certitude and judgment nevertheless belied this ambiguity.[8]

Nostrums and Quackery also revisited the problematic distinction between "patent medicines" and "proprietary medicines," which Cramp considered an artificial classification since nearly all nostrums on the market were technically proprietary while very few had actual patents. Nostrums advertised and sold directly to the public were

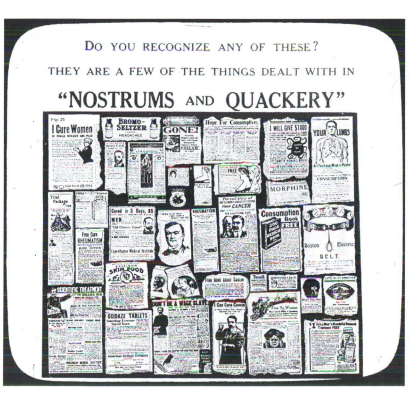

Lantern Slide #841 (ca. 1918).
(© American Medical Association. Courtesy of AMA Archives)

called patent medicines, while those advertised only directly to physicians were spoken of as proprietary medicines. Maintaining this distinction proved crucial because it suggested that only the AMA could determine which proprietary medicines were acceptable for use by physicians, while all patent medicines were deemed inherently problematic and questionable because they were advertised and sold directly to the public. As the editor of *JAMA* declared: "There is no such thing as an unobjectionable 'patent medicine' advertisement in a newspaper." Unfortunately, this hardline approach also implied that every unknowing person who used a patent medicine did so against the advice of medical professionals.[9]

The AMA's official position also belied the difficulty involved in distinguishing between patent medicines and proprietary medicines in terms of their fraudulent claims, questionable composition, and lack of therapeutic value. This created problems not just for the public but also for doctors. For example, despite the vigilance of investigators, the AMA reported that the individual members of the profession were "prescribing and using the very substances which as a combined body they condemned," while "many of the journals which they support advertised and recommended these substances." The AMA proposed many reasons for this dismal state of affairs. First, the financial power of the nostrum manufacturers continued to hold sway over many medical journals, thereby subjecting readers to advertisements for allegedly fraudulent drugs. Second, a "credulous order of mind" was blamed for the inability to distinguish evidence from mere statement, rendering "its possessor an easy victim to the lures of the promoter." The third problem, the indolence of practitioners, meant that some doctors found "it easier in treating patients to follow advice given in advertisements of proprietary drugs than to undertake the arduous task of ascertaining the condition of the patient and to base thereon a sound scientific, therapeutic treatment." Given these problems, the AMA argued that the remedy for the proprietary medicine problem seemed to lie in the hands of the members of the profession.[10]

According to Cramp, physicians also needed to address the big secret behind the popularity of patent medicines, which could be found in the fact that some patent medicines did actually contain valuable and powerful drugs that appeared to work. Cramp warned:

> The public will take these drugs in the firm belief that they are quite harmless and under the idea that, if a little is good, more is better. In other words, they get heavy therapeutic, or even semi-toxic, doses of the preparation, with the physiological results that follow such drugging. Naturally, they are greatly impressed and are apt to discount the physician's treatment, which is more conservative—naturally so because of his responsibility.[11]

Cramp insisted that until the profession resolved to believe in evidence presented by the scientific investigation of substances rather than the biased statements of nostrum agents, the problem would surely persist, and it did.

Despite Cramp's admission, the AMA proudly reported in 1917 that the effectiveness of the Propaganda Department's work had "never been more evident than during the past year." That year, for the first time ever, inquiries from the public regarding patent medicines exceeded those from physicians. This was explained as due to the "growing realization on the part of the public regarding the monstrous waste—both in money and in health—connected with the exploitation of worthless or fraudulent medicines." There were obvious reasons to draw a causal link between the propaganda work of the AMA and the increased public interest in learning more. After all, the public had been flooded with information about the patent medicine evil for much of the preceding decade. In 1913 alone, for example, 46,000 pamphlets dealing with frauds in medicine had been sold or distributed throughout the country. By 1914, the AMA was already sending out 20 different pamphlets on medical frauds, dealing with 288 preparations and individual proprietors. Over a million of these pamphlets had been put in the hands of the public by the early 1920s.[12]

The articles in *JAMA* that dealt with questionable products sold directly to physicians the "ethical" or "prescription" proprietaries as they were alternately called, were also collected every few years and published in the book titled *The Propaganda for Reform*. The first volume ran through nine editions, each edition larger than its predecessor. The AMA issued the ninth edition of Volume I in 1916, which contained practically all of the material of importance that had been published since the Propaganda Department had been created. Volume II was published in 1922 and contained additional material that had appeared in the *Journal* from 1917 onward. Despite an admitted lack of clear demarcation between proprietaries and patent medicines, the AMA continued to publish collections for each separately.

Throughout the 1920s, the AMA continued to prepare and publish articles in the *Journal*, covering a wide range of topics on medical charlatanry. During just one year, 37 articles addressed 64 allegedly fraudulent products in 21 areas (Table 4.1).

AMA leadership believed the only way to curb public consumption of these products was through education. "The education of the public is the most urgent duty of the American Medical Association," asserted AMA Secretary Frederick Green because "the support given to quacks and unscientific sects and cults is largely due to ignorance of the enormous advance in scientific medical knowledge in the past 35 years." Under the direction of Cramp, the Propaganda Department assumed responsibility for reconciling this problem.[13]

Table 4.1. Sample of Quack Topics Discussed in the *Journal of the American Medical Association* (1928)

Cure-Alls	16	Baldness cures	2
Contraceptives	9	Rheumatism cures	1
Syphilis cures	6	Obesity cures	1
Female weakness cures	4	Asthma cures	1
Gonorrhea cures	3	Purgatives	1
Alcoholic tonics	3	Abortifacients	1
Consumption cures	3	Pyorrhea remedies	1
Mouth washes	3	Diarrhea cures	1
Epilepsy cures	2	Bunion cures	1
Mineral waters	2	Stomach remedies	1

EDUCATIONAL EFFORTS

In addition to publishing a staggering array of educational articles, pamphlets, and books, the Propaganda Department appealed to physicians, health professionals, and the public alike through more formal educational channels. In 1918, for example, the Propaganda Department proudly took some credit in reporting that "the number of schools and colleges that devote a certain amount of time each session to the economic, sociologic and health phases of the 'patent medicine' evil continues to increase." Already by this time high school and college textbooks on topics including general science, home economics, hygiene, biology, and physiology were beginning to address these subjects and either used the AMA's publications or offered them as reference for supplementary reading and study. Practically all of these textbooks urged students to obtain additional information that had been prepared and issued by the AMA. In 1922, the students of a single class of one metropolitan high school reportedly sent in 130 letters of inquiry. The Propaganda Department answered each and sent educational materials as requested. More than ten years later, Cramp still received letters from students expressing their gratitude for "all of the great service" provided by the AMA in writing term papers about patent medicines and quackery. Meanwhile, educators frequently requested materials published by the AMA in the decades to come.[14]

Cramp did not just lead the antinostrum educational crusade from the comfort of his office at the AMA. He also traveled around the country to deliver public lectures and addresses on what he called the "quack menace." He accepted invitations from hundreds of groups, including women's clubs, Kiwanis clubs, churches, scientific and medical societies, and public welfare organizations, where he made stops in states around the country. Cramp also helped create a series of educational lantern slides from these presentations, which were subsequently made available for loan to physicians, public health officials, and instructors interested in giving their own illustrated talks on the nostrum evil and quackery.[15]

The AMA also took its fight against quackery on the road with a series of educational posters that covered a wider range of patent medicines and alleged forms of quackery. By the 1920s, posters covering dozens of topics were being used at health exhibits, county and state fairs, health expositions, and in high schools and colleges. In these posters, the Propaganda Department identified specific patent medicine threats, exposed and delegitimized the techniques used by unorthodox medical competitors in advertising their remedies, and urged people to rely on their AMA-member doctor for advice in navigating a treacherous medical marketplace. The AMA confidently disclaimed entire classes of drugs, including obesity cures, asthma and hay-fever drugs, cancer cure frauds, alleged deafness cures, and epilepsy cures. Other posters disavowed advertising as the tool of the quack, and attempted to undermine the authority and the appeal of the testimonial as evidence for therapeutic effectiveness.[16]

Cramp enthusiastically incorporated these posters and slides as he traveled around the country to deliver lectures on patent medicines and quackery, but he admittedly preferred the written to the spoken word and expressed his convictions more effectively in writing. He was a remarkably prolific writer, not only for *JAMA* and other AMA publications, but for many medical and lay magazines. He viewed his written work as the centerpiece of his educational efforts.[17]

Cramp frequently addressed what he considered to be a major misconception about the punitive consequences of the AMA's work in its crusade against nostrums, quackery, and pseudomedicine. In a letter to Professor William D. Cutter of the University of Southern California, he noted how many people seemed to think that the AMA had punitive powers and that the association prosecuted cases. Writing in 1933, Cramp reminded Professor Cutter that "the work in this line that the American Medical Association has been doing for over a quarter of a century—long before there were any other agencies that were interested in 'truth in advertising'—has been of an educational character purely." Cramp's insistence on the fundamentally educational purpose of the Propaganda Department often appeared to be similarly defensive.[18]

Cramp remained cautiously optimistic about the consequences of the AMA's educational work. In a letter from 1922, for example, he explained, "It is the nature of an educational campaign to produce results slowly. The Propaganda Department cannot go out into the markets and hale before the Bar of Justice those engaged in nostrum exploitation or quackery." Cramp continued, "neither does the Propaganda Department want to do such work. Man is by nature a gullible animal and this holds true in the fields of economics, politics and religion, as well as medicine. The only way of combating such gullibility is by education—a slow process, but a sure one." By emphasizing the educational role of the AMA, the responsibility for change rested with physicians and consumers who were each expected to make wise choices in

EDUCATIONAL POSTERS
ON THE NOSTRUM EVIL AND QUACKERY

The Propaganda for Reform Department of THE JOURNAL has prepared a series of educational posters on the subject of quackery and the nostrum evil. The placards measure 22 inches by 28 inches and are printed on a good grade of nonglossy bond paper. They sell for 25 cents each (postage extra) or the complete set of thirty-three posters will be sent postpaid for $7.

1.—Pulmonol.
2.—A Nostrum Tragedy in Clippings.
3.—Headache Powders.
4.—The Deadly Headache Tablet.
5.—Another Worthless Consumption Cure.
6.—Some Obesity Cures.
7.—More "Prescription Fakes."
8.—Let the Label Tell.
9.—An Obesity Cure Fraud.
10.—Testimonials Are Worthless.
11.—The "Gas-Pipe" Frauds.
12.—The Confidences of Quacks.
13.—Is Self-Drugging Dangerous?
14.—The Law as an Aid to Veracity.
15.—From the "Lie Direct" to the "Lie with Circumstance."
16—Nature's Creation.
17.—The Testimonial Industry.
18.—Doan's Kidney Pills.
19.—Beware of "Consumption Cures."
20.—Secrecy and Mystery.
21.—Pay Your Money and Take Your Choice.
22.—Some Alcohol Comparisons.
23.—Mayr's Stomach Remedy.
24.—The Federal Food and Drugs Act.
26.—Warner's Safe Remedy.
27.—Prescription Fakes.
28.—A "Rupture Cure."
29.—Some "Deafness Cures."
30.—Capitalizing the Fears of the Expectant Mother.
31.—"Epilepsy Cures."
32.—Pinkham's Vegetable Compound.
33.—Pe-Ru-Na.
34.—Hostetter's Bitters.

A SPECIAL CATALOGUE AND PRICE LIST IS ISSUED REPRODUCING THE CARDS IN MINIATURE; IT WILL BE SENT ON REQUEST

AMERICAN MEDICAL ASSOCIATION
535 NORTH DEARBORN STREET   **CHICAGO, ILL.**

"Educational Posters on the Nostrum Evil and Quackery" (ca. 1924).
(© American Medical Association. Courtesy of AMA Archives)

selecting therapies. Cramp's insistence on a strictly educational approach nevertheless underestimated the appeal of alleged quackeries for the people who used them. It incorrectly assumed that people only continued to use quack medicines because they did not know any better. The AMA could provide information but could not dictate choices.[19]

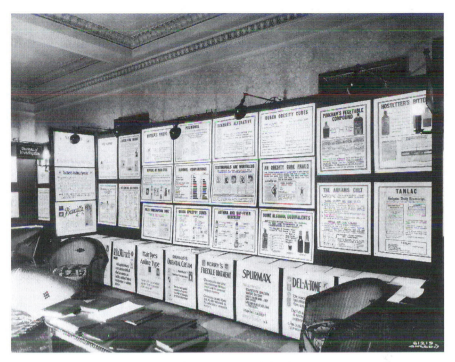

Bureau of Investigation Exhibit (1929).
(© American Medical Association. Courtesy of AMA Archives)

In 1925, the AMA's educational convictions proved instrumental in the decision to change the name of the Propaganda Department to the more descriptive Bureau of Investigation. In a candid letter to a colleague, Cramp explained that he felt the term "propaganda" had outlived its usefulness. The public had already expressed misapprehension of what constituted propaganda, and he believed the AMA had finally reached the place where their educational work had largely ceased being propaganda. The AMA House of Delegates reported that at the time that the Propaganda Department was established and "the name 'Propaganda for Reform in Proprietary Remedies' was first applied, it fully and accurately described the functions of the department that bore that name. During those years, propaganda was truly needed." But by 1925, the "acute need" had passed and the work of the Bureau of Investigation had been broadened to "cover a broader and a more general field in its attempt to give to the profession and the public information regarding nostrums, quacks, pseudomedicine and allied subjects." A professor of economics from the University of Arizona concurred: "I think your work is too scientific and unselfish to be labeled 'Propaganda.'" Responding to the suggestion that the AMA was doing itself a disservice by using it, Cramp conceded.[20]

WORK WITH GOVERNMENTAL AGENCIES

Cramp's insistence on the primarily education role of the Propaganda Department, and the renamed Bureau of Investigation, nevertheless understated the power of the AMA to shape policy and support punitive action against patent medicine manufacturers. In its work with government agencies, the Department and Bureau not only supported advertising reform but also enabled the enforcement of laws that restricted the labeling, shipment, and therapeutic claims of drugs. With this work, the AMA established a network of alliances with public and private organizations, and also bolstered the authoritative position of the profession.

Through the work of the Propaganda Department/Bureau of Investigation, the AMA capitalized on the growing bureaucratic and regulatory stature of municipal, state, and federal government in the Progressive Era and helped put countless drug manufacturers and distributors out of business. Director Cramp diligently provided letters to attorneys and representatives of various government organizations, offered data on specific concerns, and served as a witness and technical adviser on a variety of cases prosecuted by officials. Additionally, the AMA played an important part in bringing to the attention of government officials various schemes and methods deemed a menace to the public health, in violation of the law, or both. The AMA's position at the head of a network of surveillance granted it an immeasurable amount of authority and influence.[21]

The AMA worked particularly closely with the three major federal agencies that offered protection to the public in the medical or quasimedical fields. Collectively, they operated as a network of professional quackbusters. The Department of Agriculture, through its Food and Drug Administration (FDA), enforced the National Food and Drugs Act; the Post Office Department issued fraud orders debarring fraudulent schemes from the mails; and the Federal Trade Commission (FTC) investigated and took action on cases that involved or seemed to involve what were broadly spoken of as unfair trade practices. The AMA collaborated with each agency. At times, federal agencies provided the AMA with information about specific cases that the AMA had not investigated, while in other cases federal authorities received information from the AMA. Scarcely an investigation was launched by a regulatory agency without an inquiry to Cramp to see what information he had in his files.[22]

From the 1910s onward, the AMA worked extensively with the FDA, the Post Office Department, and the FTC by providing background information from its files on questionable medical concerns. The FDA had been vested with the power to enforce the Pure Food and Drugs Act, which regulated the contents of medicines and governed the claims made in or on the trade packages of foods or medicines that were shipped in interstate commerce. When such claims were judged false, misleading, or fraudulent, the manufacturers, if they were known, could be prosecuted for violating the law, and if found guilty, be either fined or forced to relabel their packages. If they put up no defense, the court ordered the shipments confiscated and destroyed. The AMA was a close ally of the FDA in this work from the beginning.

The Post Office Department, meanwhile, having jurisdiction over everything sent through the mails, prosecuted thousands of individuals and businesses that abused its services by exploiting various types of schemes deemed fraudulent. Some of the swindles documented and corroborated by material in the AMA's investigatory files, and subsequently barred from the mail, included cancer cures, bust developers, consumption cures, height increasers, obesity cures, hair growers, goiter reducers, diet systems, diabetes cures, gallstone removers, sexual rejuvenators, fake doctor diplomas, deafness treatments, and fake radium therapies.[23]

From Cramp's perspective, the FTC was a particularly important agency because it made up for the sharp limitations of the FDA and the Post Office Department. No matter how fraudulent a patent medicine may have been in its advertising, he noted that if "the manufacturer is shrewd enough—and most manufacturers of 'patent medicines' do not lack shrewdness—to make no false, misleading, or fraudulent statements on the trade package, but confines his mendacity to newspaper advertisements, radio talks, billboards, etc., he cannot be reached under the National Food and Drugs Act." The postal authorities, meanwhile, had the power of denying the use of the U.S. mail for those found guilty of obtaining money through false and fraudulent pretenses and promises but could act only in cases registered with the Post Office Department by someone who felt defrauded. The FTC, quintessentially a product of the Progressive Era, had been enacted in 1914 to make safeguards against business monopolies more effective. The government granted the five-man independent body of the FTC extensive authority to investigate, publicize, and prohibit all "unfair trade practices." Definitions of what was unfair were left deliberately vague, which allowed antinostrum crusaders to include as unfair the making of false claims or representations in the advertising of various medical treatments that covered a wide variety of alleged cures.[24]

The FTC regularly sent the AMA lists of complaints it had ordered, along with other case-related information, which Cramp considered "very helpful to the American Medical Association in its efforts to protect the public interest against the exploitation by the manufacturers of worthless or harmful nostrums." The FTC, in turn, thanked Cramp for the Bureau of Investigation's material, which constituted a "substantial aid to the Commission in advising the public of its false work in advertising." Since the commission needed medical testimony to substantiate allegations in its cases, the FTC also used the AMA as a referral service in its search for qualified authorities to testify regarding false claims, unscientific exaggerations, and therapeutic inaccuracies. Cramp, furthermore, also devoted more time to keeping physicians and the public informed about the work of the commission and how it related to the objectives of the Bureau of Investigation. In 1933 alone, for example, Cramp wrote two separate *JAMA* articles on the work of the FTC, which included over 40 examples of nostrums and quasimedical remedies investigated and prosecuted during that year. Included on the list were alleged high blood pressure remedies, bladder cures, vaginal suppositories, gallstone remedies, blood purifiers, hemorrhoid cures, aphrodisiacs, epilepsy cures, rheumatism remedies, and stomach remedies. In correspondence with FTC Commissioner William E. Humphrey, Cramp offered the hope that his modest articles would "do much to enlighten the medical profession—and through it the public—on the public service the Commission is performing."[25]

Cramp explained why these governmental bodies were so important to the consumer. While the uninformed public could develop certain protective mechanisms in the purchase of ordinary merchandise by trial and error, this was not the case with medicinal products, for "no fact is better demonstrated than that the purchaser of a medicine is wholly incompetent to tell whether it was the medicine he took or the healing power of Nature that was responsible for his recovery. The chances are at least eight to ten that Dame Nature may deserve the credit." He failed to explain how he arrived at this estimate but delivered an unambiguous message: only physicians possessed sufficient knowledge and training to prescribe effective medicines as a counterpart to the individual's natural capacity for recovery from illness or disease. This established a clear boundary set by expertise.[26]

Cramp remained sensitive to any suggestions of impropriety in this work, frequently emphasizing that he had undertaken it without any legal fees or other charges. In a five-page letter written in 1929 about the nature and extent of this work with the FTC, Cramp replied to National Better Business Bureau Representative A. E. Backman by detailing his communication on dozens of cases investigated and prosecuted from 1924 to 1928, concluding with the reminder, "I have given both my own personal time, as well as the time of the American Medical Association, without any charge."[27]

All the while, Cramp remained committed to supporting other prominent federal organizations with their investigations. If a regulatory agency launched an investigation of any sort, the Bureau of Investigation frequently was seen as the best source of information. When the U.S. Department of Agriculture (USDA) received inquiries regarding questionable patent medicines, it regularly recommended contacting the AMA, as it was not customary for the Department of Agriculture to give out information concerning the composition or quality of a drug unless proceedings involving the drug in question had been terminated in the federal courts. When postal authorities sought to proactively protect consumers against mail-order frauds, the bureau also enthusiastically provided whatever relevant documentation it possessed. Given the difficult and thankless work involving the Post Office, AMA publications offered channels for disseminating information and continued to offer a forum for extended accounts of the government's work in combating medical frauds.[28]

COLLABORATION WITH BUSINESS, VOLUNTARY, AND PROFESSIONAL ORGANIZATIONS

Cramp also promoted close interaction with state and local medical societies, health departments, women's clubs, temperance organizations, newspaper and magazine editors, advertising associations, chambers of commerce, and Better Business Bureaus by collecting and disseminating information among these groups. He even arranged to send many of these organizations advance pages of the Propaganda for Reform articles from the *Journal* each week. By diligently meeting their requests for information not only on patent medicines but also on questionable medical practitioners, publications, and institutions, Cramp orchestrated an increasingly vast network of quackery surveillance.

As the number of letters received by the Bureau of Investigation increased throughout the 1920s, a particularly large number of letters came from state medical examining boards and medical societies requesting data on individual physicians. In turn, they used this data in determining the fitness of applicants for medical licensure and society membership. In 1926, for example, the State Medical Society of Wisconsin sent a list of physicians to Cramp because it was "anxious to secure an increased membership." However, it hoped Cramp would check the list and mark those physicians who, in his estimation, were undesirable. In four short days, Cramp's reply included a statement regarding 23 physicians on whom the bureau had information. He conceded that some of the material "may not be of such a character as to warrant placing them on the list of those who should not be solicited for membership," but the candidates were variously characterized as "a patent medicine faker," associated with a clinic of "dubious character," "an advertising quack," a member of a "quack institution," "quacking for some years," "advertising a cure for cancer," and "in the 'weak men' [impotence] business." Cramp replied to hundreds of similar requests for information from medical societies across the country, always promptly.[29]

Voluntary medical organizations also benefited from the work of the Propaganda Department. When the secretary of the Montana Association for the Prevention of Tuberculosis learned of a new alleged cure, she immediately contacted Cramp to see if the AMA files contained any information on its legitimacy. She received a reply in less than a week, along with a pamphlet on quack tuberculosis cures. In a return letter to Cramp, she indicated the prestige attached to the AMA's judgment, offering thanks for the information regarding the "fake organization" that advertised the drug in question. "I do appreciate your promptness in answering my letter," she informed Cramp, adding, "I shall feel so comfortable about giving out the information coming from your organization."[30]

An especially large increase in the number of inquiries received during the late 1920s and early 1930s came from various likeminded Better Business Bureaus seeking information on quack advertisers and their sympathetic publishers. In 1932, the Bureau of Investigation furnished the Better Business Bureau of Buffalo, New York, with a "veritable encyclopedia on the subject of local quacks and locally exploited nostrums." On the basis of this information, the advertisers of Buffalo carried out an active drive against the more blatant nostrum vendors and quacks, and stimulated the local authorities to act. In this way, the Bureau of Investigation exerted a silent but far-reaching influence. By the 1930s, the AMA reported that Better Business Bureaus throughout the country, along with the National Better Business Bureau, were calling daily on the Bureau of Investigation for information regarding questionable remedies, practitioners, and institutions, with "about three letters a day" coming from these agencies. In turn, the National Better Business Bureau began furnishing periodical publishers throughout the country with bulletins of information on alleged quasiscientific or fraudulent offenders, using data furnished by the AMA.[31]

Collaborative work with a wide range of businesses, voluntary health organizations, and professional organizations illustrated how the AMA enlarged its quackery surveillance network by extending its crusade beyond questionable therapeutics to target, expose, and condemn allegedly fraudulent physicians and institutions. To effectively police professional boundaries and promote educational reform, the AMA relied on organizations to identify the breaches.

EXPANDING THE CORRESPONDENCE NETWORK

In addition to directing the massive amount of work detailed previously, Cramp personally responded to thousands of inquiries from doctors asking about nostrums that they found their patients using, as well as letters from individuals suffering from various ailments who sought information about available remedies. Letters written to the AMA, most of which were answered by the Propaganda Department/Bureau of Investigation, provide a striking indication of the broad impact of the association's work and the extent of its surveillance network. In the years immediately following the Pure Food and Drugs Act of 1906, a letter from a layperson was such an unusual event as to cause comment, but already by 1913 over 1,200 of 4,200 letters of inquiry regarding frauds in medicine had been written by curious members of the general

Table 4.2. Inquiries Received and Answered by the Bureau of Investigation

Year	Inquiries from Physicians	Inquiries from Laypersons	Total Inquiries
1918	969	858	1,827
1919	1,422	1,088	2,510
1920	1,875	1,007	2,882
1921	2,105	1,443	3.547
1922	2,646	1,970	4,616
1923	3,545	2,525	6,070
1924	3,054	2,831	5,885
1925	3,541	2,866	6,407
1926	4,112	3,645	7,757
1927	3,829	5,022	8,851
1928	4,237	5,743	9,980
1929	4,079	6,350	10,429
1930	5,556	6,687	12,243

public. By 1928, the Bureau of Investigation answered 10,000 inquiries per year from physicians and the laity (Table 4.2).[32]

A steady increase in the number of total inquiries over this period indicates not only the growing professional authority of the AMA more broadly but also the impact of the work of the Bureau of Investigation specifically. There were only two years in which the number of inquiries from physicians were fewer than the immediately preceding years, 1924 and 1927. During each of these years some of the inquiries that had previously been handled by the Bureau of Investigation were turned over to the other departments. For example, letters regarding chiropractors, osteopaths, and other "sectarian" groups were no longer answered exclusively by the Bureau of Investigation but instead were often handled by the AMA's Council on Medical Education and Hospitals. By 1924, the full effects of dramatic changes in medical education made sectarian medicine more clearly the domain of the AMA's Council on Medical Education. While the official position of the AMA toward sectarian therapeutics had long been one of suspicion at best, and outright condemnation at worst, the AMA tended to focus its attack on the educational deficiencies of sectarian groups in the 1910s and 1920s. Meanwhile, educating the public became a higher priority for the AMA, resulting in the expansion of its Bureau of Health and Public Instruction in 1927, which assumed some of the burden that the Bureau of Investigation had shouldered in responding to inquiries from educational institutions.[33]

At the same time, there was a particularly large increase in the number of inquiries from the general public, especially in the late 1920s, which can be explained by two additional parallel developments. First, the increased popularity of the AMA's consumer health magazine *Hygeia* acted as a conduit for informing the public about the services offered by the AMA in the antiquackery field. Second, the association increasingly began to use the radio during these years to acquaint the public with the achievements of scientific medicine and the work of the association. In 1928, for example, Director Cramp delivered several 15-minute talks, broadcasted from the AMA headquarters over WBBM in Chicago on subjects including medical charlatans, dangerous cosmetics, mail-order frauds, obesity cure fakes, patent medicine testimonials, and the origin and function of the Bureau of Investigation.[34]

The Bureau of Investigation considered correspondence the centerpiece of its antiquackery crusade. Inquiries from professionals and the public were considered top priorities. As Cramp explained, because the bureau's letters dealt with "the pernicious and frequently fraudulent activities of nostrum exploiters, quacks and charlatans," it was critical to exercise the utmost care to see that it made statements only "justified by the facts and supported by documentary evidence." Cramp carefully compiled and organized this evidence to effectively respond to inquiries of all sorts. As early as 1910, his office contained over 12,000 cards in a Fake File, which documented a long list of products, firms, and names of promoters. A separate Testimonial File held the names of over 13,000 American and 3,000 foreign doctors who had given testimonials for proprietary drugs. For the next 20 years, Cramp used standard three-by-five cards for an index system alphabetized by the names of products and individuals. He made additional corresponding cards for every individual who wrote to the Propaganda Department or was referred by another agency. By 1937, the Bureau of Investigation had accumulated 300,000 cards, which corresponded to over a thousand large file boxes containing correspondence and innumerable clippings from newspapers, magazines, and periodicals for various cures, remedies, treatments, institutions, and practitioners dating from 1906. This represented the most complete set of files on the subject in existence. The bureau took great pride in the fact that by 1929, this material had been used to send out more than 85,000 letters. Not one had been the subject of a suit for libel or damages.[35]

In responding to these countless inquiries, Cramp deftly expressed his humor, indignation, and passion for the cause he championed. He told historian James Harvey Young that he kept a copy of *Alice in Wonderland* on his desk, and before writing up a case he often took out the book and read a chapter to put him in the mood for the job he had to do. He pursued quackery, wrote *JAMA* editor Simmons, "with necessary caution, with courage, and with honesty of purpose." As Young put it, "thorough preparation, a fine sense of style, a recognition of the absurd, and moral conviction" made Cramp's writing effective. Although modest and sensitive, he conveyed the authority of the Propaganda Department/Bureau of

Investigation. Through his dedication, he offered an answer to virtually anyone seeking advice.[36]

"KNOCKS AND BOOSTS"

Onlookers widely praised but also vociferously criticized the work of the Propaganda Department/Bureau of Investigation. In fact, Cramp kept a special file titled Knocks and Boosts, which documented the wide range of feedback he received from doctors, patients, and various officials. The correspondence in this file, however, was predominantly praiseworthy, despite Cramp's frequent admission that his work could seem like a "thankless task." After a visit to the AMA building in 1915 by students from the University of Chicago, for example, they congratulated the Propaganda Department for "wielding a mighty influence for the public good," "the furtherance of public health and knowledge," and "the systematic handling of the organization" that seemed to "fairly reek with altruism." Additional letters from the public offered wishes for success in the AMA's good work against a "reprehensible form of duplicity" and frequently thanked Cramp for his kindness and conscientious assistance. However modest Cramp might have been, he was also appreciated for the "kind, courteous, and sincere spirit and manner" in which he provided his services. Cramp received appreciative letters from people of all walks of life, including attorneys, business owners, editors, teachers, women's organizations, hospitals, medical associations, advertising clubs, and departments of health. They all thanked Cramp for his diligence in providing invaluable information and assistance. Some expressed astonishment and delight at his comprehensive treatment of the subject.[37]

Medical society journals, lay newspapers, and magazines praised the "great service to the country rendered" by the AMA, which had "driven the enemy of the hapless sufferer to cover."[38] A Louisiana newspaper, meanwhile, concurred that the broad impact of the AMA, in conjunction with federal and state regulation, was unquestionable, but not necessarily easy to quantify, suggesting, "We no longer see the word 'cure' emblazoned on label and prominent advertisement, because the manufacturer is far too wary to expose himself to the almost certain probability of a heavy fine, for fraudulent statements as well as confiscation of his goods by Federal agents." Supporters of the AMA's campaign against nostrums and quackery firmly believed that the most effective weapon against "humbuggery" was the "limelight of exposure," through the education of the general public. As the Bunkie, Louisiana, *Recorder* concluded: "They will disappear . . . when you cease to give them financial support."[39]

On the other hand, proprietary medicine manufacturers joined forces with magazine, journal, and newspaper editors to question whether the AMA could remain objective, and thereby effective, in its propaganda campaign. Patent medicine defenders commonly argued that the AMA tried to protect its physicians more than the public. The Butterick Publishing Company, responsible for the *Delineator* magazine, warned that "The *Journal of the American Medical Association*, far from being a disinterested party, is one of the most intelligently and keenly edited magazines we know of in the interest of their particular clientele." Cramp admitted that the *Delineator* merely voiced "the general opinion on the part of the public (an opinion valiantly and vocally backed up by the 'patent medicine' interests) that the medical profession is opposed to 'patent medicines' because the sale of such products injures the physicians' business." Cramp also noted that it would be quite impossible for the average advertising agent to believe the *Journal*, or any other publication or organization, could carry out a campaign that was not based somehow or in some way on a financial return. He concluded: "One expects reasoning of this sort from the inhabitants of Moronia, and, of course, nothing else is to be expected from the 'patent medicine' people themselves. But an advertising man should have enough brains to recognize the fallacy of the argument." From Cramp's perspective, after the drug makers and their advertisers, the group to be hardest hit financially by wiping out patent medicines would be the doctors themselves. After all, he explained, "Every advertisement of a 'patent medicine' sends to the doctors' offices at least as many as it sends to the drug counter. If the medical profession were interested only in the dollars-and-cents aspect of the 'patent medicine' game, it would say to nostrum exploiters, 'Go the limit! The more victims you get, the more patients we get.' "[40]

Other critiques of AMA efforts nevertheless reflected similar doubts about the fairness and the effectiveness of the campaign. Editors of the *National Eclectic Medical Association Quarterly*, for example, sympathized with *JAMA*'s propaganda for reform strategy but lamented the journal's tendency to "criticize ruthlessly the motives of other journals and editors, even to questioning their moral attitude." Regarding the propaganda itself, the editors also suggested, "It is a well-known fact that the majority of physicians pay little heed to it, but go on in their own sweet way prescribing what they wish, and the detail man and manufacturing pharmacist still flourish." *JAMA*, meanwhile, was so strong numerically and financially from the perspective of the Eclectic journal that it considered itself "immune from molestation."[41]

Harsher critiques from the rank and file of the profession suggested the propaganda for reform campaign had become another tool unnecessarily used by autocratic AMA leaders. In 1910, the *Medical Brief* argued that "the very spirit of intolerance and petty tyranny" spread by cliquish AMA leaders was "surely alienating the confidence and fealty of the public from the doctor, and putting into the hands of his supplanters, the osteopath, the Christian Scientist, the mental healer, and the like, the very weapons with which to undermine the physician's influence and still further widen the breach." From this perspective, just as large corporations used the aggregated holdings of their stockholders to give them the necessary weight in Wall

Street to manipulate the market, so did the officers of the AMA use the membership of thousands of doctors throughout the country to give color of representation to their own schemes of political power and aggrandizement. These critics doubted the ability of the AMA to carry out a critique of drug manufacturers and sectarians with the necessary weight of impartiality and disinterestedness.[42]

Collectively, these knocks and boosts reflected the contentious nature of the AMA's work and indicated the high stakes involved. By cultivating the authority to judge the safety and effectiveness of therapies, the AMA won allies to its cause but also created enemies among proprietary drug manufacturers and sectarians. Ultimately, the work of the Propaganda Department surely discouraged the use of some remedies but it also generated reactionary responses.

SORTING OUT THE SECTARIANS

The Propaganda Department used the antinostrum crusade as a mandate to expose other approaches to therapeutics deemed quackery or "pseudomedicine," including unorthodox systems referred to as medical sects. As a result, homeopathic remedies, chiropractic and osteopathic manipulations, Christian Scientist drugless healing, naturopathic and Eclectic regimens, and several other forms of "irregular" practice served their time in the Propaganda for Reform section of the *Journal*, despite never being subjected to laboratory or clinical analyses. By dismissing other systems as ipso facto unscientific, the AMA could condemn them without even empirically examining their claims for efficacy.

The AMA still regarded homeopathic practitioners as "irregulars" in the early 1900s, but it no longer confronted them as directly and aggressively as in the past. Homeopaths almost unanimously opposed the patent-medicine menace, and some expressed sympathy for the AMA's efforts in the fight against nostrums. Other enterprising homeopaths also experienced remarkable success with their own proprietary businesses. Frederick Humphreys, one of the most successful homeopathic remedy manufacturers, had developed a method of simplifying home medication and capitalized on the growing trade in proprietaries in the last third of the nineteenth century. Humphreys' Specific Homeopathic Medicine Company broke with the homeopathic rule of administering only one medicine at a time and instead created a system for using a combination of medicines for specific diseases. At least one homeopathic colleague called his invention "homeopathic quackery." Unmoved, Humphreys brilliantly marketed two sizes of homeopathic home medicine kits. A domestic medicine guide accompanied each box, a large compendium of recommended treatments for the expensive kits and a smaller one for his cheaper cases. By the early 1890s, fifteen million copies of the latter work had appeared in five languages, 12 million of which had been distributed in the United States.[43]

In the early twentieth century, Humphreys' Specific Homeopathic Medicine Company expanded its advertising strategies by marketing independently packaged specific remedies for specific diseases or conditions. The most popular "Specific" was Humphreys' No. 77 for colds, catarrh, or "the grip." Advertisements promised that No. 77 would "keep colds away" and reassured readers that "nearly everyone" recommended it as "their own particular pet remedy." Curious consumers and medical organizations frequently wrote to the AMA for advice on Humphreys' Specifics and other homeopathic remedies. Some replies from the Propaganda Department were humorous or sarcastic. In response to an inquiry from the University of Chicago Department of Hygiene and Bacteriology, Cramp wrote, "If the patient's condition calls for 'No. 10' and that particular remedy is not at hand, I take it that two doses of No. 5 or one dose each of No. 7 and No. 3 would accomplish the same result." Subsequent replies reported that although the AMA had not analyzed Humphreys' Specifics, "it is likely, like many other homeopathic remedies that have been analyzed, the tablets will be found to consist chiefly of milk sugar." In several other responses, Cramp could not resist poking fun, surmising in one case, "If they are truly homeopathic remedies you can take the entire seventy-seven varieties and eat them with the same impunity that you would eat the same amount of milk sugar." Other letters described Humphreys' remedies as "essentially Christian Science in tablet form" and "purely psychological" in effect.[44]

Cramp's successors were more earnest in tone, partly because the AMA's official position regarding homeopathy had hardened but also because Humphreys' ran up against federal regulatory agencies in the 1930s. In 1938, when a public health educator sent an inquiry to the AMA after a pamphlet was left on her door, she asked whether any legal recourse was possible, characterizing Humphreys' manual as "vicious," "extremely dangerous," and "utterly incompetent." The Bureau of Investigation reply cited a 1931 Notice of Judgment by the Food and Drug Administration in which it had declared Humphreys' 77 misbranded under the Pure Food and Drugs Act of 1906 because of false and fraudulent claims. Humphreys' had failed to put up a defense or even appear in court, but nothing more was done than to destroy the shipment in question. Government chemists reported that the product consisted essentially of trace amounts of arsenic and extracts of plants with sugar, but the case hinged on the claim to cure all coughs. In March 1937, meanwhile, the Federal Trade Commission (FTC) brought pressure against the Humphreys' Homeopathic Company to cease representing that their product "will cure a cold or will get rid of a cold the minute one feels it coming on; or that it is a scientific remedy or that Humphreys' Remedies, as a whole, backed by a reputation for dependability of almost a hundred years, are based on modern scientific formulas." The judgment asked the company to admit that "according to the weight of scientific authority, any benefits derived from taking Humphreys' 77 for colds would be only palliative."[45]

The AMA dismissed many other sectarian therapies as unscientific, or only palliative at best. When sectarian practitioners were accused of more egregious forms of medical fraud they faced the wrath of the Propaganda Department. The AMA was particularly incensed by various sectarians described as "depraved and dirty" for exploiting cancer victims. In its early years, the Propaganda Department aggressively fought what it considered the cruelest, most heartless form of medical fraud, the cancer cure, by enlisting the support of federal authorities. One Los Angeles homeopathic doctor, S. R. Chamley, had been indicted for fraud, ordered to stop his mailings by the federal authorities, and fined. He repeatedly resumed his business, often under a different name. Chamley advertised his cancer cure as "a most wonderful, strange, but fortunate combination of several medicines, easily obtained at any large drug store." The AMA considered this the epitome of deceptive advertising designed to lure uninformed victims of cancer. The Bureau of Investigation regularly featured the Chamley case in its publications aimed at public and professional consumption.[46]

Naturopaths, meanwhile, who, according to the AMA, believed cancer could be cured "by natural processes without medicine or surgery" also earned disapproval. Naturopathic methods included a wide range of therapeutic applications considered unscientific or quasiscientific by the AMA: hydrotherapy, ozone therapy, electrotherapy, mechanotherapy, heliotherapy, and phytotherapy. One letter from the Propaganda Department surmised that naturopathic theory seemed to be made up of "about 5 per cent banalities of elementary science, and 95 per cent pseudoscientific flub-dub." From the AMA's perspective, the occasional rational or obvious thing that naturopaths propounded fooled "otherwise intelligent people into accepting the ridiculous theories which are made the basis for commercial exploitation."[47]

The Propaganda Department files overflowed with information on the man the AMA considered the most notorious naturopath in the early twentieth century, Benedict Lust, who served as president of the American School of Naturopathy and the American Naturopathic Association and owned the leading naturopathic journal, *Herald of Health & Naturopath*. In response to an inquiry about the standing of his journal in the medical world, Propaganda Department Director Cramp concluded quite simply, "It has no standing." He asserted that while Lust claimed to be opposed to the use of drugs, he was not above accepting advertisements of certain patent medicines in his *Herald of Health*. According to Cramp, Lust was "a typical representative of the cult to which he belongs." When curious patients and professionals inquired about Lust, Cramp gladly provided them with clippings from New York papers from 1910 to 1912, which documented how Lust had been convicted of practicing medicine without a license and fined $100. According to the literature in the AMA's nostrums and quackery files, Lust had either been connected with or endorsed several quasimedical fads, including a "Blood-Washing Treatment," which was "nothing more than a glorified shower bath, and could not possibly fulfill the extravagant claims made for it by Lust and other enthusiasts in the treatment of disease." Cramp reported the method consisted of nothing more marvelous than a bath spray applied over several hours.[48]

In reply to another inquiry that included a sample advertisement proclaiming the "Dignified Profession of Naturopathy," Cramp flatly responded: "The 'Dignified Profession of Naturopathy' is a euphemistic description of a quackish cult." Cramp's views on naturopathy had not softened by the early 1930s, when he suggested that if the AMA ever published an article on the accomplishments of a naturopathic doctor, the content would not be complimentary. As Cramp informed a curious citizen, "the so-called naturopathic philosophy is based on a collection of misconceptions and half assimilated facts. The claims of those who practice this method, if we may call it that, are not supported by scientific evidence. Consequently, we do not believe that a patient who consults a person practicing naturopathy will be benefited."[49]

Of all the unorthodox medical systems, however, the AMA appeared to oppose chiropractic most stridently. As a result, the Propaganda Department devoted a substantial amount of time and effort to collecting and disseminating information about chiropractors, their schools, and reports of their therapies in the press. Hundreds of clippings in Propaganda Department folders documented meetings, legislative challenges, court cases involving chiropractors, and articles reporting the death and injury of patients. Articles appearing in *JAMA* referenced this information in the form of scathing but frequently unsigned critiques. The AMA insisted that chiropractors and followers of other "medical cults" represented a threat to public safety in large part because of their "ignorance and incompetence." Cramp insisted the public was not in a position to understand the "grotesque nonsense" behind this "cult of deluded manipulators" due to the secrecy surrounding chiropractic. Consequently, the AMA countered the "chiropractic propaganda" with its own propaganda, suggesting the "chiropractic humbug" might be better called "Chiro-quack-tic" since it was simply quackery masquerading under a different name.[50]

In addition to using the same language to delegitimize sectarian practitioners and patent-medicine peddlers, the Propaganda Department/Bureau of Investigation also frequently made a direct association between their motives and techniques. A *JAMA* article noted, for example, that "Chiropractors affect, with 'patent medicine' fakers, a fine disdain for scientific medicine and the medical practitioner." They both tended to "seize with avidity on any statement made by an individual who may be presumed to have the right to put 'M.D.' after his or her name—provided that statement seems favorable to the cause." According to the AMA, there was also a common use of testimonials by chiropractors and the nostrum industry, with each employing twisted statements to make the public believe that a reputable physician supported questionable treatments. Frequently, a *JAMA* article reported, these testimonials came from an "M.D." who had never been licensed and only graduated from a sectarian medical school.[51]

JAMA articles made for advertising fodder as well. In 1914, a paid advertisement in the *Echo Enterprise*, the local paper in Hermiston, Oregon, announced in large font: "An Estimate of Chiropractic by the Journal of the A.M.A."

The advertisement read:

> Chiropractic is a freak offshoot from Osteopathy. It is the sheerest kind of quackery, practiced largely by men whose general education is as limited as their knowledge of anatomy, and who are profoundly ignorant of the fundamental sciences on which the treatment of disease in the human body depends. Chiropractic is taught—heaven save the mark!—on the mail order plan ... The so-called "colleges" of chiropractic matriculates anybody who can pay the fee. The medical and osteopathic schools require in addition to a good preliminary educational foundation, from three to four years—in some cases five—of hard study with much practical work before granting the degree of doctor of medicine or osteopathy ... Chiropractic is in no sense a profession. It is a scheme by which sharpers induce men generally of little education and with a dwarfed sense of moral obligation, to learn the tricks of a disreputable trade—quackery.
>
> —*Journal of American Medical Association*, April 11, 1914[52]

An *Echo Enterprise* reader sent a clipping of the ad to AMA headquarters, suggesting it showed the "unscrupulous methods" that osteopaths used to attract patients. In a rather reserved reply, Propaganda Department Director Cramp suggested, "The garbling of the *Journal's* editorial for the purpose of making capital for osteopathy is entirely in keeping with the professional standing of that cult." Needless to say, this reflected the unresolved and tense relationship between schools of medicine in the early twentieth century, as can be seen in additional Propaganda Department correspondence. Other osteopathic advertisements sent in to the AMA offices were labeled "drivel," a "pseudo-medical curiosity," and "outright quackery."[53]

In total, the AMA consistently condemned sectarian therapies in the same language used to deride patent medicines. It dismissed all as pseudoscientific or harmless at best, outright quackery and deluded nonsense at worst. While some orthodox practitioners certainly promoted a more broad-minded approach, the AMA unleashed the propaganda for reform with equal force against sectarians. After all, as Cramp would say, sectarians merely constituted different forms of quackery.

CONCLUSION: THE LIMITS OF REFORM

Despite the accomplishments of the AMA in its crusade against quackery, and the surveillance network it created to support the cause, Cramp frequently voiced frustration with the lack of change inspired by the work of the Propaganda Department. In a spirited reply to a doctor friend who admitted to being confused about how and why the department deemed certain things scientific and others quackery, Cramp confessed to being deeply discouraged by the writer's "total ignorance of the principles for which the *Journal* has been fighting for so many years." Cramp tried to explain. "The question as to what constitutes truthful advertising of, at least comparatively, scientific products on the one hand and what, on the other hand, constitutes false, misleading, deceptive and even fraudulent advertising of products utterly unscientific in character is very clear cut and patent." If medicinal preparations were not developed "under the conditions that conform to the general tenets of scientific work," then they fell into the category of quackery. The Propaganda Department could not guarantee that all medicines that met with the Council on Pharmacy and Chemistry's approval would in fact be therapeutically effective in all cases; they could ask only that the claims made by drug companies be based on evidence obtained under scientific conditions. Virtually all patent medicines advertised directly to consumers, by contrast, could be considered quackery.[54]

Despite Cramp's admonitions, the facts as the AMA saw them did not always represent the facts as interpreted by drug companies or consumers. Additionally, along with disseminating evidence of a reasoned, scientific character, the AMA expressed its judgments in more subjective, rhetorical form. While determinations were based predominantly on evidence gleaned from authoritative sources, AMA pronouncements also combined arbitrary labels and rhetorical flourish. The proclaimed adherence to a limited fact-based educational function in the Propaganda for Reform program also belied the activist objectives of the AMA and concealed a variety of economic, legislative, and professional advantages secured as a result of its work.

The work of the Propaganda Department, and later the Bureau of Investigation, increased the power of the AMA to influence the decisions of drug manufacturers, doctors, and consumers. The AMA identified drugs that failed to conform to the standards of scientific evidence and disseminated an enormous amount of information to the profession and the public. By working closely with educators, allied medical professions, and both public and private organizations, the AMA effectively established, sustained, and policed a nationwide surveillance network of collaborators committed to protecting consumers and working for the cause of public health. In all of these efforts, the AMA cultivated authority and exerted a tremendous amount of influence. As public deference and institutional forces legitimized the work of the AMA as arbiter of therapeutic acceptability, the association passed judgment not just on patent medicines, long derided by competing schools of medicine, but also on sectarian therapies defined as quackery or pseudomedicine. Nevertheless, the power to regulate the marketplace rested with lawmakers and enforcement agencies, and the power of choice ultimately rested with doctors and consumers.

FIVE

A NEW DEAL FOR QUACKERY

Franklin Delano Roosevelt's promise of a New Deal for Americans coincided with the first extensive national study of medical practice in the United States. The 1932 report of the Committee on the Costs of Medical Care (CCMC) originated with the work of 15 frustrated delegates at the 1926 American Medical Association (AMA) national convention who decided to investigate, and attempt to solve, the organizational sources of problems with the cost and distribution of medical care. The CCMC also provided one measure of efforts to combat quackery and redefine the boundaries of medical orthodoxy.[1]

Reports from the CCMC revealed the widespread dominance of a distinctly orthodox approach to medicine and health care. Orthodoxy had become associated with an increasingly powerful and influential AMA, a more rigorously trained cadre of M.D.s, an expansive hospital system, and a growing network of medical research that was being conducted in an array of private and public institutions across the country. At the same time, the CCMC underscored the persistence of unorthodox therapies in the medical marketplace. While efforts to establish, enlarge, and police the boundaries of therapeutic orthodoxy had helped instill a tremendous amount of confidence in the authority of physicians, Americans continued to support a wide range of alleged forms of quackery that reformers had targeted for decades. Therapeutic reformers could measure their success in the proliferation of new regulations, new institutions, and innovative therapies, but patent medicines and sectarian alternatives maintained their positions in the marketplace.[2]

The CCMC documented what it judged to be successful efforts to regulate and standardize an orthodox approach to therapeutics. The Pure Food and Drugs Act of 1906, for example, had given the *U.S. Pharmacopœia* and the *National Formulary* the legal authority to determine the standards for official medicines prescribed by physicians and dispensed by pharmacists. Both of these publications provided formulas for drug preparations with standards of identity, purity, and strength accepted by federal, state, and local governments; together they constituted a list of "official drugs." These books were supplemented by the AMA's *New and Non-Official Remedies*, published through its Council on Pharmacy and Chemistry. This publication contained the names and descriptions of articles accepted by the council after manufacturers' claims had been investigated. In 1929, this included over 600 preparations not yet considered "official" drugs by the *U.S. Pharmacopeia* or the *National Formulary*. Collectively, these reference books provided a list of medicines judged to be unadulterated and properly labeled, with statements deemed truthful regarding constituent elements and curative properties. Put simply, these drugs represented therapeutic orthodoxy.[3]

Therapeutic reformers had successfully capitalized on scientific advances to provide improved therapeutic options and an expanded institutional network, but they had been relatively ineffective in convincing the public to rely on physician expertise in responding to many illnesses. In 1932, the committee reported that of the $715 million spent annually by the American people on drugs and medicines, $165 million went to nonsecret home remedies for self-medication, while sales of predominantly secret patent medicines advertised directly to consumers amounted to an impressive $360 million. Only 27 percent of the total amount spent for medicines ($190 million of the total annual bill) consisted of physicians' prescriptions, while consumers spent another $125 million on medical services, mostly nondrug therapies, offered by sectarians.[4]

The committee noted that since only 25 percent of drugs were being consumed based on the recommendation of medical practitioners, most medicines were purchased "on the basis of such judgments as they are able to form through personal experience or the recommendations of fellow sufferers." Given that the drug industry spent an estimated $70 million annually to advertise medicines for home use, the CCMC concluded that this was part of an effort to deliberately bypass the physician and put the decision-making power in the hands of individuals. While the committee credited the AMA for its efforts to "enlighten the public on the evils of self-medication," with the work of the Propaganda Department and Bureau of Investigation, the report also asserted that the movement had been hampered by the opposition of the proprietary medicine interests and the suspicion that the AMA had "been prompted by a desire to merely increase the incomes of doctors, rather than to promote the public health." Additionally, the condemnation of patent medicines without the recommendation of adequate substitutes tended as much to hinder as promote the more rational use of drugs.[5]

Patent medicines, home remedies, and sectarian therapeutic alternatives flourished, particularly with diseases or conditions that orthodox medicine had failed to treat effectively. American Social Hygiene Association (ASHA) studies of preferred treatments for venereal diseases in the late 1920s and early 1930s, for example, showed that an average of between 40 percent and 70 percent of young men in six different U.S. cities chose self-treatment or irregular therapies over drugs provided by orthodox physicians. The ASHA explained the appeal of unorthodox remedies by noting that the old-time quack who formerly "hawked his medicine from a wagon-trail" had been replaced with the modern specialist who now "sits at a desk in his 'laboratory' or 'clinic,'" securing patients by advertisement, correspondence, and personal appeal. "Masquerading as a 'famous specialist for men,' 'specialist in blood diseases,' 'the remedy company,' 'herbalist,' 'professor,' or 'electric institute,' he reaps a full harvest from victims who are misled by his advertising matter," an ASHA pamphlet reported. In another pamphlet titled "Jerry Learns a Lesson: Keep Away from Quacks," ASHA told the story of a sick and worried man who gets taken in by "Doctor Quack" before later learning from his family doctor (who is a member of the local medical society and on the staff of two fine hospitals) that the only reliable source of treatment is offered by a fully qualified doctor competent to diagnose and treat venereal diseases.[6]

Given that physicians did not direct or control a large part of the consumption of medicines, the CCMC concluded that it was in the field of self-medication that advertising had its greatest effects on the costs of medical care. According to the committee, patent medicine advertising had become institutionalized through organizations like the Proprietary Association of America, which represented the interests of manufacturers. The Proprietary Association lobbied to influence legislation in Washington, persistently fought efforts to increase regulation, and helped members develop effective advertising strategies. The Association had aggressively challenged the efforts of the AMA to expose and restrict patent medicine advertising, and it considered the AMA a "Doctors' Trust," whose assault was "not actuated by altruistic motives, but by motives of selfishness." The AMA supported Samuel Hopkins Adams's description of the Proprietary Association as "the body for mutual help and protection of all the more powerful quacks and frauds."[7]

The CCMC, meanwhile, reported that in addition to patent medicine peddlers and the 142,000 trained and licensed physicians in active practice, there were no less than 36,000 other individuals who it considered "not well trained in the medical sciences" yet "held themselves out as able to cure disease and to treat the sick." In addition to representing nearly one-fourth of the number of practicing M.D.s, the total

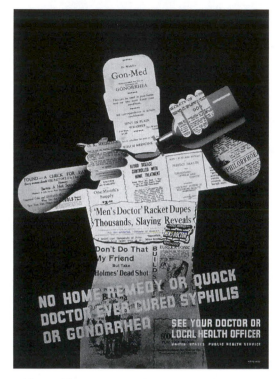

U.S. Public Health Service poster by Leonard Karsakov (ca. 1941).
(Courtesy of the National Library of Medicine)

amount spent annually for the services of sectarians, $125 million, represented about
12 percent of the of annual expenditures for the services of all physicians.

Sectarians capitalized on the authority engendered by cumulative experience, along
with the limited focus of orthodox therapeutic reformers who attempted to make distinctions between acceptable, safe, and effective drugs and medical therapies. By the
1930s, the most popular sectarians primarily offered drugless alternatives (Table 5.1).[8]

Table 5.1.   The most popular sectarian alternatives documented in *The Healing Cults* (1932).

Practitioners	Number	Amount Spent on Annually ($ million)
Osteopaths	7,650	42
Chiropractors	16,000	63
Naturopaths	2,500	10
Christian Science and New Thought Healers	10,000	10

In the CCMC's main report on sectarians, *The Healing Cults*, Dr. Louis S. Reed defined boundaries between orthodox and unorthodox medicine by employing much the same rhetoric that the AMA had used for decades. Reed asserted that sectarians exhibited common characteristics by virtue of which they could be classed as "healing cults" or "sects." First, all were allegedly founded upon and identified with certain theories or dogmas. Second, the founder of each sect launched his or her theory as an explanation for all disease and taught a procedure or method of treatment that he or she claimed to be a cure for all disease. Third, the basic theories of these groups all ran counter to the established facts of medical science. And fourth, Reed argued that medical opinion considered their claims either unsound or exaggerated. According to Reed, modern medicine had eschewed sectarianism in the process of becoming scientific. Like all science, modern medicine was "experimental and catholic," and it constantly questioned its own hypotheses, accepted only whatever was established by fact, and did not "depend on a theory." Like the AMA, Reed also generalized suspicion of medical charlatanry into a resistance to any medicine, procedure, or system of healing that was not supported by the rubric of orthodox methods.[9]

Reed also outlined the widely held belief that many people lacked the knowledge and scientific attitude necessary for the correct appraisal of the soundness of sectarian doctrines and practices, which reflected a fundamental tenet of the AMA's propaganda for reform program. According to Reed, eliminating the popular belief in the value of sectarian theories and practices, which caused people to patronize sectarians, was even more important than pushing for the legal suppression of unqualified practitioners.[10]

Beyond explaining the appeal of sectarian therapies to people who either lacked scientific knowledge or remained superstitious, reformers nevertheless failed to offer a convincing explanation for how or why alternative therapies survived on the market if they simply did not work. The editor of the *Ladies' Home Journal* offered one possible reason:

> The increasing readiness of the intelligent public not only to listen to but to adopt any new pathy or science, in which the element of drugs is omitted, spells not the ignorance or the gullibility of the public, as some physicians are ever ready and fond of designating any departure from the established school, but it spells in very plain letters a growing feeling of unrest and of distrust of the methods of the average physician, and a proclamation of individual enlightenment on this whole question.

Creating standards for orthodox drug approval, demanding laboratory and clinical evidence for effectiveness, and relegating unproven therapies to quack status proved insufficient for dictating consumer choices. This meant that however successful reformers might have been in changing regulatory standards and institutionalizing an orthodox approach to drug research and development, they remained unable to control consumption patterns.[11]

In one important sense, Reed and separate CCMC reports identified a weakness in reform strategies by suggesting that sectarians existed "on more legitimate and more substantial bases" than the orthodox profession had been willing to accept. First, Reed noted sectarian methods of treatment were useful and effective in some conditions, but orthodox practitioners had either failed to acknowledge this or make use of these methods. Furthermore, the two dominant medical sects in the early 1930s— osteopathy and chiropractic—had arisen in part as reactions against (or because of certain deficiencies in) current medical practice. As Reed suggested, for centuries drug therapy had been the dominant orthodox therapy, and this tradition militated against new methods of treating disease. Sectarians, meanwhile, had capitalized on the appeal of drugless therapies.[12]

According to the official position of the AMA's Bureau of Investigation, education had the power to change public and professional patterns of consumption. But by the 1930s, despite an impressive list of AMA publications, a broad-based indirect and direct educational campaign, an extensive antiquackery surveillance network of like-minded reformers in public and private organizations, and the steady increase in direct correspondence with professionals and the lay public, patent medicines maintained a dominant presence while sectarians held firm to their share of the market. Even though a network of reformers had successfully redefined the boundaries of therapeutic orthodoxy in many ways, the popularity of unorthodox therapies persisted.

THE NEW MUCKRAKERS

In his book *Quacks*, Dr. Charles Warner argued that the gullibility of humankind had long been the most insoluble factor in the efforts to solve the quack problem. According to Warner, quacks existed because there were always enough people who were foolish enough to believe in crooks. He identified more than 6 million deaf or partially deaf persons, 1 million tuberculosis sufferers, 0.5 million epileptics, 0.5 million cancer patients, 10 million bald men, and 20 million glasses-wearers as particularly vulnerable to quack remedies. "Until he dies, or his money runs out, the quacks keep after him," Warner explained. "They advertise for him, giving bogus testimonials for healing. They buy his name from other quacks who have taken every possible dollar from him." Nothing could be more reprehensible than defrauding the sick. Warner continued, "taking money from the afflicted, by false pretenses, especially as delay in the proper treatment of an ailment, may carry the patient past the stage where a cure might be affected." Warner and others called on the government to answer to its first duty—to protect the lives and health of its subjects—in response to this critically important problem.[13]

In his book *The Tragedy of Waste*, published in 1925, economist Stuart Chase agreed that the government had failed to protect the American consumer from predatory advertisers in the drug trade. According to Chase, nine-tenths and more of advertising was "largely competitive wrangling as the relative merits of two undistinguished and often indistinguishable compounds," whether it was "soaps, tooth powders, motor cars, tires, snappy suits, breakfast foods, patent medicines, or cigarettes." At the AMA, Arthur Cramp had similarly noted how advertising underwent a significant transition in the 1920s. The emphasis shifted from "offering copy," which presented a product straightforwardly for a reader to buy or not on its merit, to "selling copy," or the creation of desires where no craving had existed. As historian James Harvey Young puts it, patent medicine pioneers had long "sold the fear of suffering and death" and "the hope of well-being and health," but in the 1920s they cultivated the mystique of a growing cult of consumption, which capitalized on increasingly sophisticated tools designed to appeal to the emotions of consumers, developed by advertisers in collaboration with academics and psychologists.[14]

In his best-selling book *Your Money's Worth*, published in 1927, Chase collaborated with mechanical engineer Fred Schlink to argue that the government had failed to protect the American consumer from predatory advertisers in the drug trade. Chase and Schlink argued that consumers had no defense against advertising besides "a waning quality of common sense," and thus pursued their "blundering way" like "a moth about a candle." *Your Money's Worth* lamented the waste of the consumer's dollar as he or she was forced to buy in the "jungle" of competitive advertising, wasteful goods, and worthless patent medicines. Historian Charles Jackson notes that the popularity of the book was a sign that a muckraking audience might be in the making, but in 1927 it was tempered by the Ballyhoo Age enthusiasm of 1920s consumerism. The economic catastrophe of the Great Depression and concurrent collapse of confidence in the American business community ultimately made the consumer movement more viable and popular. Years later, one commentator aptly labeled *Your Money's Worth* the "*Uncle Tom's Cabin* of the consumer movement," as the Chase-Schlink volume became the prototype for several muckraking volumes to follow.[15]

Convinced that consumers needed to be equipped with accurate information about the quality of products based on scientific testing, Schlink took action in 1929. Since the government had failed to provide such protection, he and Arthur Kallet organized the Consumers' Research group to fill the void. As one of the first professional consumer-interest groups, and the ancestor of today's Consumers Union and its revered publication *Consumer Reports*, Consumers' Research began with 1,200 subscribers who paid $2 yearly for confidential mimeographed critiques of consumer goods. By 1933, regular bulletins were going out to 45,000 members. These bulletins described brand name products that had been tested by Consumers' Research so that consumers could defend themselves against the aggressions of advertising.[16]

In 1933, Schlink and Kallet also published a best-selling muckraking exposé which argued that, given the current state of the food, drug, and advertising industries, and the lax regulation of each, American consumers were little better than guinea pigs. *100,000,000 Guinea Pigs* sped through 27 printings in its first year and continued to sell well throughout the 1930s. The book was, as historian James Harvey Young puts it, "a mixture of technological analysis and fiery tract," and the "irrationality of a helter-skelter, wasteful, unplanned economic system was asserted with equal vigor." The book named actual brands, and listed their alleged crimes and frauds openly. It drew most of the information on patent medicines from pamphlets and releases that had already been published by other critics, including the AMA, regulatory agencies, and the National Better Business Bureau.[17]

The style of "guinea pig" muckraking pioneered by Schlink and Kallet, and emulated by other writers at the time, elevated the shock value of tales of fraud and deception. In the words of Young, it tended to "regard all sinners as of nearly equal culpability, condemning the big borderline advertiser exploiting body odor or bad breath with a rigor resembling that used to castigate the small operator vending a lethal radium water." Schlink and Kallet asserted, "Almost no advertising intended to influence the general public is honest in the sense that a decent scientist understands honesty." In the eyes of the law, they proclaimed, Americans were "all guinea pigs, and any scoundrel who takes it into his head to enter the drug or food business can experiment on us." While this may have been an exaggerated proclamation, it was an indication that the law had clearly failed to protect consumers in the way it had been intended.[18]

"Of all the rank flowers in the garden of rugged American individualism," Kallet and Schlink pronounced, "few have a more vile and pervasive stench than the huge $350,000,000 patent-medicine blossom." At its best, the patent medicine industry was guilty of economic fraud, selling drugs under meaningless or fantastic names, with absurd claims of therapeutic effectiveness, at anywhere from five to a thousand times their ordinary value. At its worst, the patent medicine industry was guilty of murder by selling poisons as well as persuading the poor and ignorant to rely on worthless nostrums for the treatment of diseases as dangerous as cancer and tuberculosis. What were the penalties for such murder? "No penalties whatever, even when the killing can be proved," Kallet and Schlink concluded. Under the Pure Food and Drugs Act, the courts might impose a small fine for mislabeling, but they could do nothing if a nostrum killed people but did not have technically false statements on its label.[19]

By 1932, the U.S. Food and Drug Administration (FDA) had prosecuted 18,000 cases that involved forfeiture of food and drug products, with an additional 9,000 criminal indictments. The success rates in each category were impressive, with 16,000 successful forfeiture judgments and over 7,000 criminal convictions. But as one critical review noted, the amazingly high number of guilty pleas in criminal cases (over 90 percent) and the frequent summoning of the same offender before the courts served as evidence that many firms, immune as corporations from imprisonment, regarded "the system of confiscation, suspension of sentence, and light fines as a very moderate license charge for plying their trade." In the whole history of enforcement of the act, two prison sentences had been imposed. First time offenders paid a fine not exceeding $200, and convictions for each subsequent offense were limited to fines of $300. By agreeing to slight changes in the label or formula of a drug, defendants could also often avoid the effect of even successful prosecutions, while in many other cases the goods under investigation were released under bond and surreptitiously returned to the market.[20]

The impossible task of regulating the food and drug markets ultimately fell on Walter G. Campbell, head of the FDA since 1921. He had originally been hired by Harvey Wiley as soon as the Pure Food and Drugs Act had been passed. By the early 1930s, he had only 65 inspectors to police 110,000 different products, fewer than the Department of Agriculture's program to control hog cholera and the enforcement of plant quarantine along the Mexican border. With an appropriation of about $250,000, this small corps of officials was charged with regulating the interstate commerce in food and drugs for over 100 million people, valued annually at between $15 and $20 billion. An idea of the enormity of the task is shown by the fact that the total value of the year's output of canned goods alone amounted to $745 million in 1932, while drug products exceeded $400 million. Additionally, half of the products Campbell and his inspectors faced did not even exist when the 1906 law was written, and the FDA had little authority to regulate much of the other half.[21]

Campbell was well aware of these and other longstanding problems with the original Pure Food and Drugs Act. Since the law applied primarily to what was said on drug labels, not what was actually in the bottle, government regulators were given no authority to look inside the container, let alone test the ingredients, to ensure that the contents were safe and effective. In an effort to avoid medical and scientific debates about therapeutic effectiveness, a series of court cases had also failed to definitively establish what claims could and could not be made on labels. There was still no requirement to even list the ingredients of patent medicines, unless they contained specific ingredients that had been deemed dangerous or habit-forming, including marijuana, alcohol, opium, cocaine, heroin, morphine, and a few poisons. If a bottle contained a poison not on the list of dangerous or habit-forming drugs, and if the label were blank, there was nothing the government could do to stop manufacturers from selling it and consumers from buying it. Anyone could concoct a medicine in his or her kitchen and sell it, with no testing required, as long as it did not contain one of a few listed narcotics or poisons.[22]

Perhaps the most significant weakness of the 1906 law was its failure to provide for control over false advertising. Congress had initially chosen not to invest this power with the FDA, and by 1933 the consumer was left largely unprotected from the food and drug industries. While the Federal Trade Commission (FTC) had originally been charged with responsibility over false and misleading advertising, in the Raladam case of 1931 the Supreme Court ruled the FTC could act only where false advertising was clearly injurious to competitors. So, while the Sherley Amendment provided the basis for legal action when fraudulent therapeutic claims were printed on food and drug labels, almost all forms of nonlabel advertising could be exploited with no consequence.[23]

Guinea pig muckrakers identified a number of additional problems related to advertising. Medical journals, including the *Journal of the American Medical Association (JAMA)*, continued to advertise drugs with "puffed and ridiculous statements" about the therapeutic value and promise of questionable remedies. In a 1932 issue of *JAMA*, a report on Mercurochrome, an antiseptic, by the association's Council on Pharmacy and Chemistry found that the manufacturer had made at least three untrue claims about its ability to penetrate living tissue, remain active after it dried on the skin, and remain nontoxic. Yet, in the very next issue of the *Journal*, the AMA carried a full-page ad for Mercurochrome on its back cover. In another case, ultraviolet ray lamps were advertised in the pages of *JAMA* as effective remedies for cardiac irregularity, hysteria, insomnia, sinus infections, bronchitis, asthma, nepthritis (kidney inflammation), eczema, and rheumatism, despite a lack of evidence of these effects from AMA investigations. In his exposé *Fads, Frauds and Physicians*, T. Swann Harding cited these and other ads for unproven therapies as evidence for his conclusion that "the old spirit of quackery" was "apparently still in the inner sanctum of medicine."[24]

Kallet and Schlink did not shy away from criticizing their antiquackery compatriots. While they complimented Arthur Cramp for "the able direction" of his Bureau of Investigation, and praised its reports as a valuable source of information for the "harassed consumer," muckrakers admonished the AMA for the number of questionable drugs and therapeutic devices advertised in its journal. They criticized the Post Office Department for settling too many cases without criminal action and dismissed the FTC as "unhappily dying of inaction." The sharpest rebukes were reserved for the FDA.[25]

While Kallet and Schlink admitted the 1906 law was "feeble and ineffective" as written, and that it had been further weakened by court interpretation, they nevertheless blamed the FDA for shirking its responsibility and adopting what they considered to be a pro-business and anti-consumer stance. According to critics, this leaning could be seen in the FDA's preference for small seizures of insignificant amounts of drugs over criminal actions against the perpetrators of fraud and deception, their frequent announcements of warnings to proprietary manufacturers before launching an enforcement program, their secret negotiations with manufacturers intended to promote compliance, and their preference to avoid publicity as a weapon against quackery. In criticizing FDA Chief Campbell, Kallet and Schlink rhetorically asked if anyone could be kinder than he to the quacks and crooks who purveyed cures and treatments for diseases like cancer and tuberculosis.[26]

THE FIVE-YEAR STRUGGLE FOR A NEW LAW

By the early 1930s, FDA leadership had pushed for supplementary legislation to address problems with the limited reach of the 1906 law and weak enforcement provisions for over 25 years. They acknowledged that the law was inadequate and flagrant abuses were commonplace. In the 1920s, all attempts to strengthen the law had failed. In fact, the FDA had remained on the defensive for much of the decade as a series of "ripper bills" aimed at reducing the FDA's authority had been pushed through Congress. Many were aimed at restricting the number of seizures of products judged in violation of the 1906 law. The godfather of food and drug regulation, Dr. Wiley, made his dissatisfaction with the operation of the FDA clear throughout the decade before his death in 1930. In a 1932 report on the work of the FDA, Campbell also noted that comments and inquiries revealed how a growing portion of the public expected "greater protection through the enforcement of the pure food and drug law than the legal authority conferred by that legislation will permit." He warned that it would be worthwhile to inform consumers of the law's limitations so that they might not suffer from a false sense of security.[27]

It should not be surprising that Campbell reacted with irritation when the new Assistant Secretary of Agriculture, Rexford Tugwell, offered his own unsolicited critique of the FDA in March 1933. Tugwell expressed his disapproval not with enforcement measures against fraudulent foods or drugs, but rather with a case involving a pesticide. Tugwell's office had received a letter regarding tolerance levels for lead arsenate, a poison being used to spray fruit trees. Tugwell was supposed to sign a routine reply drafted on the Department of Agriculture's letterhead, but instead he sent the unsigned letter to Campbell with a question penciled in the margin. Why, Tugwell asked, did the FDA not prohibit the use of lead arsenate altogether if it was a poison? Campbell's assistant Paul Dunbar later recalled it was like getting a "kick in the teeth" after so many long years of fighting a lone battle against pesticide residues, not to mention the ever-growing food and drug industry.[28]

When Campbell marched over to Tugwell's office the next morning, he described the weaknesses of the 1906 law. He explained how it gave him no power to make rules or declare what was safe, particularly in fields like pesticides and cosmetics, which had not been covered under the original act. Even before Franklin Delano

Roosevelt's (FDR's) inauguration, Tugwell had promised to address the problems with the FDA, which he believed had become "perverted by the attempt to protect business interests." Tugwell was also already familiar with Kallet and Schlink, and knew about their critiques of the administration. As one of the intellectual leaders of FDR's team, he had already proven himself as a shrewd tactician in proposing additional legislation during the early part of the president's famous first hundred days. Tugwell had been convinced that something needed to change, and he promised Campbell he would bring the issue directly to the White House. Within a matter of hours, Tugwell informed Campbell that he had already talked to Roosevelt, and FDR had authorized a revision of the Pure Food and Drugs Act.[29]

In hopes of riding the wave of reform during the New Deal's first hundred days, Campbell moved quickly to draft a new bill. It was ultimately designed to supplant the outdated and inadequate Pure Food and Drugs Act of 1906. He worked with other seasoned officials within the FDA and the Solicitor General's Office who had experience with inspection and enforcement. He recruited legislative writers familiar with the food and drug industries. He also sought expert advice from outside his circle, including state enforcement officials and individuals in private organizations who were interested in consumer protection. At a hearing with representatives of the food, drug, and publishing industries, members of each group expressed their reservations about making suggestions about a new law without knowing exactly what government officials had in mind. In trade papers, they voiced their displeasure with Tugwell's involvement after he chose not to stick around to hear everything they had to say but instead left a bureau chief in charge. Tugwell chose not to participate in the bill-drafting process but offered his sympathetic support.[30]

Senator Royal S. Copeland introduced the bill on June 12, 1933. It was designed "to prevent the manufacture, shipment, and sale of adulterated or misbranded food, drink, drugs, and cosmetics" and the false advertisement of each. While it embraced the intent behind the 1906 law, its major provisions addressed nearly all of the weaknesses identified by quackery critics and dramatically expanded the power of the government and the authority of the mainstream medical profession. A drug would be considered misbranded if its labeling made any therapeutic claim that, even by ambiguity or inference, was "contrary to the general agreement of medical opinion." The misbranding ban also fell on labels that gave the names of diseases, including tuberculosis, diabetes, and cancer, for which the remedies were palliative instead of cures. The bill expanded the list of dangerous drugs mentioned in the old law, required medicines containing certain narcotic and hypnotic drugs to include a warning label, and required all proprietary medicines to list the common names and quantities of all medicinal ingredients on their labels. The term "drug" would also be dramatically expanded to include not only all substances and preparations recognized by the *United States Pharmacopeia* and *National Formulary* but also all "substances, preparations, and devices intended for use in the cure, mitigation, treatment, or prevention of disease in man or other animals," as well as "all substances and preparations, other than food, and all devices, intended to affect the structure or any function of the body of man or other animals." A drug would be considered adulterated if it was dangerous to health when used according to directions. With respect to certain ailments for which the medical profession deemed self-treatment dangerous or futile, no remedies at all could be advertised to the lay public. The list included appendicitis, blood poisoning, carbuncles, sexual impotence, sinus infections, and venereal diseases. The FDA could change the list as the state of medical knowledge changed. The proposed bill also transferred the authority to regulate the advertising of food, drugs, and cosmetics from the Federal Trade Commission to the Department of Agriculture, and applied the same strict standards to the labeling of drugs and all drug advertising. Makers of proprietary drugs would also be subject to factory inspections, a permit system designed to regulate interstate shipments, and stiffer penalties including the real threat of prison for first-time offenders.[31]

Opposition to the bill came quickly and fiercely. Even the bill's sponsor came under attack. After no other Congressional sponsor had stepped in during the early drafting phase, Royal S. Copeland, a Tammany Democrat from New York, had agreed to introduce the controversial measure. Copeland had been trained as a homeopathic physician, served as health commissioner of New York City, and written a health column for the Hearst papers. All of this made him suspect according to the more extreme liberal crusaders as well as some conservatives. Copeland had demonstrated his commitment to the cause of food and drug reform by trying to plug loopholes in the 1906 law, but he later admitted he had not even read through the bill in its entirety before introducing it as the emergency session of Congress drew to a close. Critics nevertheless called the measure the Tugwell Bill, despite the convention of any bill taking its name from the person who sponsored it in Congress. Tugwell was already known as one of FDR's academic "brain trusters." Even worse, as drug trade writers noted, he had visited Russia, which made it easy to allege subversive motives for supporting the bill. The drug makers wrote that the bill would "Sovietize" drug sales. As historian Philip J. Hilts points out, the attacks on Tugwell became so frequent and extreme that lampoons appeared as well, with one suggesting that Tugwell's plan "is to abandon both the silver and gold standard . . . and issue aspirin tablets from the Federal mint." Critics warned the bill would give the Secretary of Agriculture "czaristic" discretionary powers to make regulations and interpretive decisions. At a time when other New Deal agencies were under consideration, and some industries looked toward regulatory bodies with suspicion, it was easy to accuse Tugwell of "Volsteadizing and Carrie Nationizing" the food, drug, and cosmetic industries. Years later, it was still charged that the bill had been written by inexperienced pedagogues influenced by Moscow.[32]

The critique of the bill peaked at a subcommittee meeting that Copeland held in December 1933. Representatives of the proprietary drug industry argued that the Tugwell Bill posed a grave threat. H. B. Thompson, testifying for the Proprietary Association, compared the bill to parts of *Alice in Wonderland* and insisted the only way it could be amended "was to strike out all after the enacting clause." He maintained: " . . . I have never in my life read a bill or heard of a bill so grotesque in its terms, evil in its purpose, and vicious in its possible consequences as this bill would be if enacted." Formula disclosure threatened manufacturers, opened the door to piracy, and was deemed "unreasonable, useless, unjust, and unwise." Licensing would interfere with free commerce and should be considered "a very great menace." Regarding the criminal prosecution clause of the bill, one spokesman for a proprietary group argued that the increased fines and threat of imprisonment represented punishments "severe enough to satisfy a lust for blood should one be so fastidious in his just indignation." Dr. James Beal of the National Drug Trade Conference, an organization made up of delegates from a number of national pharmaceutical associations and proprietary trade groups, objected to virtually every major feature of the Senate bill number 1944 (S.1944) from its definition of drugs to the ambiguity of terms used to differentiate palliative and curative remedies.[33]

Meanwhile, other industry spokesmen argued there was simply no need for a new law. They maintained the old one had served the purpose of controlling quackery well enough. Dr. Beal called it "the most efficient act of its kind in existence," while another called it a "monument." A new, more radical law was unnecessary to catch the few remaining charlatans. "This would be," said an advertising periodical, "like burning down the house to get rid of the mice." The irony in this position was pointed out later by Charles LaWall, a colleague of Harvey Wiley on the first drug bill, when he noted in 1937 that "the opponents of this bill have made every one of the specific objections to its passage that were made of . . . the original Hepburn Bill in 1906."[34]

Several industry spokesmen identified the dangerous consequences of the new discretionary powers that would be granted by the Tugwell bill. "Unlimited power entrusted to bureaucrats warps their judgment on the opinions they might have as normal citizens," warned William L. Daley of the National Editorial Association. Dr. Beal argued the bill placed the entire process of food, drug, and cosmetic manufacture, labeling, and shipment within the unrestrained control of the Secretary of Agriculture. A lack of clarity in terms and reliance on such an uncertain thing as "general agreement of medical opinion" also meant the standard of truth and falsity would ultimately be the opinion of the Secretary. Equally concerning was the fact that no method of appeal or review of the Secretary's provisions was provided. One editorialist warned that if the bill passed, "no manufacturer can possibly continue except by the grace of the officials in Washington." The Department of Agriculture would become a "virtual dictatorship over the trade."[35]

Other critics warned of a different power grab at play, one that involved the "allopathic medical trust," led by the American Medical Association. Dr. Aitchison, who claimed to represent 40,000 Americans but failed to reveal the nature of his National Liberties Association membership, warned that S. 1944 was one of the most diabolical bills ever laid before Congress. According to Aitchison, only "a man who is already linked up with the medical trust" could support a bill that greased his palm with "blood-soaked dollars." The AMA had nothing to do with the drafting of the bill and initially took a rather apathetic approach in choosing not to attend the December 1933 hearing. An AMA representative merely filed a brief complaining of the rule-making powers of the Secretary. Members of the proprietary medicine trade nevertheless remained convinced that Tugwell had been "duped" by the "dictators" of the AMA. Through its restrictions, they argued, the bill threatened to take away the "sacred right" of self-medication. This charge was constantly reiterated with notable examples of hyperbole, as was the case in an article from the December 1933 issue of *Good Housekeeping*, which maintained "it would be a real hardship if you or I could not take an aspirin table or mineral oil or bicarbonate of soda without a physician's prescription." While the author admitted the bill did not say that, it implied anything was possible under its provisions. According to the bill's critics, advertising restrictions would also deny the public the knowledge needed to handle simple ailments and require them to visit a physician to get medicines that would soon be stripped from the shelves of drug stores. Such charges made for effective propaganda, even if only a small number believed them.[36]

Resistance to the bill quickly outpaced the work of supporters, as existing trade organizations were transformed almost immediately into forces of opposition. While the Proprietary Association and the United Medicine Manufacturers of America proved to be the most militant, they were quickly joined by the American Newspaper Publishers Association, the National Association of Retail Druggists, and the National Publishers Association. These groups sponsored public protest meetings, paid for radio propaganda, and organized letter writing campaigns.[37]

Whereas the press had played an integral role in garnering public support for reform with the 1906 law, the importance of the advertising dollar also encouraged opposition to the bill in 1933. By the 1930s, the collective economic power of the food, drug, and advertising trades was sufficient to discourage reform measures that might anger these industries. Some patent medicine companies circulated letters to newspaper and magazine editors with the explicit warning that passage of the bill would mean a significant loss of advertising revenue. Some even revived the "red clause" from the pre-1906 days, which threatened immediate cancellation of advertising contracts if the bill passed. While proponents of the new legislation claimed that the revision was being subjected to a press blackout, the Proprietary Association sent out canned editorials against the Tugwell Bill, which showed up in newspapers around the country. The *New York Times* ran only one front-page story on the bill throughout its contentious history, and their policy was not exceptional.[38]

Confronted with such widespread opposition, Campbell went on the offensive. To rally support for the bill, he and his aides wrote articles, made radio appearances, circulated mimeographed material from field offices, mailed reprinted articles by FDA staff members, and coordinated speaking engagements around the country. To graphically illustrate the most poignant stories of quackery, Campbell and his staff created an exhibit complete with full-sized posters, bottles, labels, advertisements, and death certificates from some of the most egregious cases of food, cosmetics, and patent-medicine threats. Campbell invited senators to see the exhibit at his testimony during the December 1933 hearings, and the display was subsequently put on the road with drug unit inspectors and loaned out to any organization that requested it. The press soon dubbed the effective exhibit the Chamber of Horrors. It drew heavy crowds at expositions around the country and was made available to the public at almost every drug administration field office around the country. Among the horrors was a cosmetic called Lash Lure, an aniline eyelash dye that had caused permanent blindness in several of its victims. Crazy Water Crystals, which claimed to cure ailments brought on by constipation, high blood pressure, arthritis, liver and kidney troubles, and much more, was shown to be nothing more than an age-old but potentially dangerous laxative. The exhibit recounted deaths caused by stomach rupture and peritonitis. An analysis of Mountain Valley Mineral Water, which claimed to be an effective treatment for rheumatism, cardiac diseases, and diabetes, showed it had the same composition as the tap water where it had been manufactured, in Atlanta. Radithor, another horror, was tied to the horrible death of a Pittsburgh steel manufacturer, who had been disfigured by the proprietary radium water sold as a cure for cancer. Banbar, an alleged diabetes cure made from horsetail weed, and B & M, a horse liniment alleged to cure tuberculosis, were each accompanied by individuals' testimonials and their subsequent death certificates. The popular press widely admitted the effectiveness of the exhibit, and even Eleanor Roosevelt became a backer of the bill after making a well-publicized trip to the FDA to view the full display.[39]

While many of the horrors had also been documented and detailed by the more militant Consumers' Research group, Kallet and Schlink insisted that the bill failed to give consumers enough protection. From the consumer's perspective, Kallet maintained the bill would do little more than take "a few cartridges" from a habitual criminal, leaving him with his gun and his liberty. They conceded the bill was infinitely superior to the 1906 law. They had received hundreds of letters in support of the bill, including copies of letters sent to members of Congress and President Roosevelt himself. If no stronger law could be obtained, they recommended its passage. But they also noted that the hearings had been a platform for industry rather than the consumer. While no "ultimate consumer" had been invited to testify, spokesmen for advertising, publishing, fruit growing, food processing, cosmetic making, and pharmaceutical manufacturing had all appeared before Copeland's subcommittee to condemn the bill.[40]

In the wake of the December 1933 hearings, nearly everyone involved agreed that the bill would have to be revised. Even Copeland and Tugwell conceded that changes were necessary if the bill would have a chance of making its way through Congress to the president's desk. Over the course of the next five years, Copeland introduced five versions. Several dozen amendments were proposed and competing industry-sponsored bills introduced. Some passed one house but not the other. Protracted and acrimonious debates continued at each step. By 1937, much of the support for a new law had eroded, as repeated revisions were made in response to industry demands.[41]

Reports of a crisis in 1937 revived public interest in the debates and helped pressure Congress to move forward on the bill. Historian Philip J. Hilts maintains that this crisis was the deciding factor in the bill's eventual passage. "What seems to make a new law," Hilts asserts, "is the presence of two circumstances when a crisis occurs—a bill must *already be present* in Congress, and legislators and significant elements of the public must already *be educated and paying attention* when the crisis hits. Some say the crisis must also involve children." The case of Elixir Sulfanilamide met all of these requirements. Sulfanilamide had been hailed as a miracle medicine in the press, a chemotherapeutical breakthrough and true antibacterial that attacked and killed disease-causing bacteria. The Massengill Company of Bristol, Tennessee, started selling the drug in the summer of 1937. After salesmen for Massengill reported that doctors and patients would be happier if they could get the bad tasting medicine in a more palatable liquid form, the company decided it needed a way to repackage sulfanilamide in order to corner the market. The company's chief chemist tried a number of concoctions before settling on a combination of diethylene glycol and raspberry extract. Unaware of reports describing the toxicity of the solvent diethylene glycol, Elixir Sulfanilamide was made for appearance, fragrance, and flavor—but not for safety. At the beginning of September, Massengill packaged and shipped 240 gallons to druggists around the country, from California to Virginia. As no law required listing the solvent on the label, not one bottle did.[42]

Within a few weeks, reports of patient deaths mounted. On October 11, a Tulsa doctor sent an urgent telegram to the American Medical Association, asking for the composition of Elixir Sulfanilamide, when six of his patients died immediately after taking it. The AMA promptly informed the doctor that it had no record of the drug, and that it had not certified any liquid form of sulfa drugs. The AMA also sent a telegram to the Massengill headquarters, asking for samples. After the AMA agreed to keep the composition secret, the company complied. AMA laboratory tests quickly revealed that diethylene glycol was a highly toxic substance. Meanwhile, another doctor had called the FDA in Washington on October 14, after hearing reports of the deaths in Tulsa. The law had no explicit prohibition against dangerous substances like diethylene glycol, and no violation of its labeling requirements had occurred, but the FDA proceeded to investigate the matter on the basis that the drug had technically been misbranded. The drug had been labeled an "elixir," which according to the *United States Pharmacopeia* was a drug containing alcohol, which Elixir Sulfanilamide apparently did not.

After visiting Massengill's Tennessee plant and interviewing its lead chemist, the FDA threw its full force behind the enormous task of tracking down and seizing the shipments that had already been made. Most of the drugs had reached patients through a doctor's prescription, but some druggists had sold it over the counter to customers. Massengill dragged its feet in facilitating a recall and until prompted by the FDA on October 19, failed to send out a notice to doctors, druggists, and distributors indicating that the drug was life-threatening. By November, FDA investigators had recovered more than 90 percent of the original shipment. The administration found that 107 deaths had been reported, most of them children. The chemist who concocted the "elixir" ultimately took his own life. The doctor who owned the company admitted no responsibility for the deaths, but a prosecution for mislabeling still resulted in a $26,000 fine for Massengill. At about $240 per death, it was the largest fine ever issued by the FDA to that time.[43]

In the wake of the crisis, mail poured in to Congress and the White House, and renewed demands for a new law came from consumer groups, national women's organizations, and professional quarters. One of the most poignant letters received by FDR, written by the mother of one of the victims, begged the president to push for a law that would prevent other families from experiencing the suffering hers had. The American Medical Association issued a statement noting that the death toll suffered from taking useless quack medicines was far higher than that suffered at the hands of Elixir Sulfanilamide. After being subject to a new round of objections and proposed amendments throughout the first half of 1938, the proposed law finally passed through Congress and was signed by President Roosevelt on June 25, 1938.[44]

CONCLUSION

The long struggle to pass the Federal Food, Drug and Cosmetic Act of 1938 highlighted two concurrent tensions in the broader effort to combat quackery. First, it demonstrated how powerful interest groups could be in opposing and shaping legislative reform and regulatory efforts. The ubiquitous place of the drug industry in the broader structure of the American economy, and the tendency to tie its reform to the food industry, would prove to be particularly pivotal in future reform efforts. The five-year struggle also underscored a persistent tension between encouraging consumer protection and promoting free market principles. In this struggle, and in future endeavors, interest groups on both sides often approached reform efforts as a zero-sum game.[45]

For the most ardent foes of quackery, the act consequently represented a partial victory. Some of the most restrictive elements of the original Copeland bill had been eliminated or amended in the five-year struggle for reform. The requirement intended to force manufacturers to distinguish between palliative and curative drugs was ultimately stricken for the bill. The provision requiring full formula disclosure was omitted. The FDA would also be even more limited in its seizure power than it had been under the 1906 law. Even though the new law would better protect the consumer from false and misleading advertising, failure to provide the FDA with advertising control power restricted its charge. Manufacturers seeking to introduce new drugs into the market would have to provide evidence of safety for their products, under conditions of use prescribed in their labeling, but they were not required to prove that their products had therapeutic value.[46]

Despite its weaknesses, antiquackery crusaders conceded that the new law was still an improvement in terms of consumer protection. It banned any false and misleading statements in the labeling of a remedy, and eliminated the burden of proving fraudulent intent with respect to therapeutic claims. It required listing the common names of all active ingredients on the label. A new provision also required labels to disclose the quantity and proportion of an expanded list of 19 named drugs and their derivatives. The new law also required labels to include directions for use and warnings against dangerous uses.

The 1938 law also extended the reach of federal control of the food, drug, and cosmetic markets. The law specifically outlawed all cosmetics deemed injurious to health and brought all cosmetics except soap under the control of the FDA. It prohibited traffic in all foodstuffs deemed dangerous to health, not only those that included poisonous substances. All drugs used in the diagnosis of disease or affecting the structure or any function of the body were brought under legal control. Additionally, all therapeutic devices became subject to the same conditions of FDA regulation. The FDA also won a new tool to add to its seizures and criminal actions, the injunction.

As the next chapter will explain, the Federal Food, Drug and Cosmetic Act of 1938 also had many unforeseen consequences in the broader effort to combat quackery. As the first law to require checking drugs before they went to market, it offered protection to citizens in a field that had become notorious for predatory practices. It also created advantages for established drug companies, by making it difficult to survive in the modern pharmaceutical industry without scientists and laboratories. By requiring companies to provide scientific tests of safety for new drugs, the new law also encouraged the type of "rational therapeutics" that had been promoted by early twentieth-century opponents of quackery.

SIX

REDEFINING QUACKERY IN THE AGE OF WONDER DRUGS

The Elixir Sulfanilamide disaster played an important role in securing passage of the Federal Food, Drug and Cosmetic Act (FFDCA) of 1938. It also signaled the beginning of a chemotherapeutic revolution that dramatically changed the crusade against quackery. During the quarter century following the 1938 act, a series of laboratory discoveries ushered in a flood of new drugs that were in turn made available to consumers. With new drugs, doctors could effectively treat many fatal diseases and infections that had stubbornly resisted medical treatment for ages. At the same time, many of these drugs, like Elixir Sulfanilamide, were ultimately considered too dangerous for consumers to use on their own. This meant that access to those drugs was eventually restricted by requiring a prescription. Before 1938, the only drugs for which a person needed a prescription were certain narcotics specified in the Harrison Anti-Narcotics Act of 1914. Any other drug that a physician might prescribe could be purchased in a pharmacy without a prescription, and any prescription could be used as many different times as desired. This all changed in 1938, when the FFDCA indirectly created two different categories for non-narcotic drugs—prescription and over-the-counter. Nearly all the "wonder drugs" of the subsequent antibiotic era were made available only by prescription due to restrictions created by the FFDCA. For antiquackery crusaders, this revolution—in new drugs and new regulations—fundamentally altered the business of those pilloried as quacks as well as the techniques used to combat alleged health fraud.[1]

CHALLENGES AND OPPORTUNITIES CREATED BY NEW REGULATIONS AND NEW DRUGS

The case of sulfanilamide underscored administrative challenges that the Federal Food, Drug and Cosmetic Act had failed to explicitly outline, particularly with regard to labeling requirements and access to drugs. Everyone knew the 1938 law would restrict the range of drugs that could be offered on the market, and that it mandated that information be supplied to the consumer, but it appeared to leave the eventual choice of drugs to the consumer. At the time of the Elixir Sulfanilamide disaster, anyone could get almost any drug directly from a pharmacist without a prescription. The 1938 law did not explicitly restrict consumer access to dangerous drugs without a physician's approval. Instead, it addressed the problem with the toxicity of sulfanilamide and other drugs by requiring manufacturers to include warning labels against unsafe dosages or methods, duration of administration, or particularly unsafe cases involving children or underlying conditions.

In August 1938, the U.S. Food and Drug Administration (FDA) announced that any marketing of sulfanilamide that allowed for "indiscriminate use by the general public" would be "actionable" under the new law. This warning adhered to the labeling requirements outlined in the law. But the FDA went a step further and advised that manufacturers would be liable to prosecution unless they attached to the packages of sulfanilamide a "warning so conspicuous as to certainly attract attention" that the drug was dangerous unless used under "appropriate medical supervision." Mandating medical supervision for the appropriate use of dangerous drugs implied restricting the sale of sulfanilamide to physicians. While this did not necessarily trouble manufacturers, they worried about the possibility of being held liable for the acts of distributors, licensees, and purchasers of their products.[2]

Drug manufacturers proposed a compromise in response: require detailed labeling except in cases where the product was distributed only to professionals, when companies would be allowed to place a "warning" label on the actual product to make it clear that it was "for professional use only." This was designed to solve the problem of indiscriminate use by the lay public, but it also allowed drug companies to create a class of drugs that could not legally be sold without a prescription by putting the appropriate label on them. As historian Peter Temin points out, this had not been outlined in the 1938 law, nor is there clear evidence that this was the intent of the law. After this regulation became effective, the consumer could no longer buy some drugs without first seeing a doctor and getting his or her approval. While compliance proved to be variable from year to year, depending on the drug in question, limited

FDA resources also made it relatively easy to get away with ignoring the mandate, which could be enforced only after extensive investigation.[3]

In the absence of formal criteria, the FDA's approach to new drug regulation, which lasted well into the postwar era, placed the primary burden on the manufacturer. It required the manufacturer to provide extensive laboratory and clinical evidence on the merits and disadvantages of new drugs. The FDA also insisted that manufacturers pay careful attention to the therapeutic claims that accompanied their products, which in turn would instruct physicians on when and how to use a drug. Meanwhile, experts continued to disagree about how much evidence was needed before a new drug could be released, and FDA officials continued to complain about the quality of the scientific and clinical work presented to them. As historian Harry Marks correctly observes, determinations of safety were complex judgments, dependent upon the beliefs of those consulted as well as the available data. The viability of the new regulatory system depended on cooperation among medical researchers, the regulated industry, practicing physicians, and pharmacists. In the short term, where conflicting evidence and opinions existed, the FDA had to make individual judgments on new drugs on a case-by-case basis. For long-term assessments of therapeutic merit and safety, the FDA deferred to the scientific community and the American Medical Association's (AMA's) Council on Pharmacy and Chemistry.[4]

As early as 1939, the FDA expressed its concern about the scientific awareness and therapeutic capabilities of many physicians and pharmacists. The Elixir Sulfanilamide disaster had made clear the dangers inherent in the inappropriate medical use of drugs more broadly. Theodore Klumpp, in charge of the Drug Division at the FDA, noted that nearly all of the deaths associated with Elixir Sulfanilamide could be tied to cases in which the drug had been administered with a physician's prescription. Even more alarming, the drug had been prescribed to treat Bright's disease, mercury poisoning, renal problems, and backaches. None of these conditions had a remote connection to the infectious diseases for which sulfanilamide was known to work. The FDA hoped to improve the quality of therapeutic practice by requiring more information be given to physicians about the relative merits of different drugs through labeling requirements and its own ongoing announcements and reports, but by and large FDA officials had no power to challenge physicians who used drugs without regard to agency-approved indications. In general, the FDA dealt with the problem of inappropriate use by focusing on clarifying the terms on the drug label.[5]

Relying on the compliance of physicians and pharmacists revealed its own set of problems. One of the early FDA cases brought against pharmacists involved the repackaging of another sulfa drug, sulfathiazole, for self-medication, despite the fact that it had been shipped to druggists bearing the warning that it was for use "only by or on the prescription of a physician." Following reports that Sullivan's Pharmacy in Columbus, Georgia, was selling sulfathiazole at a dime a tablet, two

FDA inspectors posed as would-be customers and, without prescriptions, successfully purchased the drug. In each case, the druggist took a dozen pills from a bottle, put them in a small box, and handed them to the undercover inspector in exchange for money. All that was written on the box was the misspelled name of the drug—"Sulfothiazal." The bottle from which the pharmacist had taken the tablets, meanwhile, included the prescription-only warning and a further caution that physicians should familiarize themselves with the use of sulfathiazole before administering it. The label explained that some people might experience severe toxic reactions, so daily blood and urine examinations were suggested to check on dangerous abnormalities that might develop.[6]

After making its way through district and circuit court, the case ended up at the Supreme Court in 1948. In a divided opinion, the court reversed an earlier ruling that the 1938 law did not apply in the Sullivan case because the selling of the drug had been solely intrastate. Even though the sale in question did not technically fall under the 1938 law's interstate commerce stipulation, the Supreme Court ruled that it came within the law's provision forbidding the retailer from altering the packaging or labeling of the drug in a way that resulted in misbranding. According to the law, the alteration or removal of labels was prohibited. Unlike the earlier circuit court decision, the Supreme Court did not address whether the drug should have been sold by prescription. Nevertheless, with the support of the highest court in the land, the FDA subsequently accelerated its campaign against the sale of hazardous drugs without prescriptions, in the interest of protecting consumers.[7]

By this time, FDA inspectors had discovered another way in which prescription drugs were being abused: the indiscriminate and unauthorized refilling of prescriptions by pharmacists. Investigations revealed that this practice was most widespread with one of the dangerous and habit-forming drugs specifically mentioned in the 1938 law. Barbiturates, depressants of the central nervous system, had appeared on the market early in the century, and medical researchers had quickly taken note of an increasing rate of barbiturate addiction. They were used primarily to treat epilepsy, certain nervous conditions, and sleep disorders. But the quantity of barbiturates being produced and consumed seemed to clearly surpass legitimate needs. By 1948, drug manufacturers produced 24 sleeping pills a month for every man, woman, and child in the country. The annual FDA report for 1951 revealed that approximately 75 percent of the criminal actions alleging violations that year were directed against illegal sales of prescription drugs; in about 90 percent of the cases, the drugs sold or refilled without prescription included barbiturates and amphetamines. Meanwhile, FDA inspectors discovered tragic case histories that confirmed reports of increased deaths from accidental overdose and suicide due to barbiturate use. After a woman in the Midwest had been admitted to a hospital, a check on the source of her barbiturate supply found that she had a prescription for 30 capsules refilled 16 times within three months. Another woman, arrested for drunkenness, was found to be a barbiturate addict who on a single sleeping-pill prescription issued in August 1944 had obtained refills continuously for the next four years without further physician's orders. An FDA inspector found that another woman who had overdosed had received a total of 7,000 barbiturate capsules via mail, from a prescription written at a pharmacy in a state where she no longer lived. The dealer was fined $2,000, given a suspended one-year prison sentence, and placed on probation for three years. The Sullivan decision emboldened the FDA to take action.[8]

In October 1948, Commissioner Paul Dunbar announced a controversial new FDA policy. All prescription refills would henceforth be considered illegal unless they had been specifically authorized by a physician. After consulting the laws of various states and foreign nations, as well as scholarly works on the matter, the FDA concluded that the unauthorized refilling of prescriptions by pharmacists amounted to over-the-counter selling of drugs that had been labeled for sale only by prescription. The organized pharmacy lobby pushed back. Spokesmen maintained that most prescription refills dealt with safe drugs, and refilling amounted to 40 percent of their total prescription business. Given that the legal control of pharmacy had traditionally been instituted at the state level, they also worried that federal intervention by the FDA would irreparably damage the sacred physician-pharmacist-patient relationship. In April 1949, a pharmacist member of the House of Representatives sponsored a proposed law on their behalf. It would exempt all products dispensed upon prescription from the jurisdiction of the FDA. FDA officials quickly met with leaders of the National Association of Retail Druggists to work out a compromise.[9]

In 1950, Congressman Carl Durham and Senator Hubert Humphrey, both pharmacists, introduced an amendment to the Federal Food, Drug and Cosmetic Act, which was designed to clarify ambiguities regarding the prescription versus over-the-counter distinction and the question of prescription refills. A House of Representatives committee report noted that the existing law had problematically allowed the manufacturer to decide whether a drug was sold by prescription or over the counter. This had led to confusion. The same drug could be classified differently by manufacturers and could even be labeled differently in the same shipment. A pharmacist could be prosecuted for selling a drug labeled for prescription use only, but if the FDA disagreed with the designation of the drug, it had to sue the manufacturer to change it. The draft amendment submitted to the House was meant to ban unsafe prescription refills, and it included three different classifications of drugs that would require a physician's authorization.[10]

To many pharmacists, physicians, and drug makers, this type of control threatened the decision-making authority of medical professionals and the autonomy of medical practice more broadly. In the words of James Hoge, of the Proprietary Association, granting the FDA the authority to separate over-the-counter drugs from prescription drugs meant introducing "a plan for the regulation of the drug industry to an extent never heretofore proposed or contemplated." Charles Wesley Dunn, general counsel for the American Pharmaceutical Manufacturers' Association, warned that the measure vested in the government significant bureaucratic control of the drug industry and the medical profession. He argued the bill represented "an important step toward socialized medicine, and that control will be exercised by an executive who is the Government leader for socialized medicine." Dunn was referring to Oscar R. Ewing, who also served as official spokesman for President Truman's proposed national health insurance legislation. A minority report from the House supported these concerns and argued that the bill jeopardized the right of self-medication. In congressional testimony, meanwhile, others repeated Hoge's warning that the bill could be "a handmaiden of socialized medicine" that would raise the costs of drugs and increase agitation for government relief.[11]

By the time the Durham-Humphrey Act was passed, in October 1951, the FDA's authority to distinguish between prescription and over-the-counter drugs had been removed from the amendment. Dangerous drugs, habit-forming drugs, and new drugs cleared by the FDA as prescription-only items, nevertheless, now had to bear the prescription-only label and could not be refilled by pharmacists without physician authorization. The act also included an objective definition of prescription drugs as any drug intended for human use that "because of its toxicity or other potentiality for harmful effect, or the method of its use, or the collateral measures necessary for its use, is not safe for use except under the supervision of a practitioner licensed by law to administer such a drug." Reference to the efficacy of a drug, which had been included in the House revisions, had been eliminated. The authority to decide whether a drug was available by prescription or over the counter was left with manufacturers. If the FDA disagreed, the issue had to be settled in court.[12]

The Durham-Humphrey Amendment represented the culmination of a decade-long debate between regulators and the drug industry. It transformed the prescription drug market, and enshrined the distinction between prescription and over-the-counter drugs. The origins of today's prescription drug market, the "stunning change in the way drugs were to be sold," and the power it granted manufacturers to shape the drug market and consumer access, has been seen as an arbitrary creation by historian Peter Temin. Temin argues that in the course of enforcing the provisions of the 1938 law, regulators made an administrative decision to create a new class of drugs. Government policymakers had lost faith in the ability of the consumer to make decisions about the use of dangerous drugs, and they decided to supplant the earlier open-market drug economy. Harry Marks argues that the drug industry played a more significant role in this process. Industry representatives defended the authority of manufacturers to make decisions about labeling on the basis of their expertise, and both regulators and the regulated agreed on a standard for ensuring the safety of drugs.

At the same time, the regulated industry imparted ideological significance to the prescription drug regulations during the Cold War, in a successful campaign to use anti-socialist rhetoric to maximize the industry's control. The industry's success, Marks concludes, depended at least partly on the "powerful appeal of anti-statist and anticommunist rhetoric in postwar America."[13]

While it may be true that the codification of the prescription and over-the-counter drug categories owed itself to a combination of bureaucratic decisions and self-interested political wrangling, each of these explanations ignores how the antiquackery campaign conducted by therapeutic reformers also influenced the structure of regulation before and after World War II. The most ardent critics of quackery had long argued that consumer ignorance could be blamed for the persistence of alleged nostrums and medical charlatans. Despite extensive educational campaigns, which had been conducted in the hope of exposing the inner workings of quackery, consumers continued to patronize alleged quacks. The regulatory structure that had evolved prior to 1938, meanwhile, came to rest on the belief that medical science offered the tools to distinguish between quack and legitimate therapeutic practices. If no scientific evidence existed to support the safety and efficacy of a given therapy, it was most often judged to be quackery, especially if marketed directly to unknowing consumers. Antiquack crusaders instructed consumers to rely on physicians to make informed therapeutic choices, rooted in laboratory and clinical evidence. Ethical pharmaceutical manufacturers, meanwhile, distinguished their wares from nostrums on the basis of their scientific validity. Despite competing priorities, the 1938 law nevertheless provided an opportunity for regulators and some of the regulated (established pharmaceutical manufacturers primarily) to unite against a common enemy, the quack, in the name of safety and consumer protection. Regulators and regulated shared a common objective (which had been made more prominent in the age of wonder drugs) to deliver on the immense promises offered by the unfolding therapeutic revolution. They also shared a common intellectual and institutional background in many cases, and a common goal to address the emerging problems in a dramatically changing drug industry.

CHANGES IN THE DRUG TRADE

The chemotherapeutic revolution that followed the quarter century after 1938 fundamentally changed the drug market in substance and structure. Other sulfonamides quickly followed the original sulfa drugs, and the wartime development of penicillin helped the American pharmaceutical industry come of age. Penicillin was followed by other antibiotics like streptomycin, antimalarials, synthetic vitamins, antihistamines, tranquilizers, vaccines, and other potent therapeutic agents for the treatment of an equally long list of diseases and conditions. Previously life-threatening infections, venereal diseases, tuberculosis, malaria, yellow fever, cholera, typhus and typhoid, polio, and measles could now be treated and controlled. Partial relief could be offered for sufferers of arthritis, asthma, hypertension, skin affections, nervous disorders, gastrointestinal diseases, and mental illnesses. The drugs discovered during this revolution therefore came to dominate the market. The FDA's annual report of 1956 noted that 90 percent of the prescriptions written by doctors that year called for drugs that had not been commercially available when the 1938 law went into effect.[14]

Consequently, as historian James Harvey Young notes, pharmaceutical manufacturers accelerated a trend already started, by streamlining their production of new and potent chemical agents, while reducing production of plant-based botanical medicines. One pharmaceutical firm, Smith Kline & French, had marketed over 15,000 products during the 1920s, but by the late 1950s their line had been cut to under 60. Actual production of new pharmaceuticals still nevertheless grew dramatically. While Americans had spent less than $200 million for prescription medicines in the 1930s, by 1957 the total had grown to $2 billion.[15]

The chemotherapeutic revolution also combined with stricter laws to upset one of the fundamental distinctions between quackery and legitimate medicine that reformers had ceaselessly fought to create for decades. The most ardent members of the anti-quackery network had condemned virtually all forms of patent medicines that were advertised and sold directly to the public. This longstanding distinction became outmoded as new over-the-counter pharmaceuticals were increasingly advertised directly to consumers through the press, magazines, radio, and television. Pharmaceutical companies also launched their own proprietary remedies and acquired well-established proprietary firms that had developed a reputation for being brand name specialties. Large corporations that marketed both prescription and over-the-counter drugs, and focused on specific specialties, came to dominate the drug trade. As more dramatic and spectacular prescription pharmaceuticals were developed, proprietary companies also began marketing prescription drugs or purchased pharmaceutical concerns. Meanwhile, some proprietaries conscientiously set out to undergird their age-old claims for efficacy with scientific evidence as well, while others introduced new ingredients or changed their outdated formulas. As firms diversified and merged into large corporations making and marketing drug products of all types, the drug industry heralded a revolution in medical economics as well as therapeutics. By 1956, five companies controlled over two-fifths of the proprietary market. By 1959, of the 409 most prescribed drugs, 83 percent were brand-name specialties, while only 17 percent were generic-name drugs.[16]

As the prescription pharmaceutical business boomed, proprietary medicine makers and secret-formula patent medicine companies began to lose their share of the overall drug market. Early in the century, proprietaries outsold prescription drugs by over two to one, but by the late 1930s sales of the two types had evened out. After two decades of the chemotherapeutic revolution, the prescription drug market had become three times as large as the proprietary market. New over-the-counter pharmaceuticals also gained business at a rate that surpassed old-line proprietaries. Over time, the self-medication business continued to shrink following the 1938 law and became increasingly confined to the treatment of minor ailments. According to a Census of Manufacturers report in 1954, analgesics (mainly aspirin), laxatives, vitamins, cold and cough preparations, antacids and stomach remedies, antiseptics, and liniments topped the list.[17]

QUACKERY AND SELF-MEDICATION

Most major proprietors heeded the FDA's warnings and scrutinized the labels of drugs aimed at direct consumer sale. According to the estimate of one trade editor, 97 percent of the labels used in the drug industry were modified. Even the Proprietary Association, the longstanding defender of proprietors (including some of the patent medicine variety as far as the AMA was concerned) took steps to comply. In 1939, James F. Hoge, counsel for the Proprietary Association, warned that any manufacturer who tried to "play hide-and-seek" with the new law would "pay dearly for his fun." The association subsequently policed the copy of its members, tightened its own code of advertising practices, and sponsored laboratory research on the botanical ingredients of many proprietary formulas. In an address before the association in 1947, Charles Crawford complimented members on "an impressive record of the number and extent of improvements you have made over the years." The FDA commissioner's annual report from 1940 noted that widespread changes in labeling were also often accompanied by radical changes in the composition of some proprietaries along with sharp reduction in dosages for those containing potentially dangerous ingredients. This led the commissioner to conclude that the public benefit of the new act could not be measured wholly in terms of legal actions. In cases where proprietary manufacturers did not comply, the FDA turned all three of its weapons—seizures, injunctions, and criminal actions—on offenders.[18]

The FDA commissioner's report from 1941 revealed the extent of the problems that remained. That year, there were 218 total seizures and 91 criminal prosecutions involving drugs or drug products, excluding therapeutic devices. These numbers were similar to earlier years, despite the fact that the FDA had been mandated to devote attention to 3,785 manufacturers, with 1,866 factory inspections and the examination of 6,276 interstate samples. In the self-medication field, this included a survey of cold and headache preparations containing acetanilide or acetophenetidin. Twelve of these products were seized because recommended dosages could result in the ingestion of dangerous quantities of these ingredients. Ten additional preparations were seized due to inadequate warning statements or failure to declare the

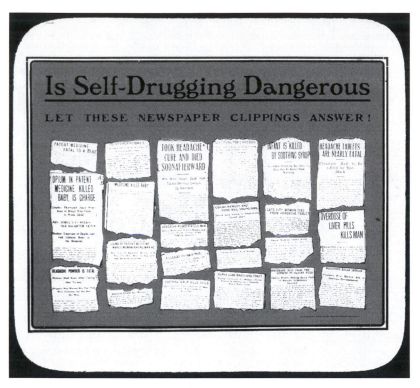

Lantern Slide #2 (ca. 1918).
(© American Medical Association. Courtesy of AMA Archives)

presence of these ingredients. Several of these preparations were also shipped in bulk and repackaged; they were judged to be in violation of the act because the repacker failed to label the goods properly after their receipt. Three seizures were made of remedies for chronic alcoholism containing emetine; four of inhalants containing an excessive quantity of epinephrine; five of weight-loss preparations containing drugs such as thyroid extract in dangerous amounts, or containing a laxative and failing to list its presence on the label; six of a dangerous abortifacient; and seven of a mineral water dangerous because of its high fluorine content. All told, actions directed against "dangerous drug preparations" resulted in 67 seizures and 12 prosecutions. In 1940, there had been only 25 seizures and 1 prosecution for dangerous drugs. Drug products considered misbranded due to false and misleading therapeutic claims or inadequate warning statements constituted the basis for the bulk of the remaining number. In the realm of therapeutic devices, the FDA took action against a wide range of contraptions, including an inhalant device for asthma, a rectal dilator, nipple shields, bust developers, intrauterine pessaries, and battery and coil devices for applying an electrical current to various bodily orifices.[19]

The continued investigation of self-medication products was nevertheless made more difficult as the onslaught of new wonder drugs placed a major drain on resources. The massive effort to locate and remove one of the new prescription wonder drugs from the market in 1941 underscored how self-medication products could be deprioritized. In December 1940, thousands of sulfathiazole tablets had been contaminated with as much as 60 percent phenobarbital, a highly potent sedative, and placed on the market. A laboratory analysis by one of the manufacturers confirmed a physician's complaint made that same month, but the FDA did not take action until March 1941, when the Massachusetts State Department of Public Health issued another complaint directly to the administration. The effort to recover 122,600 tablets from 800 primary shipments consumed the equivalent of 3,205 workdays; 12,187 visits to distributors, doctors, and druggists (excluding an additional 25,000 known visits by cooperating agencies); and the examination of approximately 1,593,000 invoices and 592,000 prescriptions. Only 22,324 tablets were recovered, the rest presumed to have been consumed or voluntarily destroyed. It proved to be impossible to definitively ascertain the source of the contamination. The new-drug application under which sulfathiazole's distribution had been authorized was revoked, and the procedure for administration of the new-drug section of the act was revised. The review of applications now called for "a full description of the methods used in, and the facilities and controls used for, the manufacturing, processing, and packing" of each new drug.[20]

Despite the obvious dangers of powerful new products of the chemotherapeutic revolution, in the battle to make self-medication safe in the early years after the Food, Drug and Cosmetic Act, the FDA framed the war on quackery as one directed against "the careless or unscrupulous fringe." As Commissioner Crawford defined it in 1947, "In this group are some who are clearly dishonest, some who are choice crackpots, and some who are grossly negligent in the conduct of their affairs." Young has characterized the FDA's efforts to stop "fringe operators" as a sort of cat and mouse game played at tortoise speed. Perennial targets of FDA regulators sought loopholes in the law, which they exploited until taken to court. Nostrum vendors, old and new, meanwhile, changed their techniques to exploit their wares within the confines of stricter labeling regulations, and challenged the FDA in court more tenaciously.[21]

The FDA used labeling restrictions as a primary tool in going after "fringe operators." One provision in the act classified labels as misleading if they failed to reveal certain types of "material facts." In interpreting this, the FDA included in its definition of material facts the fact of a difference of opinion among qualified experts as to the truth of a representation, "if there is a material weight of opinion contrary to such representation." Drug manufacturers tried to avoid the provision by either not making curative claims on the label or restricting claims to advertising materials.

Another provision in the 1938 law required labels to bear "adequate directions for use," including proper warnings to the would-be self-doser. If the drug might be unsafe for children, or dangerous in too large or too many doses, or risky if the user suffered from a given ailment, the label had to say so. The FDA also deemed directions inadequate if the label failed to provide directions for use in all conditions for which the drug or device was "prescribed, recommended, or suggested in its labeling, or in its advertising." In an effort to proactively guide manufacturers, the FDA also prepared a long list of warning statements appropriate for laxatives, nose drops, douches, cough remedies, liniments, pain killers, and other popular proprietary products.[22]

To establish the legality of various labeling provisions, and close loopholes exploited by self-medication specialists, cases had to be tested in the courts. The first court test for the "adequate directions for use" section of the law involved a California man named Chester Walker Colgrove, who sold his petroleum-based Colusa Natural Oil in two-ounce bottles for $3.00. The label for the topical ointment and capsules stated that they were to be used for the treatment of a variety of skin ailments including psoriasis, eczema, leg ulcers, and athlete's foot. The FDA believed that the statements on the labels, along with accompanying before-and-after pictures in advertising materials, were false and misleading, and did not provide directions for use in all conditions for which the drug was recommended. A jury found Colgrove guilty of misbranding and fined him $1,500.[23]

To adhere to the letter of the law, Colgrove removed his therapeutic claims from the labels and instead elaborated on the uses of Colusa Natural Oil in circulars which he packed with shipments of the drugs. In the subsequent seizure trial, seven well-qualified medical and chemical experts testified for the government. Colgrove produced 30 witnesses, including 14 lay witnesses and satisfied users, and 14 doctors who testified by deposition, one 83-year-old physician from Houston who personally appeared before the court, and one chemist who testified regarding the physical properties of Colusa Oil. While Colgrove maintained that a conflict of medical opinion clearly existed, the judge found "no credible or adequate scientific or medical foundation for any claim" that Colgrove's oil would cure the four diseases specifically identified. The questions of whether a drug was effective in curing or giving some relief from the disease for which it was recommended was looked upon as a demonstrable fact. Between 1944 and 1946, the FDA executed 125 seizures of Colusa Natural Oil. The FDA hoped that another loophole had been closed, but Colgrove was far from finished.[24]

The new labels for Colusa Natural Oil listed directions but no diseases. Mention of psoriasis, eczema, leg ulcers, and athlete's foot was confined to advertisements. Colgrove also went a step further. He included glowing endorsements from doctors in the new ads and supplied newspapers with detailed instructions of what he wanted printed. He then ordered extra copies of the ads to be delivered to druggists who sold

Colusa Oil. The government asked a court for an injunction to stop Colgrove from distributing his oil on the basis that it was misbranded because labels failed to fully explain how a drug should be taken for ailments specified in advertising. The judge agreed and ordered Colgrove to cease this practice until the case was tried in court. Ultimately, Colgrove was fined $9,000 and given a two-year suspended jail sentence along with five years of probation.[25]

A series of other cases allowed the FDA to stretch the adequate directions for use clause and obstruct the loophole exploited by companies that limited therapeutic claims to advertisements and accompanying material. In the case of one "perennial litigant," Ada Alberty, who sold a variety of nutritional products for an even longer list of diseases and ailments, a court ruled more explicitly that the intent behind the adequate directions for use requirement must be understood within the context of the law's goal to protect public health. As drugs were intended as remedies for bodily ailments, the court ruled that no drug could be "said to contain in its labeling adequate directions for its use unless every ailment of the body for which it is, through any means, held out to the public as an efficacious remedy to be listed in the labeling, together with instructions to the user concerning the quantity and frequency of dosage recommended for each particular ailment."[26]

The Supreme Court addressed the "accompaniment" problem by making similar references to public health objectives in cases involving other techniques that "fringe operators" employed in an effort to skirt the law. Health lecturers, for example, frequently sold their wares by including labels that did not clearly violate the 1938 provisions. Health lecturer Lelord Kordel, for example, sold books and circulars that included therapeutic advice separate from his actual merchandise, often displayed on a rack near the counter where his products were sold. Medical device manufacturers, meanwhile, often shipped their machines and advertisements separately. Fred Urbeteit, a Florida naturopath, shipped his sinuothermic machines to chiropractors from Florida to Ohio, but the literature that ended up in the waiting rooms of chiropractors, including a simulated newspaper complete with testimonials praising the success of Dr. Urbeteit's methods, was shipped separately. Meanwhile, in the Kordel case, a Wisconsin court had ruled that the test of "accompanying" under the law was one of commercial connection, not of physical continuity, and the manufacturer was found guilty of misbranding. In the Urbeteit case, a judge subsequently ruled in favor of the defendant because he could not see that advertising literature accompanied the machines. Ultimately, the Supreme Court concurred in the Kordel case and reversed the Urbeteit decision, ruling that loopholes must not undermine the purpose of the 1938 law—to protect public health. In the absence of adequate directions of use, each violated the law.[27]

The focus on labeling provisions created other opportunities for FDA inspectors, but at times also required laborious investigations. One case that typified the long and slow process involved an "unlicensed, diploma-mill doctor" who reportedly sold a highly dangerous abortifacient paste for the early termination of pregnancies. The revival of these corrosive products increased dramatically during the war. The FDA had determined that no adequate directions could be written that would make the medications safe. The doctor in question had supplied the paste for both self-medication and professional use. Interstate shipments had reportedly been made under various names. To apply the law, FDA inspectors had to get proof that the doctor made or caused such shipments. Four inspectors, working in pairs, set up a day-and-night vigil that led to numerous high-speed chases after the doctor left his office, armed with packages. Several times the doctor outdistanced the inspectors on icy Chicago streets. Finally, one morning, at 3:30 a.m., after trailing the doctor to a postal station with the headlights of the government's car turned off, one of the inspectors witnessed the doctor as he dropped a package in the chute. That package bore an interstate address. At the destination, another inspector obtained a sample upon delivery. With only one package in evidence, however, the investigation continued for another two weeks before investigators intercepted another late night delivery. The FDA indicted the doctor on charges of having shipped a misbranded drug interstate since it did not bear adequate directions for use. He was tried, found guilty, and sentenced to two years in prison. The FDA brought similar actions against the makers of Leunbach's Paste, Dependon Intra Uterin Paste, Interferin, and others.[28]

CONCLUSION

After a decade of successful court cases, one scholar confidently overstated that the law had left "no apparent loopholes through which the nostrum maker can make unfounded claims." Vincent Kleinfeld, in charge of litigation under the Federal Food, Drug and Cosmetic Act over which the Department of Justice had jurisdiction, asserted that a careful study of the legislative history revealed the extremely liberal manner in which many of the provisions of the act had been construed. The "extraordinarily vigilant yet level-headed manner in which the statute had been administered" had resulted in an attitude of real respect toward and confidence in the FDA on the part of Congress, the courts, the affected industries, the press, and the consuming public. Consequently, the greater part of the regulated industry had come to realize that the act protected not merely the average consumer but also the typical manufacturer or distributor who attempted to "bring before the public safe, wholesome, and honestly labeled products, thus building invaluable good will and undoubtedly thereby increasing financial returns."[29]

The FDA's George Larrick offered a more sober analysis of lingering problems with enforcement. One problem area, travelling pitchmen, had increasingly gained the agency's attention and proved difficult to prosecute in many cases. The FDA referred to these self-billed lecturers as "spielers." Under FDA pressure, many had abandoned labeling claims and even ceased sending circulars to outlets selling their products. Instead, they simply recommended their products from the lecture plat-form. In some cases, lecturers rented out auditoriums and took in as much as $25,000 a week in fees and sales. In other cases, nostrum vendors recruited teams of salesmen to sell products door-to-door. To avoid FDA prosecution, many printed no claims on the bottles of drugs sold as cure-alls. FDA investigators sometimes posed as customers and secretly recorded the spiels of pitchmen, subsequently using their promises as evidence to win court cases. Other times, it proved more difficult to pros-ecute fringe operators on the basis of their therapeutic claims because they moved into gray areas where medical science had little to offer, or scientific opinion remained divided. Such was the case with arthritis remedies, nutritional products, and remedies for the common cold.[30]

Limited penalties and a lack of resources also hampered the FDA in fighting quackery. First-time offenders could be subject to imprisonment for up to one year and fined up to $1,000, but there were no limits set on minimum penalties. Throughout the 1940s, fines remained in the neighborhood of $100 to $200 for the most part, and in some cases were as low as $1. The average fine in 1950 was $565, but in more than half of the cases terminated, the fines were $300 or less. That year, only 60 of 363 cases were closed with fines of $1,000 or higher. Jail senten-ces were imposed in 17 of those cases, involving 22 defendants. The sentences ranged from one hour to four years and averaged 11 months, but 14 of those sentences were suspended. A lack of resources, meanwhile, limited the number of cases that could be brought before the court. At the start of the 1950s, the appropriations and staff, never adequate to the task, had remained at approximately the same levels prevailing in 1938. At the 1953 inspection rate, Commissioner Larrick predicted it would take the agency 10 years to inspect every food, drug, and cosmetic establishment—not including retail stores—with a staff of just over 200 inspectors.[31]

This meant that while antiquackery reformers could justifiably celebrate some of the effects of legislative reform, combined with pharmaceutical advances, they never-theless remained unsatisfied. Fighting quackery remained only one part of the FDA's mandate, and there were clearly not enough inspectors to do the job. Given the dra-matic changes in the structure of the drug industry, and market volatility, it also remained hard to identify the border between legitimate proprietaries and nostrums at one extreme, and the boundary dividing ethical drugs and proprietaries at the other end of the spectrum. Even the most used and safest drugs could still be dangerous and illegal in the hands of the wrong people. Nevertheless, the FDA tirelessly continued its work.

SEVEN

REVIVING THE ANTIQUACKERY CRUSADE IN THE 1950s AND 1960s

Each generation needs to learn anew the why and wherefore of its institutions and blessings; otherwise they are taken for granted. Today, the right of the public to pure foods, effective drugs, safe cosmetics, and truthful labels has become generally accepted. It was not always so. We need to be reminded of Dr. Wiley and his 23-year struggle to obtain our first Federal pure food and drug law. It helps us understand and appreciate the value of the protective laws we now have, and the truly wonderful progress made by our food, drug, and cosmetic industries in this half century. It also helps us understand our problems of today and our obligations to insure that food and drug products of today and tomorrow will continue to be the best in the world.

—FDA Commissioner George Larrick (1956)[1]

In 1956, members of the antiquackery network used the 50-year anniversary of the Pure Food and Drugs Act as an occasion to celebrate the accomplishments of a half-century of regulatory work. Few questioned the parallel progress they had witnessed in terms of scientific and regulatory advances in the drug field in the first half of the century. Less sanguine observers nevertheless expressed a common concern about the negative consequences of changes brought by the chemotherapeutic revolution. In the regulatory field, a dearth of money and personnel meant that protection tools had lagged behind the growth and progress made by the drug industry. At the U.S. Food and Drug Administration (FDA), little had changed in terms of the size, scope, and character of its operation since the enactment of the 1938 law. In the meantime, the volume and variety of drug production, along with the complex task of drug evaluation, had grown by leaps and bounds. While scientific advances had dramatically increased the number of disease-specific drug therapies, the absence of specific therapies for a number of prominent diseases left the market open to those who would capitalize on the lack of knowledge or understanding among patients and physicians alike. Medical researchers and regulators had more tools than ever to invalidate the effectiveness of alleged quack remedies, but an enormous difficulty remained in the attempt to present scientific evidence in matters of medical judgment to the public. A related unresolved tension persisted in the dual charge of regulators to protect consumers and promote free enterprise.[2]

PERSISTENT PROBLEMS

In referring to the 1955 report of the Citizens Advisory Committee, FDA Commissioner Larrick suggested that consumer protection under federal law had for years been "lagging behind the growth and progress made by the drug industry." In his 1956 annual report, Larrick recounted the range of problems—besides fighting quackery—that still confronted the FDA. A rash of accidental poisonings among children who ate aspirin tablets, obtained from packages left carelessly within their reach, had prompted the FDA to ask drug manufacturers to use conspicuous package warning that such drugs should be kept out of the reach of children. Meanwhile, 20 drug recalls had been supervised by the FDA in the preceding year due to an array of compliance problems. In some cases, the potency of the drug did not correspond to the information on the label. In other cases, injectibles were not sterile. In one case, new toxicity studies revealed damaging effects to small laboratory animals not included in earlier reports. The illegal sale of dangerous prescription drugs also continued to present a serious threat. Barbiturates (for sleep) and amphetamines (stimulants) were most commonly encountered in an expansive network of bootleg operations. In 1956 alone, criminal prosecutions were filed against 114 drug stores, pharmacists, lunch counter and tavern operator employees, filling station loiterers, and peddlers.[3]

In the public proclamations of reformers, fringe quack operators nevertheless continued to present the gravest threats to public health and safety. Commissioner Larrick lamented how each annual report from the FDA represented "another chapter in the continuing war against worthless medicines," which reappeared "year after year in new or continued attempts to victimize the public." The 1954 and 1955 annual reports of the FDA outlined an injunction case that banned shipments of a hormone product misbranded with sexual rejuvenation claims but that—after laboratory tests—was subsequently found to be inert. A proclaimed ulcer remedy, promoted in popular magazines, had to be seized after manufacturers attempted to import the product from overseas before a new-drug application had been filed with the FDA. Manufacturers of an antacid, who merely promised "temporary relief of excess gastric acidity" on their drug's label, faced criminal action and FDA seizures due to blatant claims, in full-page newspaper ads, that a regimen of their pills could cure an array of intestinal and stomach disorders. Among the 51 medicines seized in 1956 for false and misleading claims were articles composed of dried alfalfa, cereal grass, apple derivatives, buckwheat flowers, powdered pumice, sulfates, papaya, and royal jelly (said to be a special bee food for productive and long-living queen bees), which collectively bore claims for the treatment or prevention of almost every disease imaginable. Without evidence for the efficacy of these ingredients, in most cases the FDA emerged victorious when challenged at trial.[4]

The FDA also faced the difficult challenge of presenting convincing scientific evidence in matters of medical judgment, in a wholly defensible form, in court cases vigorously defended by "fringe operators." In a long-delayed case against a mineral water manufacturer, whose product was advertised for the treatment of kidney disorders and arthritis, the government charged that it would not be efficacious for these conditions. When the case was finally decided in 1956, the jury did not confirm the FDA's charges. The FDA lost another case in a district court trial that involved an alleged diabetes remedy on the grounds that a 1923 patent had established the validity of its efficacy. An appellate court eventually reversed the decision on the grounds that insulin offered the only effective measure available to control the disease.[5]

The public face of the FDA's legal battles, which dominated national press headlines in the 1950s, involved two other cases that hinged on disputes over the extent of scientific evidence for the efficacy of an arthritis therapy and an alleged cure for cancer. The Tri-Wonda case involved a three-drug combination arthritis therapy that had been around since the 1920s. The principal ingredients included a combination of acids, a laxative, and a preparation containing a single vitamin and added flavoring. The government presented arthritis specialists who testified not only from expert knowledge but also from clinical trials they themselves had conducted, which proved that the drug was worthless for treating arthritis. The defense provided its own witnesses, including a pharmacologist and three general practitioners, who testified that clinical trials they had conducted proved the value of the medication. Seven full weeks of trial were needed to hear all that had to be said about the drug. After three years of appeals, the FDA eventually succeeded in its attempt to limit the maker's claims, and Tri-Wonda was removed from the market. The protracted battle nevertheless highlighted the difficulty involved in establishing definitive scientific proof where the causes of the diseases in question remained poorly understood.[6]

The case against Harry Hoxsey, more than any other in the 1950s, stimulated a surge of media coverage for the FDA during the late 1950s and early 1960s and placed the issue of scientific evidence center stage. Hoxsey had been selling his cancer remedy since the 1920s. In 1950, the government sought to enjoin Hoxsey from shipping his medicines for the treatment of internal cancers. In developing their case, FDA officials focused on demonstrating the ineffectiveness of Hoxsey's medicines, while disproving his claims that patients had been cured. At the trial, Dr. David I. Macht, a distinguished specialist in pharmacological and experimental therapeutics from Johns Hopkins testified that there was "absolutely no basis" for the effectiveness of any of these substances in cancer treatment. Another specialist testified that the potassium iodide in Hoxsey's concoction would actually speed up the growth of cancer. Still another cancer research scientist testified that an experiment conducted for the FDA had not cured mice but instead increased the size of malignant growths upon autopsy. In tracking down case histories of scores of Hoxsey's patients, many of whom had been featured in Hoxsey's testimonial-filled pamphlets, FDA inspectors found a pattern. In selecting 16 cases, they argued that all of Hoxsey's proclaimed "cures" fell into three classes: (1) the patient had never had cancer, although he or she was treated for it at the Dallas clinic; (2) the patient had been cured of cancer by proper surgical or radiation treatment before consulting Hoxsey; or (3) the patient either still had cancer or had since died of the disease.[7]

Hoxsey never took the stand and based his defense mainly on the testimonials of his own medical experts and successfully treated patients. Of Hoxsey's 11 patients who testified that they had been cured of internal cancer, the government argued the only evidence that three ever had the disease was their own affirmation. In four other cases, the government introduced rebuttal testimony to show that the patients had been cured before consulting Hoxsey. In the four remaining cases, the sole evidence that the patients indeed had cancer was the testimony of Hoxsey's medical director, an osteopath who had seen only a couple of dozen cancer patients before joining Hoxsey's staff in 1946. Dr. Durkee acknowledged he had seen some 35 to 50 patients a day in Hoxsey's clinic, where he examined each patient for an average of five to 10 minutes and made his diagnosis in most cases without a biopsy.

Despite the evidence presented by the government, Judge Atwell ruled in favor of Hoxsey and refused to grant the injunction. He could not agree that the weight of evidence established the ineffectiveness of Hoxsey's treatment and ruled that it was neither injurious nor futile. Its "percentage of efficient and beneficial treatments," the judge decided, was "reasonably comparable to the efficiency and success of surgery and radium." The FDA, suspecting that Atwell himself had once been a Hoxsey patient, was not surprised by the decision. Nor did the prosecutor surrender. Upon appeal, the circuit court agreed that the "overwhelming weight of disinterested testimony" showed that only a biopsy could provide an accurate diagnosis, and only surgery or radiation therapy could effect a cure. With the injunction in place, Hoxsey went on the offensive in an effort to restore his good name. He went on extensive lecture tours, paid a ghostwriter to author his autobiography (which he sent to every U.S. senator and representative), worked to expand his clinics to other states, and joined other foes of the FDA and the American Medical Association (AMA) in accusing these organizations of conspiring to stifle medical freedom. By 1956, one estimate put his annual gross income at $1.5 million, paid by some 8,000 patients.[8]

In April 1956, the FDA took an unprecedented step by issuing a warning that Hoxsey's methods were "worthless" and "imminently dangerous," complete with press releases; warning notices issued to farm, lodge, and church periodicals; and the circulation of public posters. The basis for issuing the warning could be found in a provision of the 1938 law that authorized the dissemination of information regarding drugs in cases that involved an imminent danger to health or gross deception to the consumer. Prior to 1956, this provision had been primarily used to warn people about the dangers of using new prescription drugs without the supervision of physicians. The crux of the FDA argument about the need for a public warning about Hoxsey rested on the belief that death from cancer was "inevitable when cancer patients fail to obtain proper medical treatment because of the lure of a painless cure 'without the use of surgery, x-ray, or radium' as claimed by Hoxsey." The FDA proclaimed, "Those afflicted by cancer are warned not to be misled by the false promise that the Hoxsey cancer treatment will cure or alleviate their condition. Cancer can be cured only through surgery or radiation." The FDA explicitly outlined this position in posters displayed in 46,000 post offices and postal substations across the country.[9]

Many of those who responded to the FDA's 1956 public warning supported Hoxsey and his viewpoints. As historian David Cantor has skillfully demonstrated, most of the people who wrote to the FDA (for reasons other than seeking further information) attacked the administration for its campaign. A few wrote in support of the warning. Others provided information on their experiences with physicians and with Hoxsey. Many complained about the treatment they received from orthodox doctors. Even more commended Hoxsey for the hope he provided patients. Several letters also included a critique of quackery within mainstream medicine. One writer maintained that orthodox treatments were "the most damnable quackery ever invented by the devil," while another concluded that "a quack is one who cuts and bleeds and burns and collects, while knowing and admitting that the method of treatment being used offers no hope for the patient." Others associated quackery with financial corruption and deceit. These writers characterized the AMA as "money grubbers" and "poorly educated MDs." Hoxsey supporters argued, by contrast, that in many ways he was the antithesis of the quack. He had invited his harshest critics to test his treatments. He was generous, honest, open, and charitable. Some argued

Public Beware!

WARNING AGAINST THE HOXSEY CANCER TREATMENT

Sufferers from cancer, their families, physicians, and all concerned with the care of cancer patients are hereby advised and warned that the Hoxsey treatment for internal cancer has been found worthless by two Federal courts.

The Hoxsey treatment costs $400, plus $60 in additional fees—expenditures which will yield nothing of value in the care of cancer. It consists essentially of simple drugs which are worthless for treating cancer.

The Food and Drug Administration conducted a thorough investigation of the Hoxsey treatment and the cases which were claimed to be cured. Not a single verified cure of internal cancer by this treatment has been found.

Those afflicted with cancer are warned not to be misled by the false promise that the Hoxsey cancer treatment will cure or alleviate their condition. Cancer can be cured only through surgery or radiation. Death from cancer is inevitable when cancer patients fail to obtain proper medical treatment because of the lure of a painless cure "without the use of surgery, x-ray, or radium" as claimed by Hoxsey.

Anyone planning to try this treatment should get the facts about it.

For further information write to:
U. S. DEPARTMENT OF HEALTH, EDUCATION, AND WELFARE
Food and Drug Administration
Washington 25, D. C.

U.S. Food and Drug Administration poster (1957).
(Courtesy of the National Library of Medicine)

the label of "quack" had become an indiscriminant epithet applied to anyone who did not take orders from the AMA or FDA.[10]

If critics attacked the FDA for promoting orthodox quackery and the commercial interests of the "medical trust," they also directly questioned the FDA's assertion that the Hoxsey treatments were worthless. In most cases, they relied on empirical evidence, in the form of their own experiences and those of friends and family. Some confirmed their own observations of a cure with the observation of an orthodox physician. Others reported cures they had heard from trusted colleagues and pastors. They also wrote of cures reported in magazine articles, circulars, sermons, meetings organized by Hoxsey and his supporters, and on the radio. Hoxsey's critics dismissed these forms of evidence as anecdotal and unreliable fodder for the ignorant. Hoxsey's supporters revealed a much more complicated process by which they often ascertained the credibility of arguments based on the integrity and reputation of the source.[11]

This process by which people arrived at individual decisions about the effectiveness or ineffectiveness of alleged quack medicines, and the reliability they attached to the source of information, represented an ongoing challenge for the FDA. However much FDA insiders admitted their frustration in cases where the preponderance of evidence clearly rested with the prosecution, they acknowledged the appeal of lay witnesses and the continued distrust of medical experts. Albert Holland, medical director of the FDA, identified a related problem in prosecuting cases where a judge or jury were ill-equipped to answer questions involving competing medical evidence. When a specific effective therapy did not exist for a given medical condition, Holland acknowledged its absence was "an invitation to those who would capitalize on the lack of full understanding of the disease or syndrome both on the party of the patient and the unknowledgeable physician." The Hoxsey case highlighted a dilemma. Clinical data was time consuming and extremely expensive to gather, but FDA legal advisors also understood it offered "perhaps the most convincing type of evidence that [could] be used." Without testing the actual effects of various drugs in question, it would be difficult for the government to convincingly show that the claimed therapeutic effects were not true.[12]

In the anniversary year of 1956, Commissioner Larrick pointed to victories against Hoxsey and others as evidence of the FDA's adaptability. He insisted the problems ahead would be no more difficult than the ones already solved. He argued that cooperation with the drug industry represented the best path forward, to ensure not only the maximum voluntary compliance with the law but also the most stringent scientific evaluation of the safety and effectiveness of drugs. Other FDA insiders remained less optimistic about the future. They bemoaned the laborious nature of investigations and court cases. They remained disillusioned about the persistence of quackery, especially in fields like cancer and arthritis remedies. Some argued that the only way to solve future problems would be to tighten legislative restrictions, work more closely with public and private antiquackery forces, and expand the anti-quackery network against offenders even further.

ANTIQUACKERY FORCES UNITE

In the late 1950s, a new wave of muckraking journalists zeroed in on what many considered a scandalous revival of quackery. Despite the widely publicized efforts of the antiquackery network, the situation appeared to be getting worse overall. In a typical exposé from 1957, a series of articles in the *New York Post* reported the nation's annual nostrum bill had topped $1 billion. According to author James Cook, this included not just extreme examples like Hoxsey's "witch-doctor brew" but also a wide range of over-the-counter drugs, including cold remedies that did not cure colds, "old-fashioned bromides and anti-histaminics" masquerading as "the new 'tranquilizer' drugs," and an assortment of vitamin and mineral mixtures that claimed to cure a wide range of diseases but actually cured none. In his illuminating book the following year, *Remedies and Rackets*, Cook asserted America now contained "170,000,000 Guinea Pigs." He wondered if regulators were bold enough to combat the "quackery, hijinks, and razzle-dazzle" that played consumers for suckers.[13]

"Just how gullible is the American public?" asked a *Chicago Sun Times Magazine* article in 1959. Norma Lee Browning informed readers that Americans were wasting approximately "$500,000,000 a year on a fantastic assortment of high pressure health gimmicks calculated to put pep in your step, sparkle in your eye, and hustle in your muscle, besides curing everything from baldness to bunions." The AMA attributed $500 million just to false and misleading offers for vitamins, minerals, and food supplements. The American Cancer Society, meanwhile, said cancer quacks were taking in $10 to $50 million annually. A congressional committee reported that weight reducing frauds were a $100 million a year business. The Arthritis and Rheumatism Foundation maintained that 45 percent of the 11 million people with arthritis in the United States were lured into wasting more than $250 million annually on misrepresented products. The FDA figured that bogus cures and fake medical devices duped the public out of an additional $250 million annually. According to the journal *Medical Economics*, this put the total quack take at over $1 billion by 1960. *Time* magazine reported that a huge portion of this money—an estimated $500 million—was being spent by "a duped public on misrepresented drugs or remedies sold door to door," where the hapless victim had no protection from federal and state laws. *Time* lamented how millions had fallen for quackery partly because of this lack of protection, but also largely because their physicians had simply failed to offer a cure for what ailed them.[14]

Members of the antiquackery surveillance network also acknowledged the extent of the problem. In 1958, the Post Office Department reported that mail frauds were at their "highest level in history." Postmaster Arthur Summerfield estimated the American public was spending $10 million each month on false medical cures ordered through radio, television, magazine, and newspaper advertisements. The National Better Business Bureau, meanwhile, reported receiving 10 times as many quackery complaints as came in two years earlier. In the March 1958 issue of the *Journal of the American Pharmaceutical Association,* an editorial asserted, "Vicious and cruel medical hoaxes are being perpetuated on a gullible public at the highest rate in history." The author compared the quack to the robber, kidnapper, and murderer, and suggested the patent medicine man of 50 or 100 years before was a neophyte in bilking his ignorant and trusting customers when compared to the modern charlatan.[15]

As early as 1960, the *Wall Street Journal* reported that the "Crusade on Quacks" had been accelerated. The article also identified a particular irony. "The further researchers advance the frontiers of knowledge," Jonathan Spivak noted, "the tougher it becomes to distinguish the quack from the scientist who has made a useful discovery." Making this distinction required resources. Private voluntary health organizations responded. The American Cancer Society established its own Committee on Quackery, published regular reports on the status of unorthodox therapies, and circulated thousands of pamphlets detailing the dangers of cancer quacks to prospective patients. The federally funded National Cancer Institute complemented this effort by exhibiting a series of its own warning posters about cancer quacks. The Arthritis and Rheumatism Foundation sponsored the first extensive national study of arthritis, published by Ruth Walrad in 1960, and used it as a platform for extending its publicity campaign with press releases, speaking tours, product bulletins, and the expansion of local chapters nationwide.[16]

Other longtime leaders in the crusade against quackery took similar steps to intensify their efforts. Riding the wave of publicity generated by the Hoxsey trial, FDA appropriations finally began to steadily increase after years of struggling with inadequate resources. The FDA moved quickly to expand its educational and regulatory campaign against medical quackery. The inspection staff in 1956 numbered 250; in 1957, it was increased to 300. Congress also approved a 20 percent increase in appropriations that same year. By mid-1957, the agency could report "more defendants . . . serving jail sentences for false curative claims than at any time in FDA history."[17]

With the appointment of Wallace F. Janssen as the director of the new Division of Public Information, press releases increased and thousands of educational pamphlets blanketed the country. "Your Money and Your Life: An FDA Catalog of Fakes and Swindles in the Health Field," provided A to Z coverage of dozens of quack remedies from air purifiers to wrinkle removers. Commissioner Larrick warned, "In by-gone days the masked man who held up the lonely traveler would demand 'Your money or your life!' Today, when it comes to the safety and integrity of foods and drugs we do not always have that alternative. It can be: 'Your money *and* your life!' " A new Secretary of the Department of Health, Education, and Welfare, Arthur Flemming, agreed. He made headlines by holding press conferences pointing out the dangers of quackery in the nutrition and weight-loss fields.[18]

In 1959, the AMA launched its own $50,000 campaign against fraudulent food supplement promotions and weight-loss medications, concentrating on the door-to-door peddlers who evaded authorities. The work of the AMA in this area included the distribution of thousands of kits containing pamphlets, reference lists, and information on how to obtain free literature, exhibits, and films from the AMA. The Bureau of Investigation updated, reissued, and created thousands of educational pamphlets on other topics as well. The bureau toured exhibits designed to warn the public about the dangers of "Mechanical Quackery," charlatans intent on "Fooling the Fat," and the tactics employed by "Modern Medical Pitchmen." Meanwhile, in the pages of *Today's Health*, successor to *Hygeia* as the AMA's popular magazine for interested consumers the AMA placed more emphasis on antiquackery themes than it ever had before. The association even produced and distributed 150 copies of its own film on the dangers of quackery in the nutritional field, called *The Medicine Man*. Between 1958 and 1963, the film was shown 14,000 times, including 1,043 telecasts.[19]

Key figures in the antiquackery surveillance network decided an even closer collaboration among regulatory, professional, and voluntary agencies would be necessary to more effectively educate the public and enforce the laws designed to protect consumers. Given the perceived "revival" or "boom" in quackery identified at the end of the 1950s, some of the longtime rivals believed a more united show of force was required. They hoped a united educational campaign might awaken the public to the magnitude of the threat in a way that separate warnings had apparently failed to do.[20]

The AMA's Oliver Field and the FDA's Wallace Janssen played particularly pivotal roles in the push to renew the collaborative venture. Under the joint sponsorship of the AMA and FDA, the First National Congress on Medical Quackery met in Washington D.C. in the fall of 1961, as part of a united effort to launch a "vigorous, multi-faceted attack on medical quackery." In early October, the *Chicago Sun-Times*, and scores of newspapers around the country, announced that the nation's "big guns" had been called up for the war on medical quacks. The many-sided attack to be forged at the conference included 700 men and women from the Post Office Department, the Federal Trade Commission (FTC), the FDA, the AMA, the Department of Justice, the American Cancer Society, the Arthritis and Rheumatism Foundation, the National Better Business Bureau, state medical societies and licensing boards, research institutes, women's clubs, medical and pharmacy schools, and health insurance companies. The goal was to attract attention to the gravity of the problem and attempt for the first time a coordinated campaign against the quacks. As the AMA

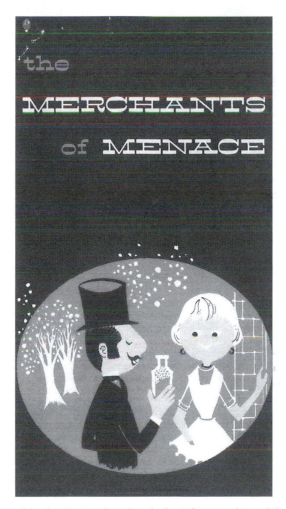

Pamphlet created by the AMA and used as the basis for a traveling exhibit (ca. 1960).
(© American Medical Association. Courtesy of AMA Archives)

press release stated, "recognizing that medical quacks and charlatans thrive in the dark shadows of public ignorance, the Department [of Investigation] felt the meeting could be an effective way of throwing the spotlight on this problem." In a separate FDA press release a few days before the meeting, the secretary of health, education, and welfare, Abraham Ribicoff, explained: "It is highly appropriate for organized medicine and Government agencies to work together on this problem. Quackery is a menace to the public health. It is a kind of criminal activity that deserves close attention. This conference will provide an opportunity to exchange information on better methods of law enforcement, and to alert the public to the prevalence of quackery."[21]

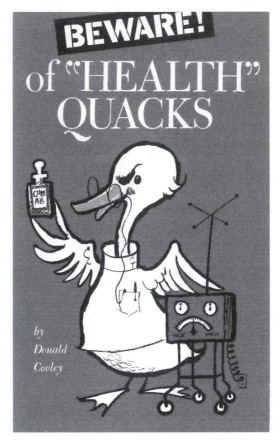

Pamphlet created by Donald Cooley and distributed by the AMA by the thousands (1962).
(Courtesy of American Medical Association Archives)

Delegates at the congress studied exhibits demonstrating an array of mechanical devices and assorted "merchants of menace." They could try on a therapeutic collar that allegedly cured disease by magnetizing the blood. An interactive exhibit allowed attendees to push a doorbell and hear the pitch of a salesman touting a surefire vitamin-enriched panacea. They could relax in an "orgone energy" unit that resembled a wooden hut, where they were "exposed" to an "invisible energy field" that painlessly targeted aches, pains, and assorted ills. Countless pills and potions with shrewd therapeutic claims also lined exhibit hallways.[22]

Delegates listened to a day and half of speeches made by representatives from the most prominent organizations opposed to medical quackery. Director of the AMA's Legal and Socio-Economic Division, C. Joseph Stetler, began the meeting by restating the hope the organizers shared—that the congress would "be the beginning of a

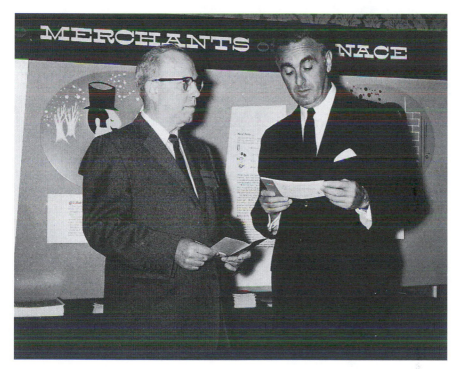

AMA President Leonard W. Larson and Secretary of Health, Education, and Welfare Abraham Ribicoff at the 1961 congress. (© American Medical Association. Courtesy of AMA Archives)

hard-hitting and revitalized crusade by private and governmental agencies against the hucksters of pseudo-medicine." AMA President Leonard W. Larson insisted that contrary to stereotypes, quackery in the 1960s was modern, commercial, cosmopolitan, and "almost respectable" for some. Larson believed the congress faced a difficult challenge in stripping off this "mask of respectability . . . to show the public the vicious, scheming villainy beneath." By operating "just within the bounds of the law—but well outside the realm of human decency and honesty," Stetler explained, quacks had made "slippery targets for law enforcement agencies." Secretary Ribicoff echoed these sentiments. He noted how quackery had become more sophisticated. He lamented that "despite our system of education (not as good as we want it to be, but more universal than any other), despite our high standards of living, despite, even, the basic laws in this field and the Government agency that enforces them, today quackery is flourishing."[23]

Given the extent of the problem, Larson and many other speakers recommended education as the best tool, even if they differed on tactics and points of emphasis. Larson asserted, "We must educate the public thoroughly and effectively. We must wage psychological as well as scientific warfare. We must not only prove the worthlessness of quackery, but we also must establish confidence in sound medical and health care." Dr. L. Henry Garland of the American Cancer Society agreed that information remained the most valuable commodity. He recommended a combination of public education, professional education, and continued research. Commissioner Larrick called on health and nutrition educators at all levels to stem the tide of quackery.[24]

Other speakers offered more specific strategies for combating quackery effectively. While Inspector Duffy agreed that education was key, he also firmly believed that there was "nothing so educational as a stretch in jail—or a stiff fine which takes the profit out of profiteers—to halt the advance of medical quacks." The FTC's Paul Rand Dixon insisted that changes in legislation were needed to give agencies like the FTC and FDA the power they needed to adequately protect the public. The AMA's Morris Fishbein called on newspapers and periodicals to reject advertisements that claimed cures for any number of dangerous conditions. AMA Department of Investigation Director Field argued that conventional antiquackery forces would need the help of all interested people—consumer groups, educational groups, religious organizations, and educators to accomplish his tripartite goal of increased public awareness, strengthened regulations, and a clearer means of "distinguishing between the legitimate medical practitioner and the one who pretends to be one." Believing that "the keys of hope, fear, longing and desperation influence human action more profoundly than do reason, education, or social mores," Dr. William H. Gordon, a Texas physician and veteran of the anti-quackery crusade, worried about the effectiveness of all of these measures.[25]

All of the speakers at the congress nevertheless believed it was possible to reduce the costs of quackery—in terms of money and lives lost, disillusionment encouraged, or treatment delayed. Gordon concluded that the elimination of quackery would be accomplished only "when the charlatans are removed." Larson acknowledged, "I do not believe for an instant that quackery will go up in smoke just because we thunder at it or grumble that it must be destroyed." To successfully "rout quackery," he believed supporters must "first loosen its stranglehold on the public's imagination and pocketbook." Meanwhile, Herbert J. Miller and William Goodrich joined Ribicoff and Larson in predicting eventual eradication. Many others suggested that a complete victory might never be won.[26]

While participants failed to emerge with a clear agenda for the future war against quackery, the congress unquestionably accomplished its goal of bringing its message to American consumers from coast to coast, and even overseas. Associated Press (AP) and United Press International (UPI) articles detailing the primary conference messages were published in more than a thousand dailies. All major radio and television networks carried news reports, and many also did special programs. The popular magazine *This Week* published a feature article by AMA President Larson simultaneous with the congress, in which he urged readers to join the "new war against quacks." Many national magazines sent writers to the congress and published articles the following year.[27]

While nearly all of the press coverage emphasized the spirit of unity and co-operation championed at the meeting, some members of the antiquackery surveil-lance network disagreed on what shape regulatory reform should take. There was general consensus on the urgent need for more funds on the federal, state, and local level to fight quacks. But physicians at the congress generally took the position that there was no need for drastic new federal legislation to deal with quackery. What was needed, they insisted, was better enforcement of laws already on the books. FDA Commissioner Larrick disagreed. He insisted the FDA urgently needed more power to wage its antiquackery fight. In fact, Larrick revealed that the administration was already drafting a new law that would give the agency the authority to rule on the efficacy as well as the safety of all drugs. This kind of legislation, Larrick said, would "very definitely" help in the quackery fight because it would throw the burden of proof on the quacks instead of the FDA. They would be barred from distributing any cure-alls until they had proved the drugs were effective. As it stood in 1961, the FDA had to show that quack drugs were worthless or harmful before it could act to protect the public.[28]

Stetler, the congress chairman and head of the AMA's Legal and Socio-Economic Division, sharply disputed Larrick's claim that the new authority was needed to fight quackery. He served notice that the AMA would fight Larrick's proposal on the grounds that decisions should be left to private physicians. In an editorial published in *Medical World News*, Morris Fishbein charged that giving efficacy authority to the FDA would mean that "hundreds of people" would die unnecessarily while government bureaucrats pondered whether a new drug was sufficiently effective to be released. "I doubt any new legislation is necessary," maintained Fishbein. "Our present agencies, given adequate funds for the employment of necessary scientific and investigative personnel, and given the courage that they need by the full support of the higher echelons of our democracy, would probably eliminate most of the char-latans and quacks now prevailing in the United States."[29]

The concerns of Stetler and Field highlighted a deeper divide within the anti-quackery network on matters of drug evaluation. The AMA's Council on Drugs (pre-viously the Council of Pharmacy and Chemistry) had provided public information and professional judgment about the efficacy and safety of new drugs for decades. The AMA's publication, *New and Non-Official Remedies*, had offered a guide to new medications to tens of thousands of physicians over that same period. The 1938 Federal Food, Drug, and Cosmetic Act undercut this independent function by mandating a more active role for the FDA in evaluating new drugs. But even after this time, the AMA continued to carry out its separate, arguably complementary functions. Initially, the FDA and AMA continued to maintain an amicable working relationship during this period and regularly exchanged information and insights. In the 1950s, this began to change. While the FDA developed its own novel principles of drug evaluation and introduced new tools for monitoring drugs after they were approved, the AMA continued to assert its role in the drug review field while simultaneously ramping down its drug evaluation operations. The AMA may have seen the writing on the wall, as it decided to stop distributing *New and Non-official Remedies* at no cost to physicians as early as 1952. The AMA also came under fire from the mid-1950s onward as it began what Daniel Carpenter describes as "a slow departure from the activity of dispassionate, institutionalized pharmaceutical evaluation" and began openly embracing drug advertising in *JAMA*. When the excesses of the pharmaceutical industry became front-page news in 1960 due to a controversial congressional investigation that would culminate with a dramatic legislative proposal that ultimately changed the medical marketplace for decades to come, tensions between the FDA and the AMA were heightened, even as they joined forces in launching a new war on quackery.[30]

NEW DRUGS, KEFAUVER, AND THALIDOMIDE

While the FDA had deservedly earned a reputation for conducting what Commissioner Larrick called a "hot war against medical quackery" in the late 1950s, the administration had also, less publicly, dramatically increased its investment in protecting the public from unsafe and ineffective drugs through other channels. The struggle to enforce laws against the "fringe operators" captured headlines in popular publications and industry trade reports, and the FDA cultivated a wave of media coverage with its press releases and public education campaigns. But Commissioner Larrick consistently made a distinction between the agency's "old business" of combating the customary quack and its "new business" of regulating the modern drug market, at least when addressing fellow regulators and industry insiders. This meant that while most of the public continued to associate the work of the FDA with its policing duties as de facto quackbuster, the administration quietly spent more time and money investigating the booming pharmaceutical industry. A common goal of preventing fraud transcended the divide between this old and new business, as did the focus on tightening control over new drugs.[31]

In identifying problems with the new business of pharmaceuticals, the FDA tended to not generally cast blame on the drug industry as a whole. In fact, reformers frequently acknowledged the value of working proactively and cooperatively with drug manufacturers. They noted how regulations had helped draw competitors together, in the research laboratory and in opposition to the most egregious lawbreakers. As Commissioner Larrick saw it, the philosophy of the FDA was to bring about cooperatively with industry the maximum voluntary compliance with the law. To this end, the doors of the FDA were open to any representative of industry who wanted to discuss the requirements of the law. Another FDA official argued that such cooperation between the pharmaceutical industry and regulators had exerted a "profound [positive] influence on the country's industrial and social development."[32]

Ever since the 1938 law had first granted the FDA the authority to ensure the safety of all new drugs before they were marketed to the public, the administration had used the requirement of a new drug application as a tool for controlling the pharmaceutical industry and fringe operators alike. The new drug application (NDA), or lack thereof, offered inspectors a crucial device in developing cases against homespun remedies sold outside mainstream channels, but the NDA also allowed the FDA, as gatekeeper for the flow of new pharmaceuticals, to more broadly influence the way research was conducted and how drugs were marketed. Without the proper research, no NDA would be issued. Without proper labeling, an NDA would be denied. For enforcement purposes, the regulation of labeling also assumed primary importance in the postapproval activity of the FDA. As FDA Medical Director Holland saw it, product labeling was "inseparably linked to safety," for it was "only through truthful informative labeling that the physician becomes aware of the usefulness, the limitations, and the potential side effects and contraindications to its use." The regulation of the label could therefore be used to ensure that a drug was not only safe but also worked in the way it claimed to.[33]

In 1955 and 1956, the FDA changed its rules for the NDA in an effort to bring the old regime of inspection in line with the new regime of pharmacological science. Whereas the new drug section of the 1938 law had primarily required a demonstration that drugs would be "safe for use," the revised NDA allowed for the summary rejection of any new drug application that did not contain full, detailed reports from extensive experiments confirming safety as well as the therapeutic effects claimed in the application. The revised NDA thereby made it possible for the FDA to govern clinical experimentation and its reporting, require that drug companies essentially hand over their data for analysis, and compel the reporting of therapeutic results. The FDA also became more active in seizing products that were being marketed without a new drug application. As the 1950s drew to a close, the FDA increasingly destroyed product lines, shut down labs and factories, and issued drug recalls, often due to the lack of an effective or amended NDA.[34]

It was within this context that Tennessee Senator Estes Kefauver commenced hearings on pharmaceutical production, pricing, and profits before his Subcommittee on Antitrust and Monopoly in December 1959. By that time, Kefauver had become one of the most popular politicians in the country, due in no small part to his nationally televised hearings on organized crime and his 1951 best-selling book *Crime in America*. By the late 1950s, he had turned his attention to what he saw as a pattern of anticompetitive and inflationary behavior in the steel and auto-mobile industries. As part of his inquiry into the ability of large corporations to manipulate prices, consumers, and politics, Kefauver widened his exploration to other manufacturing sectors of the economy and thereby turned national attention to the details of the pharmaceutical industry. What he and his staff found was striking. Of 25 industrial sectors considered, the drug industry had by far the highest profit rate. When the manufacturing cost of common medications was compared to the retail price, investigators discovered markups of 1,000 percent or more. Kefauver used these statistics and others in confirming an already established concern about inflation in drug prices.[35]

By the spring of 1961, Kefauver was finally ready to introduce a number of different policy solutions in the form of an omnibus bill, S.1552. The bill addressed the problem of pricing and profits primarily by incorporating a number of patent provisions designed to increase competition and expand the availability of generic drugs. The bill was also intended to address a number of other issues that had come to light in the course of the hearings. Testimony revealed the extent of problems with the general overpromotion and misuse of drugs. The hearings also confirmed that many pharmaceutical ads were misleading and based on little or no evidence. Testimony from Commissioner Larrick revealed the growing number of recalled drugs that had been pulled from the market after the initial approval process. Kefauver concluded that the power granted to the FDA to evaluate the effectiveness as well as the safety of medicines before they made it to the market, and to tie that power to the new drug application process and postmarket evaluation, would codify existing practice and offer the best chance of rectifying these evils. He also hoped it would prevent consumers from wasting their money on worthless pharmaceuticals.[36]

Throughout 1961 and into the spring of 1962, the bill received favorable media coverage and popular support, but opposition thwarted S.1552. While not one of Kefauver's witnesses denied either that efficacy regulation was in practice or that it was legitimate and legally permissible, the American Medical Association stubbornly opposed the new efficacy requirement on the grounds that it would rob doctors of their authority. In their eyes, allowing the government to determine whether a drug was effective or ineffective set a dangerous precedent. The Pharmaceutical Manufacturers' Association opposed the patent system changes as onerous and overly intrusive. In the Senate, Republicans Everett Dirksen of Illinois and Roman Hruska of Nebraska personified the AMA-PMA alliance and managed to skillfully emasculate Kefauver's measure in committee. Meanwhile, a lack of support from President Kennedy and the White House staff deflated Kefauver's initiative.[37]

As the Elixir Sulfanilamide tragedy helped turn the tide in favor of the 1938 act, so did another drug crisis bust the stalemate over Kefauver's proposed legislation. The story of the thalidomide disaster began almost two years before Morton Mintz's momentous story about it appeared on the front page of the Sunday edition of the *Washington Post* on July 15, 1962. In September 1960, the William S. Merrell Company of Cincinnati, Ohio, had submitted a new drug application for thalido-mide (trade name Kevadon), a sedative designed to supplant widely used barbiturate-based sleep medications. In her first review of a new drug application as an FDA medical officer, Frances Kelsey identified serious problems with the drug, which had been tied to an epidemic of birth defects in Europe and Australia. It had in fact already been withdrawn from the European market. Mintz's story proclaimed Kelsey the "heroine of the FDA" and credited her with keeping an extremely danger-ous drug off the market. On Monday, follow-up stories appeared in the *Los Angeles Times*, the *New York Times*, and the *Chicago Tribune*. Kefauver, whose staff had delib-erately leaked the details of the Kelsey story to Mintz, wasted no time in taking advan-tage of the news. The Senate introduced Kelsey in Congress on July 18, 1962, along with Larrick and other FDA officials. Kefauver then called upon President Kennedy to award Kelsey a national medal of service, which was presented in a highly publi-cized White House ceremony on August 7. President Kennedy then signed Public Law 87-781, the Drug Amendments of 1962, into law on October 10, with Frances Kelsey standing behind him.[38]

The Drug Amendments of 1962 contained key provisions that not only governed pharmaceutical regulation for decades to come but also helped establish a new basis for the long battle to combat medical quackery. First, the amendments required evi-dence of safety and "effectiveness" in the form of "adequate and well-controlled inves-tigations" before any new drug, not just prescription products, could enter the market. It remained to be determined what constituted the terms outlined in the pro-visions, but all drugs, for the first time, were formally required to have the effect they purported to have. This requirement gave sharper teeth to FDA authority that had been previously implied but not legally empowered. Second, the sponsor of a drug formally assumed the burden of proof for new drug applications moving forward. This meant no drug promoter could sell a product without meeting this rigorous pro-vision, without facing action from the FDA. Ultimately, this prevented a number of controversial new drugs (which may have been marketed to pharmacists and doctors with impunity under earlier provisions) from making it to market in the closing dec-ades of the century. Third, the amendments gave FDA inspectors new authority to inspect company records regarding drug development, clinical testing, and produc-tion, in addition to sampling drug and monitoring manufacturing activities. In theory, this authority prevented drug makers from operating under the "dark shadows of public ignorance" that antiquackery critics had long condemned. In practice, these provisions gave the FDA an unprecedented amount of power in shaping the drug market for the rest of the century. For those who had been engaged in a decades-long fight against what they defined as medical quackery, this, along with the show of unity demonstrated at the National Congress on Medical Quackery, created a palpable sense of optimism moving forward.[39]

A QUALIFIED OPTIMISM

The optimism and unity shown at the first National Congress on Medical Quackery inspired a series of meetings at the state level, from California to Missouri and Pennsylvania to Connecticut. In summarizing the proceedings of the first Pennsylvania Congress to Combat Health Quackery in 1962, Secretary of Health C. L. Wilbar repeated what quickly became an almost standard script among opponents of quackery. He praised the work of the AMA and FDA in fighting hard against the "unscrupulous operators in quackery." He identified some of the methods to be used in the fight. He implored attendees to clean up their own professions, to speak up against quackery, to take advantage of every opportunity to educate consumers about quackery, and to support the efforts of government and private agencies. But he also echoed a common concern that it was often "impossible to differentiate between the legitimate and the fraud." Wilbar embraced scientific inquiry and evaluation as the best solution to the problem. He believed that positive change depended on a concerted and coordinated educational campaign.[40]

At the Connecticut State Congress on Medical Quackery in September 1962, National Better Business Bureau Vice President Irving Ladimer similarly articulated a tempered optimism in the fight against quackery moving forward. Ladimer asked why it was "that despite a more sophisticated consumer, a more alert profession, a host of Federal and State agencies regulating advertising, labeling and communication, and a stronger structure of self-regulation," that deception and bilking of the public continued. He observed that the "fundamental come-on" of quackery still managed to enchant, captivate, and ensnare the public. He offered several explanations for this. First and foremost, he cited what he considered the "average consumer's pitiable lack of scientific knowledge in most matters pertaining to health." Other factors included a general inability to accept the fact that there were certain diseases for which no cure was yet known to medical science; the perpetual search for the "fountain of youth" that seemed to permeate society; and the eagerness of the afflicted to believe the promises of the "quick, easy, 'miracle' remedy." Collectively, these and other related factors had helped create "a climate in which false, deceptive or fraudulent promotions" flourished. Here, he blamed the media for assuming little responsibility in protecting their audiences from fraud. He blamed consumers for the naïve belief that if something was printed about a medical treatment "it must be true!" Ladimer failed to acknowledge that antiquackery pioneers had been making these same arguments for decades.[41]

Ladimer also conceded that antiquackery forces may have oversold the country on the extent and effectiveness of the ability of the government to control the problem. He worried that the new powers granted to the FDA by the 1962 Drug Amendments might result in a post-thalidomide false confidence among consumers that "everything on the market must be O.K." Ladimer suggested this could be disastrous. He echoed a widely held belief that there would "never be a sufficiently large staff to watch each dereliction." Antiquackery forces could not rely wholly on government policing. Consumer vigilance and self-regulation would also be critical elements of a successful campaign.[42]

Just as antiquackery forces had campaigned for increased consumer vigilance for decades, so had they issued appeals for "rigorous self-discipline" among professionals. As part of the renewed crusade embodied by various congresses on medical quackery, the National Better Business Bureau argued that "self-regulation, self-control and discipline" were the best way for businesses to "reduce the fleecing of the public as well as avoid criticism and the likelihood of outside restraint." Antiquackery crusaders increasingly made similar pleas for self-policing and self-discipline among medical professionals of all varieties. Nurses received instructions on how to guide their patients away from quackery and into the competent hands of physicians, by bolstering their faith in the medical profession and its recent advances and by telling patients how to recognize quackery. Local and state medical societies called on their members to take responsibility for educating their patients and policing their ranks. The American Pharmaceutical Association, meanwhile, organized a symposium on the pharmacist's role in protecting the public from quacks and quackery, and devoted an entire issue of its journal to the subject. As part of an effort to inform and instruct pharmacists on how they could facilitate investigations and the enforcement of antiquackery laws, the FDA's deputy director of the Bureau of Enforcement argued that the "pharmacist's number one job" in this fight should be "to recognize quackery in all its forms and to oppose it and debunk it at every opportunity both professionally and privately." Calls for self-regulation were also extended to publishers and broadcasters. Warren Braren, of the National Association of Broadcasters, for example, embraced the authority granted the FDA by the 1962 Drug Amendments by arguing that a product should not be advertised if it had not been proven safe and effective for the condition for which it was sold.[43]

While these calls for self-regulation collectively signaled a rallying cry for disparate groups, they nevertheless revealed underlying tensions within the antiquackery network. Some framed self-regulation as a necessary complement to government intervention. Many others warned self-regulation was even more important in protecting the free-enterprise system from further government encroachment.[44]

A series of national congresses, and widespread media coverage, highlighted the successes in the renewed antiquackery crusade for the remainder of the decade, but

they also underscored a number of seemingly insurmountable problems. At the
Second National Congress on Medical Quackery in 1963, representatives from the
FDA, FTC, and Post Office Department outlined the positive results of increased
regulatory activity. Regulators detailed successful prosecutions against the manufacturers of worthless medical devices, vitamin regimens, cosmetic formulas, dangerous
obesity drugs, and fraudulent arthritis panaceas. They also bemoaned the limited size
of their legal and scientific staffs in this effort, while the "insidious growth of quackery" became "more difficult to apprehend and prosecute" with every passing day.
Congress attendees expressed nearly universal agreement that education was the best
weapon, in the long run, against quackery, but an equally strong consensus was
reached on the generally "inadequate, non-specific, and nebulous" educational efforts
already in place. This meant that while educators agreed that a comprehensive program of general health education was needed, there was little agreement on how to
reach specific goals.[45]

When "old friends and fellow warriors" met at the Third National Congress on
Medical Quackery in October 1966, to continue the "battle of governmental and private agencies against the purveyors of false hopes and nostrums," new AMA President
Charles L. Hudson focused his introductory remarks on the subject of the "medical
cults" that had received only marginal attention at previous congresses when compared to the fringe operators targeted by regulatory agencies. Hudson noted how
the AMA had laid the groundwork for discussions at the Third National Congress
by publishing an article in *Journal of the American Medical Association (JAMA)* on
the lack of qualifications at schools of chiropractic. A booklet was also included in
the congress packet for attendees, titled *Chiropractic: The Unscientific Cult.* Hudson
identified two principal challenges in the campaign against chiropractic. First, it
would be difficult to "strip the mask of respectability" off of chiropractic quackery
and show the public the "vicious, scheming villain underneath it." Second, it would
be challenging to not only "prove the worthlessness of quackery" but at the same time
to "establish confidence in sound medical and health care."[46]

Though united in their fight against a shared enemy, the generals disagreed about
the relative roles of government regulation, self-regulation, and education in the war
on quackery. John W. Knutson, president of the National Health Council (a federation of national professional and voluntary organizations), underscored these tensions
in his opening address at the 1966 congress. He acknowledged improvements in collective efforts to alert and educate the general public but doubted that the effort since
the 1961 conference had "reduced the relative extent of the medical quackery problem." He explained this was partly due to limited resources, rapidly changing technology, and the ability of quacks to "use one of the most fundamental and most
cherished characteristics of our democracy to further his own ends . . . faith in your
fellow man." The primary reason for limited success, however, was a lack of

regulatory teeth behind the movement. "I deem it impractical and unrealistic," Knutson asserted, "to expect a public education program to keep pace and properly prepare the public to exercise discriminating judgment in what is true, what is false, what has been adequately tested, what is promising, and what is worthless." The increasing requirement for highly specialized knowledge to make such judgments convinced Knutson and others that governmental agencies must be provided with the regulatory powers and the enforcement capability to ensure that "the quacks, the crooks, and the experts in chicanery" would be required to fulfill the same standards of testing as those who worked in the drug business with integrity and honesty. Without that kind of protection, and without increased restrictions on the potential and actual quack, Knutson predicted that conference-goers would be "indulging in a lot of self-righteous indignation at the next National Congress on Quackery." No one doubted the value of laws and educational campaigns in the fight, but agreement on the proper balance of each remained elusive.[47]

At the fourth, and final, Congress on Health Quackery in the 1960s, held two years later in 1968, James Harvey Young offered an historian's perspective on the work that had been done since the first congress seven years earlier. Young noted that given the long history of quackery, it was unlikely that the battle would be won decisively. In fact, he observed that there had been periods when "new laws, scientific advances, and too optimistic a view of man's inherent reason and goodness" had made people drop their guard, and quackery had surged forward with new vigor. The team of "experienced fraud fighters" that had inspired the first meetings in 1961 had by 1968 already been dismantled. Legal cases became increasingly difficult and costly to prosecute, and fewer of them had been begun. The FDA spent more and more time evaluating prescription pharmaceuticals. One new drug application alone could run over 4,000 pages and eat up 200 days to evaluate. It should have been no surprise that the FDA cut back on publication of its long-running Notices of Judgment, which had served a decades-long role of alerting the public and professionals to some of the most egregious alleged frauds.[48]

CONCLUSION

For new AMA President Dwight L. Wilbur, it remained a puzzle that defied logic that in a nation where science had advanced to the point where Americans stood at the threshold of the moon, people would pay good money to sit on the dirt floor of a farmer's barn because he announced that radioactivity in his earth would cure cancer. He felt it impossible to understand the businessman or his university-educated wife who would totally ignore the millions of words spoken and written by competent medical and scientific authorities on nutrition, exercise, and weight control, but would leap to buy a paperback book that purported to show how to lose magnificent amounts of weight without giving up a single dessert or changing a single eating habit. It was even more incomprehensible to Wilbur that thousands of people would not let anyone but a bonded and certified technician touch their television set, would insist that the school board maintain a strict certification program for teachers, would refuse to take their car to any repairman except the dealership where they bought it, or check all door-to-door salesmen through their Better Business Bureau before buying a product, but when they came down with the flu, or got a recurring headache, or had indigestion they would go looking for the help of a chiropractor.[49]

By and large, members of the antiquackery network at the end of the 1960s failed to see any contradiction between their belief in the gullibility, ignorance, or delusion of the consuming public and their faith in the power of education to enlighten the masses. AMA leadership remained convinced that "the undiscerning, the uninformed, the unsuspecting and the desperate" could be spared the costs of quackery through an expanded educational campaign. From the antiquackery crusader's perspective, people could simply not be rational, conscientious, well-informed, and scientifically literate, and still willingly choose a quack over a qualified, expertly trained physician. And yet, intelligent people apparently did just that.

EIGHT

REDEFINING QUACKERY IN THE
CLOSING DECADES OF THE
TWENTIETH CENTURY

Americans, generally being an optimistic people, have believed that problems are for solving. Early in this century, when quackery came to be recognized as a major problem in the health field, many observers predicted its certain death. Common sense, increasing education, the truths of science, and laws aimed at securing honest labeling would drive quackery from the marketplace. Especially as modern medicine developed and conquered one disease after another, anything so outmoded and unneeded as quackery would shortly wither away. But this has not happened. Quite the contrary! Health quackery today is a multibillion-dollar business, and its future prospects look brighter still.

—James Harvey Young (1976)[1]

On the morning of May 31, 1984, a congressional hearing proclaimed that quackery had become a $25 billion problem. The meeting of the Subcommittee on Health and Long-Term Care, chaired by Congressman Claude Pepper, marked the conclusion of a four-year investigation into quackery and its impacts on senior citizens. The Pepper Committee estimated that older adults spent $10 billion per year on quackery, and that the nation as a whole probably wasted $25 billion. Pepper declared that quackery should be considered a national scandal. "Federal efforts against quackery are minimal and appear to be diminishing," he announced. "States are also non-responsive . . . I should say we invited the Department of Justice to send witnesses to testify before us here today. They declined the invitation." Pepper lamented, "the Department of Justice, apparently under the impression that quackery is still something practiced by medicine men out of covered wagons, reported, 'The typical medical quackery case . . . does not lend itself to Federal criminal prosecution.'" Accordingly, the Department of Justice (DOJ) said its role and experience in this area was "very limited." Meanwhile, by 1984 the U.S. Food and Drug Administration (FDA) was devoting less than 1 percent of its resources to this kind of fraud. A spokesman at the FDA had stated the previous year that the agency was "simply overmatched . . . there are too many quacks, too skillful at the quick change of address and the product name for the cumbersome procedures of the FDA." A subsequent congressional report charged, "it is clear that preventing and controlling health fraud and quackery is not an FDA priority." The Federal Trade Commission (FTC) also seemed strangely paralyzed, overburdened by its broader mandate to regulate massive businesses and hindered by its restrictive mission to deal only with matters involving interstate commerce. In Pepper's opinion, the only agency of the federal government worth commending was the U.S. Postal Service, which had proven the most alert in trying to detect crime, punish those who were responsible, and prevent repeat offenders.[2]

The Pepper Committee found that quackery had become a big business due to its immense profitability and apparent lack of risk. In many cases, a web of phony practitioners, charitable foundations, and clinics worked together to perpetrate the most egregious schemes, identifying the desperate, and even arranging travel and accommodations to facilitate the fleecing that they perpetrated. The "inventiveness of the quacks" was judged to be "as unlimited as their callousness and greed." Phony products included cancer cures made from ground up diamonds, a tonic made from horse warts suspended in sour milk, and serums drawn from human urine and fecal matter. The committee identified promoters who advised people with arthritis to bury themselves in the earth, sit in an abandoned mine, or stand naked under a 1,000-watt bulb during the full moon. Raw brain matter was being promoted as a cure for Alzheimer's disease. Raw eye extracts were prescribed for blindness, and raw heart concentrate was suggested for heart disease. More than 75 percent of the products analyzed by the committee were found to be dangerous or potentially hazardous. Fewer than 5 percent of the products were deemed fit for use.[3]

Why had quackery remained such a booming business in the wake of the 1960s, a time when reform-minded optimists had united in their commitment to squashing it once and for all? An FDA-contracted report from 1972 offered some potential answers. The 426-page report, entitled "A Study of Health Practices and Opinions," found that millions of Americans were using worthless, unnecessary, and potentially dangerous amounts of quack remedies. The most egregious forms of quackery included health-food fads, fraudulent cures for arthritis and cancer, and supplements that were readily available in most drug stores and health-food stores. Thirty-five million adults were using vitamin and mineral supplements without the advice of a doctor. One-fifth of the public was convinced that cancer, arthritis, and other diseases were caused at least in part by vitamin and mineral deficiencies. The report concluded that there was "an enormous waste of money, not to mention adverse health effects, from misguided consumer experimentation with health products." This news—that millions of Americans were being duped by fraudulent panaceas—affirmed what antiquackery crusaders had reported for decades.[4]

Through extensive questionnaires and follow-up interviews, the report offered an unprecedented amount of data on the health attitudes and beliefs of Americans. This included key insights into the widespread continued use of health practices deemed quackery by medical professionals. The study found a striking "absence of logic or system," for example, in how Americans acted in health matters. People reported that they would often try medications or treatments, whether they believed in them or not, because they were "worth a try." The long-held generalization that fallacious health practices most often resulted from specific faulty beliefs, which could be changed with proper education, was also not supported. In fact, few people reported having an organized set of health beliefs, which led the authors to conclude that it was natural that many health attitudes would be ill informed and inconsistent. The report found a "widespread lack of understanding of the potential dangers of ineffective treatment," and a marked tendency for people to rely on their own judgment over that of a physician.[5]

Many of those surveyed reported a lack of trust in the medical profession, which had a clear impact on the decisions they made regarding medical care. More than one-third of those interviewed, representing some 44 million people, said they would go on using a medicine a doctor had told them was worthless if they thought it was helping them. More than 10 percent said they would try a treatment that a friend said had helped them, even if a doctor said it was ineffective. Regarding cancer, 42 percent of those interviewed said they would not accept the unanimous judgment of doctors and other scientists who asserted that a certain cancer "cure" was worthless, if they had heard from the patients of a few doctors that it helped them. Only 45 percent of the total sample thought a medicine condemned by medical experts should be banned by law.[6]

While many people made decisions that clearly went against the advice of doctors, those surveyed reported a surprising amount of trust in advertisements for drugs. Regulators may have been shocked to learn that three in eight people believed that advertisers in the health field were so rigorously policed and regulated that serious distortions and fabrications were very unlikely or impossible. Substantial numbers believed that quackery was easy to recognize. They referred to popular portrayals of "quacks" as objects of humor and maintained they were blatantly weird, preposterous, or hucksterish. These views confirmed a fear expressed by many antiquack crusaders in the wake of the passage of the Kefauver-Harris Drug Amendments of 1962 that consumers would suffer from a false sense of security.[7]

While newspapers largely printed the results of the study without substantial comment, the report did not go unchallenged. Sardonic reporter Nicholas von Hoffman took issue with what he called the "disgusting conviction" expressed in what the report referred to as "rampant empiricism." The report dismissed "rampant empiricism" as "a very literal belief that individual response to treatment is entirely unpredictable." The report's authors maintained this misconception had led many consumers to justify "any 'treatment' or regimen, no matter how outlandish, on the grounds that it may work for them although it does not work for anyone else." Von Hoffman argued this made it sound like the medical establishment would "rather have you die while exhibiting a proper respect for medical expertise than cure yourself by your own 'outlandish' methods." He retorted, "How any lay person could think up treatments more outlandish, painful and unsuccessful than some the medical profession has concocted—say, for cancer or bad backs—isn't discussed." Von Hoffman concluded that the mandate to follow a physician's advice was particularly problematic given the average doctor's lack of knowledge about alternatives available to consumers in fields like nutrition. He maintained that the paternalism of medical professionals in their war against quackery, combined with proposals for increased regulation and enforcement, offered another example of a parallel question asked in the contemporaneous abortion controversy: did Americans even have a right to control their own bodies?[8]

Another study, published in June 1972, found that, at least for the moment, consumers remained in control of their decisions, even if their choices continued to mystify mainstream medical professionals. The study of El Paso, Texas, residents by sociologists Julian B. Roebuck and Bruce Hunter found that many people remained unaware of the actions of antiquackery crusaders and, even when aware of the adverse judgments they had issued, might still reject the label of quackery or the sanctions associated with it. Almost 50 percent of respondents used friends and family as the chief source of information when choosing a doctor, with just over 5 percent reporting that they consulted groups like the American Medical Association (AMA), FDA, commercial associations, and the scientific community. When choosing to evaluate a specific medical therapy, respondents relied even more heavily on the mass media (41 percent) than family and friends (36 percent), while "established authoritative bodies" like the FDA were the least chosen (2 percent). Respondents demonstrated a general lack of knowledge about the various types of unorthodox healers that were frequently targeted as quacks by groups like the AMA, but nevertheless expressed a willingness to try their services if they had not yet done so. When asked about specific remedies and healers categorized as quackery by "formal sanctioning bodies," 30 percent expressed a great deal of confidence in their effectiveness. This led the authors to conclude that the "scientific and medical establishment" had failed at "promulgating and enforcing normative controls relating to health-care quackery." As the FDA report had also indicated, many consumers embraced the broader movement for their empowerment and combined it with a spirit of experimentalism.[9]

These studies underscored several reasons for quackery's apparent proliferation in the 1970s and 1980s. Alleged quacks effectively used advertising to their full advantage by capitalizing on public faith in truthful marketing, while an underfunded and understaffed bureaucracy could not keep pace with policing and prosecuting alleged offenders. Meanwhile, Americans grew disillusioned about the value of and intent of bureaucratic efforts more broadly, and were drawn to the antiestablishment rhetoric of many alternatives outside mainstream medicine. The educational strategy of antiquackery forces also remained ineffective. These failures and others inspired a backlash against antiquackery forces. Empowered consumers were willing to fight to defend their freedom of choice in medical matters, to the dismay of those who worked the hardest to rid the market of remedies and "cures" that had been deemed fraudulent. Meanwhile, some of the most prominent leaders in the antiquackery network began to slowly retreat from the full-scale assault they had ordered in the 1960s.

A SELLER'S MARKET

Consumers of health-related products faced a dilemma in the 1970s and 1980s. They were increasingly barraged with conflicting messages about health. Advertising played a particularly pivotal role in creating confusion. Living in the land of medical plenty, Americans reported feeling dissatisfied, unhappy, and anxious. Some blamed advertisers. Consumers had "been made that way by design of a great American institution," one critic observed. The advertising industry's purpose, critics charged, was to "build American industry by attacking the individual and collective American psyche." Already by 1970, the average citizen was reportedly being subjected to 1,500 advertising messages a day in newspapers, magazines, signs, radio, TV, and mail totaling an annual investment of $16 billion. That equaled approximately $90 for every man, woman, and child in the country. Advertising for headache remedies alone topped $100 million a year and appeared to be growing.[10]

In 1973, Guenter B. Risse, a physician and historian at the University of Wisconsin–Madison's medical school, argued that quacks proliferated at least partly because of a false sense of security created by consumer protection groups like the FDA and FTC. "People assume that what advertisers tell them must be true or that these claims couldn't be made," Risse explained. It seemed society was letting advertisers, not medical science, tell it what was normal and abnormal. In antiquackery

texts intended to clarify the evolving relationship between quackery and the consumer, health scientists observed evidence of peoples' noncritical, even fantastic faith
in the published word. Authors noted the dilemma faced by people who were
expected to make distinctions between the legitimate and fraudulent, especially since
similar advertising techniques were used by each. In cases where medical science had
not found a cure for an illness—cancer, arthritis, backaches, and so on—Risse
believed anxious "straw-grabbers" increasingly turned to the quack who "fraudulently
or through ignorance" provided hope.[11]

According to another critic, promoters of quackery had "mastered the art of
manipulating the media." While people wrongly thought that health claims in ads
must be true or they "wouldn't be allowed," a false claim was against the law only if
it appeared in an advertisement or on a product label. To skirt the law, health products were increasingly peddled in articles and books, on the radio, and on television
talk shows. Essentially, the media became the label. Frequently, magazines featured
advertisements for various vitamins and drugs that had been hailed in seemingly
objective and scientific articles. Promoters learned quickly to make false, unfounded,
or exaggerated claims for health products and services, and they got away with it by
putting the claims under the umbrella of freedom of the press. They also learned to
manipulate the media by exploiting its affinity for sensationalism. This included
nationally syndicated newspapers, magazines, and newsletters that promoted psychic
healers, miracle cures, or wondrous new weight-loss diets, as well as a constant barrage
of accusations of a conspiracy on the part of the medical establishment to suppress
cures for often fatal diseases such as cancer.[12]

The impact of advertising on consumer decision making could be seen most
clearly in the field of nutritional solutions to health problems, which increasingly
became a dominant feature of unorthodoxy for years to come. Critics of "nutritional
myths" noted that advertising in this field had become increasingly sophisticated.
Advertisers even recruited doctors to craft clever ads that "made pseudoscience sound
like science." The 1972 study of health practices and opinions reported that when it
came to self-treatment with vitamins and supplements, many consumers adhered to
a set of doctrines widely promoted in advertising copy. One in four Americans had
been on a diet in the preceding three years, half of them without a doctor's recommendation, and 3 million had tried over-the-counter preparations that claimed to
help the user eat less. Twenty-six percent had used nutritional supplements expect-
ing specific observable health benefits, without a physician's advice. Three-quarters
of the American public believed that extra vitamin pills would provide more pep
and energy, a finding the study said was "the most common of the misconceptions
investigated." As historian James Harvey Young notes, "the warning words of scientific nutritionists, dieticians, consumerists, and regulators, however, were out-
weighed a thousand or more to one by the printed and oral verbiage of

pitchmen." The vitamin and supplement industry boomed. An array of drugs, devices, dietary regimens, and advice books continued to promise an easier solution to obesity and other nutritionally related health problems than medical science could offer.[13]

Meanwhile, efforts to regulate the growing vitamin and supplement industry consistently failed. In 1962, the FDA announced its plans to update the regulations for food supplements that had first been put in place after passage of the 1938 law. After months of hearings and an accumulated congressional record of 32,000 pages, no new law was passed. In 1973, the FDA again proposed reforms designed to rationalize the promotion of vitamins and supplements. Almost immediately, the health-food and vitamin industry, led by the National Health Federation (NHF), charged the FDA with threatening the "medical freedom" of consumers. Despite efforts by the FDA to reassure people that regulation was intended only to "require full and honest labeling and fair promotion of vitamin and mineral products," the NHF effectively stoked fears that the government intended to eliminate certain vitamins from the marketplace or, if available, limit access via prescriptions and higher costs. Opponents of the FDA proposal flooded Congress with some 2 million letters.[14]

In a stunning turn, the bill introduced in the ninety-third Congress not only negated the FDA's attempt to tighten controls but also proposed to cut back the agency's regulatory authority to a pre-1938 level. After the bill stalled, a revised version, attached as a rider to the Health Research and Health Services Act, passed in 1976. Despite strong opposition from a wide range of groups, including the American Society of Clinical Nutrition, the Committee on Nutrition of the American Academy of Pediatrics, the American Association of Retired Persons, Consumers Union, and Ralph Nader's associates and supporters, the 1976 amendment became the first retrogressive step in federal legislation respecting self-treatment options since the initial Pure Food and Drugs Act of 1906. FDA Commissioner Alexander Schmidt called the bill a "charlatan's dream." As far as supporters of the legislation were concerned, the amendments represented a step in the direction of medical freedom. Consumer health specialist William T. Jarvis lamented, "When the public is convinced it cannot trust conventional health products and services, its alternative is to turn to the substitutes offered by quackery. It is easy to see why the salesman of unproven health products and services have formed organizations which lobby for 'health freedom'—which in reality is a hunting license for quackery."[15]

While the impact of lobbying by the National Health Federation and their supporters should not be underestimated, the broader climate of disillusionment with government also played a role in weakening regulations in the supplement trade. Writing in 1977, historian James Harvey Young observed that Vietnam and

Watergate had each encouraged a widespread disenchantment with bureaucracy, including its regulatory function. Other contemporary observers identified a parallel lack of faith in science to solve some of the world's most important problems. The sounding of environmental alarms in the 1970s further fueled critiques of the role of science in society and highlighted some of the problems it could create. When combined with a lack of consumer literacy regarding medicine and science generally, critics charged, it was no surprise that people embraced alternative worldviews.[16]

Consumer advocates expressed widespread disappointment with the state of regulatory oversight in the 1970s. In the antiquackery field, regulatory agencies could make a strong case that insufficient funding and manpower had made it difficult to accomplish the broad task assigned them by Congress. The Post Office investigated some 200 incidents of mail-order quackery each year, but the understaffed agency was forced to settle about six out of seven with an agreement to discontinue the questioned practice. Of all the regulatory agencies, perhaps none was more maligned than the "malingering" Federal Trade Commission, "whose sloth and concern with trivia" had earned it the nickname "the little old Lady from Pennsylvania Avenue." Consumer advocate Ralph Nader's "Raiders," disgusted with the FTC's neglect of consumer interests, lambasted the commission in a 1970 report, calling it a "self-parody of bureaucracy, fat with cronyism, torpid thru an in-breeding unusual even for Washington, manipulated by the agents of commercial predators and impervious to governmental and citizen's monitoring." Meanwhile, the 1962 Kefauver-Harris requirement to demonstrate the effectiveness of drugs before they went to market had provided the FDA with new tools in combating quackery, but this had also vastly increased the FDA's obligations in other areas. Congress had also mandated a retrospective review of the unwieldy over-the-counter drug market to ensure safety, efficacy, and truthfulness on labels. Amidst its accumulating duties, the FDA had deprioritized its crusade against quackery.[17]

Congressman Pepper hoped to highlight the negative consequences of this regulatory retreat with his 1984 hearing on quackery. In the wake of the hearing, Pepper introduced three bills intended to strengthen the government's authority to control health fraud. The National Health Federation, with the support of more than a hundred local chapters and 25,000 members, lobbied aggressively against each bill, referring to the proposals as "lysenkoism." NHF President Maureen Salaman reportedly went so far as to buy a plane ticket on a flight with Congressman Pepper, arranging to have seat next to him so that she could "bend his ear" all the way to his destination. After failing to pass the bills during the ninety-eighth Congress, Pepper decided not to reintroduce them. It remained to be seen if the "serious effort to reeducate the public concerning the hazards of quackery," which Pepper had also recommended, would be enough to make a difference.[18]

THE LIMITS OF THE CONSUMER
EDUCATION STRATEGY

For decades, antiquackery crusaders had believed that aside from regulatory re-form, education offered the "only effective countermeasure to quackery," especially if ignorance, superstition, and fear were the primary reasons people chose to patronize quacks and purchase questionable medical products. Educational strategies had been based on the assumption that behavior could be changed if the reasons behind those behaviors could be effectively addressed. Reformers also believed that orthodox medi-cal science would be able to sort out the valuable from the spurious, using the newest investigative techniques, incorporating what was useful and exposing what was not so that the fringe would gradually wither away. By the mid-1970s, each of these assump-tions had come under fire. People in and out of the antiquackery network began to argue that earlier educational campaigns—like mainstream medicine more broadly—had failed to adequately address important philosophical, metaphysical, and psycho-logical factors that influenced the health and decisions of consumers.[19]

Many advocates of the holistic health movement in the 1970s argued that "holism" offered something that mainstream medicine did not. Holistic health practi-tioners often concentrated on the spiritual, offered therapeutic applications of holistic ideas, and privileged the individual patient in a way that conventional physicians often could not, given the ontological basis of an orthodoxy rooted in scientific authority and primarily committed to surgical and drug interventions. Advocates of holistic health included the nonmaterial as influences in health and disease, and offered therapeutic alternatives that addressed spiritual, psychic, and emotional imbal-ance. In 1981, professor of psychiatry and medicine George Engel lamented that, by contrast, the "biomedical model" left "no room within its framework for the social, psychological, and behavioral dimensions of illness" that had been so widely empha-sized in the 1960s and 1970s. As biomedicine failed to translate a more holistic definition of health into therapeutic applications, the medical profession continued to endure harsh criticism for its reductionist philosophy. Physicians faced widespread public demands for health-care reform, and patients turned increasingly to the holistic health movement for alternatives.[20]

Equating many holistic health practices with quackery posed a problem in the edu-cational campaign of reformers. As Stephen Barrett, of the Lehigh Valley Committee Against Health Fraud noted, the very word "quack" could "help his camouflage by making us think of an outlandish character selling snake oil from the back of a covered wagon—and of course no intelligent person would buy snake oil nowadays, would he?" Maybe snake oil was not selling well in the 1970s, but Barrett observed that acupuncture, "organic" food, diet fads, megavitamins, spinal manipulations, and alleged cancer cures abounded. In his mind, each of these represented different forms of quackery. And herein was part of the problem for quackbusters like Barrett. On the one hand, they proclaimed that quackery was everywhere. On the other hand, they admitted the modern quack was not easy to spot. The quack frequently wore the cloak of science. He used "scientific" terms. He wrote with scientific references. He was even introduced on talk shows as the "scientist ahead of his time." The common characteristic in all forms of quackery, Barrett and others argued, was deception. For the person who already used these approaches, as part of a broader holistic approach to health, the argument that "they were being deceived" likely had little effect. What Barrett and others labeled quackery was becoming mainstreamed.[21]

Antiquackery crusaders also struggled to convince people that holistic health practices and other alleged forms of quackery did not in fact work, as a growing number of users proclaimed their success. When asked why many people developed confidence in the types of doctors and drugs that quackbusters considered unscientific quackery, Barrett noted that because most ailments were "self-limiting," they would improve with any treatment at all. "Good doctors rarely take credit for what nature does, while unscientific practitioners usually do," he explained. The placebo effect could also mislead patients. "If a person thinks he has been helped by something, he may feel relief from his pain or other discomfort," even if the treatment modality in question had no direct correlation to recuperation. As Raymond O. West, an epidemiologist at the Loma Linda University School of Public Health explained, "Here is an important reason why quackery seems to succeed. If [a treatment] has the patient's confidence, he feels better. Thus 'immune milk,' at seventy cents a quart, honey and apple-cider vinegar, concentrated seawater at $3.00 a pint, copper bracelets, magic spikes, vibrators, Z-rays, and alfalfa teas—all these have had their proponents; all have seemed to work for some expectant sufferers, but the end thereof can be a way of death." Even for those placebos with no dangerous side effects, the critic of quackery maintained these therapies represented a grave risk: perhaps the greatest risk of all could be found in the legitimate, scientifically validated orthodox therapies it denied people.[22]

As an educational tool, the explanation for the placebo effect had two primary weaknesses. First, if some kinds of alleged quackery sometimes seemed to be successful, the placebo argument likely had an effect only on those people who had not used the therapies in question. In the FDA's 1972 study of health practices and behaviors, large majorities reported being satisfied with the results they thought they obtained, regardless of what antiquackery professionals claimed. Meanwhile, the placebo argument also appeared to be weak given the lack of scientific evidence for the effectiveness of many over-the-counter and prescription drugs that had *not* been categorized as worthless or fraudulent by antiquackery forces. Regulators, scientists, physicians, and drug manufacturers failed to agree on the best way to determine the effectiveness of the hundreds of thousands of over-the-counter proprietaries on the market. Nearly all of them agreed that clinical research concerning efficacy was inadequate. At a symposium focused on "the efficacy of self-medication" in 1972, attended by a score of industry, university, and governmental scientists and officials, nearly all agreed that a large measure of consumer satisfaction in using over-the-counter drugs derived from the placebo effect. Meanwhile, a 1978 Office of Technology Assessment (OTA) report found "only 10 to 20 percent of procedures currently used in medical practice have been shown to be efficacious by controlled clinical trial." While this may have been an unfair critique given that the premarketing demonstration of efficacy for prescription drugs was required only after the 1962 Kefauver-Harris Amendments, and controlled clinical trials had gained prominence only in the preceding 20 years, the evidence served to effectively undercut antiquackery crusaders' own arguments.[23]

BACKLASH

The 1970s also witnessed an unprecedented backlash against the drug industry, the medical profession, and other members of the antiquackery surveillance network. Some antiquackery educators attributed the problem to a cresting "wave of hostility toward the Establishment and the crusade for a counterculture." A growing awareness of the risks involved with mainstream modern medicine also helped shift attention further away from the dangers of alleged forms of quackery and onto the pharmaceutical and over-the-counter drug industries. Reports showed that 2.5 million prescriptions were written in 1974, at a cost of $10 billion. Many, it turned out, were fraught with previously unacknowledged dangers. Studies revealed that two drugs, each safe and useful by itself, could be life threatening when simultaneously taken. Even the most valuable drugs could cause adverse reactions, which were responsible for 28 percent of hospitalizations. One out of every seven days of hospitalization, in fact, resulted from "therapeutic misadventure." A Department of Health, Education, and Welfare publication even raised the question of whether drug therapy could be doing more harm than good. Other reports documented the disturbing overuse and overprescription of antibiotics, despite revelations of their impact as a dangerous environmental pollutant. Some of the most scathing critiques of the drug industry, regulators, and the American Medical Association were provided by muckraking journalists like Morton Mintz, who documented what he called "the irrational and massive use of prescription drugs which may be worthless, injurious, or even fatal."[24]

In the 1970s, the medical profession was subjected to greater scrutiny than perhaps any time in the twentieth century. Critics argued that doctors had forgone the needs of patients. Even spokespersons for the profession admitted that susceptibility to the lures of the quack could be partially explained by the brevity of contact and impersonality that had come to characterize the relationship between patients and physicians. Medical professionals also struggled to address the growing sense that in many cases, medicine actually did more harm than good. A committee of the New Hampshire Medical Society reported such a distrust by patients that people considered their "reliance upon nostrums and quack administrations" more valuable than any learned professional. The power and money image of organized medicine further contributed to the alienation of many. A common response was turning away from the qualified physician.[25]

By the mid-1970s, the AMA struggled to maintain its position as the spokesperson for organized professional medicine as it came under attack from all sides. Widely criticized for its conservatism and opposition to health-care reform at the legislative level, the AMA had grown accustomed to critiques from congressional representatives, consumer advocates, and others outside the organization. Meanwhile, the U.S. Postal Service and the Internal Revenue Service had launched independent investigations of the association for underpaying its bills. The FTC had also filed its own complaint against the AMA, alleging that the association had illegally restrained competition among medical doctors by preventing members from advertising the types and prices of services they offered to the public.[26]

In May 1975, amidst mounting challenges, the AMA fired some 70 employees and undertook a major reorganization, which included the unceremonious closure of the Department of Investigation (formerly named the Bureau of Investigation and Propaganda Department). The AMA explained that the structure of councils and committees had outlived its usefulness, while many of the activities of the Department of Investigation had gradually been adopted or facilitated by other existing departments focused on medical education, consumer issues, and scientific matters. The responsibilities of the Council on Quackery were merged with the AMA's Council on Scientific Affairs, which self-consciously decided to avoid "tackling anything sharply controversial." The AMA continued some of its antiquackery activity for years to come, but with no department solely dedicated to the antiquackery cause, and activities sharply curtailed, the AMA gradually abandoned its role as the foremost clearinghouse on quackery-related material in the country, and de facto leader of the antiquackery surveillance network.[27]

In the wake of the AMA reorganization, the situation only got worse when a doctor, who claimed to work in the AMA's Chicago offices for about 10 years, began leaking confidential AMA documents to federal officials and news outlets around the country. One set of documents revealed how the AMA, which publicly asserted its independence from the nation's $8.4 billion-a-year pharmaceutical industry, included representatives of drug companies in its private policymaking discussions. Another packet revealed how the AMA and drug companies joined forces to kill 1970 legislation designed to provide patients with less expensive medicines. Additional documents revealed how money made its way circuitously from Chicago to

the coffers of congressional representatives who favored the AMA, despite the illegal-
ity of direct political contributions from the association. The source, named Sore
Throat because of the similarity of his role to that of Watergate's still unidentified
Deep Throat, denied that revenge was the reason for his revelations. "The AMA,"
Sore Throat told *Time* correspondent Marguerite Michaels, "is a health monopoly
that caters to vested interests rather than devoting itself to the betterment of health
care." He hoped revealing is secrets would lead to the formation of a new organization
to do what the AMA had stopped doing: "promoting the science and art of medicine
and the betterment of public health."[28]

In October 1975, Sore Throat dispatched a new set of documents that he said supported his contention that the AMA was more interested in reducing competition
than providing the public with adequate care. The documents outlined several aspects
of the AMA's campaign against the chiropractic profession, which had prompted the
House Oversight and Investigation subcommittee to conclude that the AMA's
crusade may violate antitrust laws. Many of the documents stated the intent by the
AMA to eliminate the chiropractic profession or outlined plans to carry out that
intent via harassment, delicensing, and inducement of the boycotting of chiropractic
services. In response, a spokesman for the AMA called the approximately 20,000
active chiropractors, licensed in all 50 states, a "medical threat to the American people," but added "in no way have we violated the antitrust law." For several years to
come, the AMA would remain mired in lawsuits related to chiropractic. The protracted battle culminated in 1987, in what chiropractors referred to as "the case of
the century," when a U.S. District Court found the AMA and many of its associates
guilty of a conspiracy against chiropractors and found them to be in violation of
federal antitrust laws. The permanent injunction issued against the AMA required
JAMA to publish the court's judgment. In 1990, the U.S. Supreme Court let this
decision stand without comment.[29]

While the case of chiropractic was considered by many to be a public relations disaster for the AMA, an even more divisive unorthodox therapy underscored the backlash against the medical establishment in the 1970s and early 1980s—the case of
Laetrile. Laetrile has been called the most controversial and economically successful
unorthodox cancer remedy of the twentieth century. It was derived from apricot ker-
nels, and proponents of Laetrile alternately billed it as l-mandelonitrile beta glucuro-
nide (the compound from which its name was derived), amygdalin (a substance
commonly found in the pits of many fruits), or vitamin B-17. In 1970, the FDA
initially approved and then withdrew an application for an Investigational New
Drug permit for Laetrile (required before clinical trials could begin) because research
with animals had shown that it was not likely to be effective as an anticancer agent.
Uncertainty about the chemical identity of the drug also made questionable the
results that might be obtained.[30]

During the period of intense public and legislative interest in Laetrile that followed the FDA's reversal, promoters of Laetrile blamed a conspiracy among leaders in industry, government, and orthodox medicine. The AMA, the American Cancer Society, the Surgeon General, and an overwhelming majority of the nation's most qualified experts in the field did not recognize Laetrile as effective. Proponents of Laetrile gathered their own medical and scientific experts and had them testify, along with patients who felt they had been cured by Laetrile, before state legislatures, in hopes of being granted an exception to federal law. Largely sympathetic national media coverage helped Laetrile gain momentum. With little objective scientific evidence available to convince state legislators and the public that the drug was ineffective, and no results from rigorous, controlled clinical trials published, in 1977 Oklahoma became the first of 24 states to enjoin the FDA from impeding or preventing the importation and interstate transportation of Laetrile. In most cases, use was restricted to terminally ill cancer patients, and only with an affidavit from a practicing physician.[31]

Given that nearly all of the evidence for the safety and effectiveness of the drug in humans was testimonial or anecdotal, the National Cancer Institute (NCI) of the National Institutes of Health (NIH), the principal cancer research organization of the federal government, increasingly came under pressure from legislators and segments of orthodox medicine to undertake clinical studies. NCI had initially balked. Laetrile had already been repeatedly screened in test animals. Most of the test results were negative. Some showed marginal levels of activity that could not be reproduced. A clear showing of success in animals had traditionally served as a precursor to clinical testing. There were also ethical objections in some corners to the prospect of offering cancer patients a drug for which no anticancer activity had been convincingly demonstrated in studies to that point. Many people in and out of government objected to spending public funds on what they believed to be a worthless treatment. Others argued there were humanitarian reasons to conduct a trial since thousands of cancer patients were being exposed to a drug with "no known effectiveness, dubious safety, and poor manufacturing quality."[32]

In 1980, the NCI finally supported a multi-institutional investigation of Laetrile led by a distinguished cancer researcher at the Mayo Clinic. The final report of the trial made clear that in the group of 178 patients, Laetrile produced no discernible benefit, as measured by tumor size or prolongation of survival. More than three-quarters of the patients had died by the end of the study, and their survival times seemed fully consistent with those of patients receiving no treatment. Additionally, several patients had symptoms suggestive of cyanide toxicity or blood cyanide levels that approached the toxic range, a known side effect of Laetrile. Critics of Laetrile argued that the study demonstrated that it could not be considered either safe or effective. Laetrile promoters maintained that it was not administered properly in the study, that degraded Laetrile had been used, and that the researchers had stacked

LAETRILE WARNING

Cancer patients and their families are warned that:

LAETRILE IS WORTHLESS

Whether sold as a drug (amygdalin) or as a "vitamin" (B-17), Laetrile is worthless in the prevention, treatment or cure of cancer. The substance has no therapeutic or nutritional value.

LAETRILE IS DANGEROUS

Laetrile can be fatal for cancer patients who delay or give up regular medical treatment and take Laetrile instead.

Laetrile contains cyanide and can cause poisoning and death when taken by mouth. One infant is known dead of cyanide poisoning after swallowing fewer than five Laetrile tablets. At least 16 other deaths have been documented from ingestion of Laetrile ingredients (apricot and similar fruit pits).

Laetrile is especially hazardous if the injection form is taken by mouth. This can cause sudden death.

LAETRILE MAY BE CONTAMINATED

Laetrile is not routinely subject to FDA inspection for quality and purity as are all other drugs.
Analysis has shown some Laetrile to contain toxic contaminants. Ampules of Laetrile for injection have been found with mold and other adulterants which can be dangerous when injected.

Those who persist in the use of Laetrile or its ingredients should:

○ Be prepared to deal promptly with *acute* cyanide poisoning if the oral product is used. Vigorous medical treatment must be started immediately or death can result.

○ Watch for early symptoms of *chronic* cyanide poisoning, including weakness in the arms and legs and disorders of the nervous system.

○ Keep the drug out of reach of children.

GET THE FACTS

For full details about the hazards of Laetrile, see your family physician or a cancer specialist, or write the Food and Drug Administration, Laetrile, HFG-20, 5600 Fishers Lane, Rockville, Maryland 20857.

Donald Kennedy
Commissioner of Food and Drugs

Food and Drug Administration Pamphlet (1979).
(Courtesy of American Medical Association Archives)

the deck to ensure its failure. Nevertheless, in 1984 a district court dissolved all injunctions against the FDA, and the government began enforcing the statute against Laetrile as an unapproved drug. The FDA also prepared leaflets, published articles in the FDA *Drug Bulletin* (which was sent to more than a million health professionals), and issued a special widely disseminated public warning, only the second time in the FDA's history that such a warning had been issued. Laetrile seldom made the news in years to come, although it remained one of the most popular substances used by alleged cancer quacks. In 2001, an article in the *Los Angeles Times* reported that Laetrile had begun a revival or sorts, with more than 2,000 websites featuring the drug, most commonly sold as amgydalin or vitamin B17.[33]

At the 1984 Pepper Committee hearing on quackery, discussed at the beginning of this chapter, FDA associate commissioner of health affairs, Stuart L. Nightingale, addressed some of the important policy questions raised by the Laetrile experience. He suggested that the Laetrile phenomenon may have been preventable had its traffic been prosecuted vigorously at its inception. The fact that Laetrile continued to be traded and promoted without FDA approval throughout the 1970s indicated that the system could bend, if not break, in the presence of public pressure and skilled promotion. The debate, after all, had been settled, in the minds of most observers, only after a government-funded clinical trial revealed that Laetrile was neither safe nor effective. At the same time, Nightingale warned that another medical fraud of the same magnitude was likely on the horizon, if not already present. The widespread public interest in Laetrile and sympathetic media coverage of the case were harbingers of things to come.[34]

The AMA arguably would have been the ideal candidate for undertaking a campaign to address the problems outlined in the 1984 congressional report on quackery, but the multifaceted backlash against the association along with the closure of the Department of Investigation had marked the beginning of its gradual retreat from its decades-long position of leadership in the antiquackery network. Inspired in large part by the Laetrile case, a new generation of fraud fighters assumed responsibility for continuing the battle. Dr. Stephen Barrett, a psychiatrist, has been credited as the originator of the idea to establish private organizations dedicated to the antiquackery cause. Inspired by James Harvey Young's book *The Medical Messiahs*, which he described as a chronicle of "government efforts to control health hucksters," and a 1969 antichiropractic book written by a member of the AMA's Committee on Quackery, Barrett incorporated the Lehigh Valley Committee Against Health Fraud in 1970. Barrett eventually joined the AMA's Committee on Quackery and became a nationally known consumer advocate, author, and lecturer on the subject of health fraud in the 1970s. He also collaborated with two of the other most prominent antiquackery groups formed independently in California in the second half of the 1970s, amidst the mounting Laetrile controversy. Dr. William Jarvis, professor of preventive medicine at the Loma Linda University School of Medicine and member of the California attorney general's task force on health fraud, helped organize a group in southern California, while University of California–Berkeley's Dr. Thomas Jukes and oncologist-hematologist Dr. Wallace Sampson formulated plans to organize a group with similar objectives in northern California. In 1978, these groups merged to become the California Council against Health Fraud. By 1984, the council had expanded to the point that a majority of its members resided outside California, so the decision was made to change the name and scope of the organization. By the late 1980s, the renamed and re-energized National Council against Health Fraud (NCAHF) boasted 2,300 members.[35]

The NCAHF—self-identified as "Quackbusters Incorporated"—was made up primarily of physicians, scientists, and educators committed "to exposing medical fraud schemes, alerting governmental agencies to scams, and writing newsletters about the

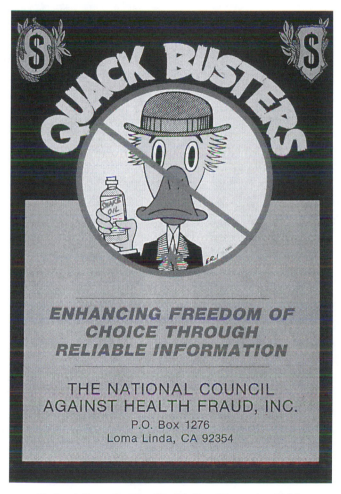

National Council against Health Fraud Poster (ca. 1986).
(Courtesy of the National Library of Medicine and Stephen Barrett, M.D.)

dangers of permitting such practices to proliferate." With this work, and a tiny annual
budget of $50,000 collected from small member donations, the NCAHF, more than
any other group, assumed responsibility for leading the antiquackery fight following
the closure of the AMA's Department of Investigation. "Sometimes you wonder
why you do this; but if someone isn't willing to stand up against quackery and fight
for truth and honesty, then society is in a lot of trouble," Jarvis observed. Under the
council's watch, some of the tactics and terms of the decades-long antiquackery
crusade would remain the same, while others would fundamentally change as the
twentieth century came to a close.[36]

MEDICAL QUACKERY, HEALTH FRAUD, AND ALTERNATIVE MEDICINE

In 1990, the results of a government study presaged a fundamental shift in the
enduring crusade against quackery. The federal Office of Technology Assessment
(OTA) report titled "Unconventional Cancer Treatments" had been published in
response to mounting debate surrounding the latest in a long line of controversial
cancer therapies. The OTA report began with the admission that an "objective,
informed examination of unconventional treatments" was difficult, if not impossible.
The "war over cancer therapies," which had been widely publicized in the American
media over the preceding decade, was described as a highly polarized situation in
which both sides had often described the opposition as a "malevolent monolith."
The report found that "the cancer establishment" had characterized alternative and
adjunctive cancer therapies as "the work of quacks preying on desperate and credulous
cancer victims," while the proponents of alternative cancer therapies had depicted
established therapies as "the 'cut, burn, and poison' therapies of a cynical and
profit-driven conspiracy." According to the OTA Summary, the acrimonious debate
between unconventional and mainstream communities reached well beyond scientific
arguments into social, legal, and consumer issues. Sides had been closely drawn, and
the rhetoric was often bitter and confrontational. The report concluded that "little
or no constructive dialog has yet taken place."[37]

In his critique of the OTA report, the chairman of the NCAHF board, Wallace
Sampson, insisted the very terms used had distorted the issues. Sampson argued that
in using the term "unconventional," the report had adopted the language of an
unwritten *Dictionary of the Absurd*, which had been created by proponents of quackery as a set of "euphemisms to disguise unproven, disproved, erroneous, anomalous,
ineffective or fraudulent practices." Sampson explained, "In one linguistic feat,
the 'holistic' movement labeled rational 'biomedicine' as 'reductionist' and rational
thinking as 'linear.' Unscientific thinking became 'nonlinear.' The term 'holistic'

diminished the status of measurement and rationality and inserted spirit, mind, and consciousness into medicine." He argued quackery and fraud were being obscured by euphemisms that included "unconventional" and "alternative." As far as he and other quackbusters were concerned, these terms indicated a fool's choice. Meanwhile, "unconventional" and "alternative" had not even been clearly defined by proponents. In the OTA report, "unconventional" was used to describe ineffective cancer therapies that until then had been considered quackery by Sampson and most other antiquackery crusaders.[38]

At the same time, many involved in the antiquackery cause had advocated their own linguistic shift, equally wrought with problems, by embracing the term "health fraud" over "quackery." At the Pepper Committee hearing, associate commissioner of health affairs Nightingale informed the chairman that the FDA had self-consciously embraced the term "health fraud" over "quackery," which they considered "less comprehensive." A book on dubious cancer treatments published by the American Cancer Society in 1991 referred to health fraud as the "avant-garde term for quackery," more useful because it carried "a more negative social stigma" than did quackery. The advantages of the term must have been readily apparent to the leadership in the National Council against Health Fraud as well. Health fraud was free of the past baggage associated with quackery and appeared to elevate the discussion. The term also led to some confusion, however, as it increasingly became associated with entirely different subjects in public discourse such as Medicare billing scams, counterfeit pharmaceuticals, misconduct in medical research, and illicit drugs. These were the types of health fraud that increasingly captured headlines as the twentieth century drew to a close.[39]

Quackery still had its own problems with definitions. William Jarvis, then president of the NCAHF, noted that one definition of a quack—"a pretender to medical skills"—often meant someone who practiced medicine without a license. But he also estimated that some 60 percent of cancer quacks alone were licensed practitioners. Another definition of quackery put the emphasis on fraudulent representation, but this also had its faults. "Many quacks do not intentionally pervert the truth as much as they perversely believe in falsity almost as a sort of religion. In this sense, not all quacks are frauds, and not all frauds are quacks," Jarvis observed. Taking misinformation as the crucial ingredient in quackery also had its problems. Jarvis considered the use of placebos (without the patient's knowledge) a part of a physician's proper management of a patient. The NACHF ultimately adopted the definition of a quack used by the 1984 Pepper Committee—"anyone who promotes medical schemes or remedies known to be false, or which are unproven, for a profit"—which offered the means of distinguishing innovative and legitimate experimental medical care from quackery, according to the council's president.[40]

In the closing decade of the twentieth century, professional opponents of health fraud chose to focus primarily on two issues, each framed by this definition of quackery: opposition to increasingly popular medical therapies that they believed had not been definitively proven (most of which fell under the category of alternative medicine, which they considered a misnomer); and improving the regulation of health products (almost exclusively over-the-counter items) and health services (by and large those provided by alternative practitioners). But whereas federal policies had predominantly been used in the past to support the objectives of antiquackery forces— first with the Pure Food and Drugs Act of 1906, then with the Federal Food, Drug and Cosmetic Act of 1938, and later with the Kefauver-Harris Amendments in 1962—the 1990s brought a remarkable series of developments that undermined or frustrated these efforts.[41]

In 1991, the creation of a new federal agency, dedicated to the study of what it called unorthodox medical practices, came as a shock to many in the antiquackery camp. In November 1991, the Senate Appropriations Committee responsible for funding the National Institutes of Health declared itself "not satisfied that the conventional medical community as symbolized at the NIH has fully explored the potential that exists in unconventional medical practices." To "more adequately explore these unconventional medical practices," the committee requested that the NIH establish an advisory panel to "to fully investigate and validate these practices . . . to screen and select the procedures for investigation and to recommend a research program to fully test the most promising unconventional medical practices." With little support from leaders at the NIH, and an initial budget of $2 million, the Office for the Study of Unconventional Medical Practices (OSUMP) became the first government-sponsored organization devoted to the study of alternative medicine. Given the historical conflict between the forces against quackery and the diverse ranks of alternative medicine, the creation of the office represented a major shift in federal policy.[42]

In July 1992, *Newsweek* reported that "in an unprecedented Washington sanctioned version of East meets West" the newly convened office was finally "getting serious" about scientifically evaluating treatments that were "once regarded as way out." Investigative journalist Daniel Glick explained how the medical establishment had for years shunned "alternative medicine" while insurance companies refused to pay for it and federal officials harassed its practitioners. "It's like the Berlin wall coming down," explained Dr. Dean Ornish of the University of California–San Francisco. According to Glick: "Like supplicants before the altar of medical respectability, rolfers, acupuncturists, homeopaths, herbalists, therapeutic-touch practitioners, massage therapists and others" had besieged the NIH with requests to have their healing arts scrutinized by the scientific method, and now the task of figuring out just how to study these therapies had come to the fore. The *Newsweek* article closed by suggesting: "If science can separate the charlatans and profiteers from the true healers, the search may unearth a truly radical cure—keeping people healthier and lowering the bill at the same time."[43]

Describing how the NIH, "the country's pocketbook for biomedical research and long a stern protector of the most rigorous brand of science, is about to start venturing into the realm of alternative medicine," *New York Times* reporter Natalie Angier noted that some researchers had already hailed this initiative as "visionary," while others "likened it to governance by horoscope." Those who favored the office argued that it could help validate some commonly used but marginalized remedies that people had sworn by for hundreds if not thousands of years, by focusing on the therapies that were most useful and how they worked in the body. Supporters also noted that alternative therapies were often much less invasive than conventional medical approaches and were often far less expensive—an important consideration in a time of exploding health costs. "I think it's a great idea that the NIH is going to do this, and I support them 110 percent," said Dr. Halsted R. Holman, a professor of medicine at the Stanford University School of Medicine. "It's unfortunate that a lot of these therapies are viewed as alternative, because it puts a stamp of craziness on things that are potentially valid." Dr. Jennifer Jacobs, a member of the office's ad hoc advisory panel, hoped the office would at last give her and her homeopathic colleagues the financial support to prove the worthiness of their treatments and the science behind their approach. "We can treat illnesses for which modern medicine doesn't have the answer, like chronic fatigue, menstrual problems, arthritis," she said. According to Jacobs, homeopaths had not been able to document this on a large scale primarily because of a lack of funding for research.[44]

Critics in the antiquackery camp warned of a threefold danger in alternative medicine—wasting money on patently useless therapies, subjecting oneself to potentially dangerous unregulated and untested practices, and potentially dismissing or neglecting regular medicine in the process. Stephen Barrett explained, "Quackery isn't about selling products and services—it's about selling misbeliefs. If you are not sick, these misbeliefs may not cause you serious harm. But if you are sick, they may kill you." Barrett and other quackbusters dismissed homeopathy as the "ultimate fake." NCAHF founder William Jarvis maintained that proponents of homeopathy were either "stupid" or "deliberately fraudulent." He criticized acupuncture as a practiced "based on primitive and fanciful concepts of health and disease that bear no relationship to present scientific knowledge." Jarvis rejected macrobiotics as "not only unproven but a bizarre and dangerous diet for sick people." He considered aromatherapy "crazy." "If you are going to claim that something is safe and effective for human disease, you need to have proof," he insisted.[45]

In 1993, a landmark report in the *New England Journal of Medicine* found that "unconventional medicine" in fact already had an "enormous presence" in the U.S. health-care system, whether it had been proven or not. Specifically, the survey found that a full one-third of adults in the United States (34 percent) had used at least one alternative therapy. The report provided another startling finding: "The estimated number of visits made in 1990 to providers of unconventional therapy was greater than the number of total visits to primary care doctors nationwide, and the amount spent out of pocket on unconventional therapy was comparable to the amount spent out of pocket by Americans for all hospitalizations." This included an estimated 425 million visits by Americans to alternative medicine providers (10 percent more than the 388 million visits to primary care physicians). Expenditures associated with the use of unconventional therapies, meanwhile, amounted to approximately $13.7 billion, three-quarters of which was paid out of pocket. This was more than the $12.8 billion spent out of pocket annually for hospital care.[46]

The fact that the 1990 study defined unconventional therapies as those "neither taught widely in US medical schools nor generally available in US hospitals" implied how marginalized unorthodox therapies had been and highlighted the novelty of the government-supported research program for the new NIH office. For the purposes of the study, "unconventional medicine" referred to 16 interventions found to be representative of unconventional therapies used commonly in the United States on the basis of pilot research. This included lifestyle choices such as special diets, mind-body techniques including meditation and self-help groups, as well as alternative systems of medicine including chiropractic and homeopathy. An accompanying article, in the same issue of the *New England Journal of Medicine*, noted that roughly one-third of the studied unconventional practices entailed theories that were considered "patently unscientific and in direct competition with conventional medicine, for example, chiropractic, spiritual healing, herbal medicine, 'energy healing' (with crystals and machines), homeopathy, and acupuncture." The author maintained that some of these treatments were "probably quackery," some of them were "just the American version of the health spa," and others could be considered lifestyle choices more than therapeutic interventions.[47]

The *New England Journal of Medicine* study was published at the peak of a related legislative struggle that had begun with the hope of strengthening the ability of federal agencies to combat health fraud, but ultimately had the opposite outcome. In the early 1990s, two bills had been introduced in Congress in the hopes of tightening control over the largely unregulated vitamin and supplement industries; increasing the FDA's enforcement powers; raising penalties for violating the Food, Drug and Cosmetic Act; and restricting advertising materials and labels. In response, the health-food industry and supportive consumers across the country led a massive campaign that urged Congress to "preserve the consumer's freedom of choice to choose dietary supplements." Industry leaders warned retailers that they would be put out of business if Congress granted the FDA increased regulatory powers. Industry-backed consumer alerts warned that vitamins and supplements would be stripped from the shelves of drugs stores and health-food stores, and made available only by prescription. The end result was passage of the Dietary Supplement Health and Education Act (DSHEA) of 1994, which substantially weakened FDA oversight.[48]

The DSHEA broadly defined a dietary supplement as any product "intended to supplement the diet" that included one or more of the following ingredients: vitamins, minerals, herbs or other botanicals, amino acids, or other dietary substance used to supplement the diet by increasing total dietary intake. Products meeting this definition had to bear nutritional labeling and could not include health claims that made any explicit reference to any diseases. As long as they existed before 1984, they were allowed to make general claims about the product's effect on the body without any evidence. This allowed supplements to be advertised as drug-like products while avoiding the strict premarket FDA review that conventional drug products had to endure. Since manufacturers did not have to submit safety information for supplements, this also placed the burden of proof on the FDA, forcing the agency to rely on adverse event reports, product sampling, information in the scientific literature, and other sources of evidence of danger.[49]

The cost-benefit analysis of the DSHEA revealed underlying philosophical, political, and economic priorities that had shaped the campaign against quackery for much of the twentieth century. Supporters argued that dietary supplements offered an inexpensive means to promote health, were less dangerous and harmful than drugs, and empowered consumers to make choices related to preventive health care. Other supporters embraced the libertarian ideal of a free-market philosophy. They believed that while the government could try to educate consumers, it was up to people to make their own decisions about how to spend their money. Some more vociferous supporters also denigrated the FDA as an overly intrusive enemy bent on controlling the medical marketplace. Critics, by contrast, identified a wide range of unreasonable risks associated with the new regulatory regime. In terms of health costs, critics noted that some dietary supplements had already been proven unhealthy or dangerous, while others were fraudulent. They warned that people would be wasting their money, abandoning their physicians, and even risking their lives. They believed that outlandish claims of some manufacturers would provide false hope and in the most extreme cases might encourage the rejection of modern medicine, increased paranoia, and "irrational anti-government ideas." While the potential for these effects continued to be debated for years to come, one thing was clear: the DSHEA played a central role in the subsequent explosion of the supplement industry. In 1995, the stock of publicly traded supplement companies increased in volume by 80 percent. The overall market grew by about 15 percent within two years.[50]

The NCAHF's Barrett warned that economic and political priorities made it easy to forget that it had taken a tragedy—the poisoning caused by the use of an elixir of sulfanilamide—to prompt Congress to pass the Food, Drug and Cosmetic Act of

1938, while it took reports of birth defects among the children of women who took thalidomide during pregnancy to secure passage of the Kefauver-Harris Amendments in 1962. He predicted that the combination of Congress's lack of interest in protecting consumers and general public ignorance about the potential dangers of these products might ultimately have similarly disastrous consequences.[51]

In the 1990s, consumer protection remained a major concern for quackbusters like Barrett as the network of reformers and regulators became fragmented and preoccupied with other pressing issues. Many of the same players continued their educational and regulatory efforts, including Better Business Bureaus, nongovernmental or voluntary health agencies, and state and federal agencies. The AMA continued to act as a resource in some cases, but its policies and activity in the field of health fraud remained limited. After nearly two decades without a national conference dedicated to the subject of quackery, members of the antiquackery network finally met in the 1980s in a series of National Health Fraud Conferences in an effort to coordinate activities and share information. The agencies assigned the task of policing quackery remained understaffed, circumscribed in authority, and overburdened with a heavy load of other responsibilities. The FDA possessed tools to act against promoters of dangerous or ineffective drugs and devices, including product seizures and injunctions, but given the financial and resource burden of court cases, the agency rarely used criminal prosecution to go after suspected quacks. The FTC retained its authority to act against false and misleading advertising, but the agency handled only five or six cases a year involving alleged health frauds. Stephen Barrett, who had already written 25 books on the subject of health fraud by 1990, warned, "Since government action against quackery is limited, individuals wishing to protect themselves must be vigilant" by relying on their own judgment. His list of the most prevalent and persistent forms of quackery included worthless remedies for cancer and arthritis, the false claims of chiropractic treatments, ineffective homeopathic remedies, fraudulent weight-reducing schemes, the overselling of vitamins and supplements, and other dubious mail-order schemes to defraud consumers.[52]

Antiquackery groups continued to exploit many of the old tools used to combat health fraud. They published and promoted reference works, consumer guides, magazine articles, and newsletters designed to keep interested readers abreast of the latest schemes and scandals. One of the more popular compendiums by Barrett and Jarvis of the NCAHF, *The Health Robbers: A Close Look at Quackery in America*, topped 500 pages in its 1993 third edition and included an introduction by popular advice columnist Ann Landers. Jarvis also edited the bimonthly *NCAHF Newsletter*, which offered some of the most scathing analyses of alleged quackery available to consumers. Council member Barrett reportedly used whole networks of volunteer undercover operatives to infiltrate unorthodox groups for the NCAHF. Barrett published the results of these studies in his monthly newsletter *Nutrition Forum*. He also used the accumulated evidence as the grist for successful court actions, U.S. Postal Service mail fraud convictions, and FTC probes of questionable marketing techniques at health-food stores. Although antiquackery forces may have been fewer in number compared to earlier decades, they remained equally persistent and no more restrained.[53]

To these old-school techniques and tactics, the NCAHF's Barrett added the popular website Quackwatch in December 1996. Although Quackwatch operated on a shoestring budget funded mainly by small donations and profits from the sale of Barrett's books, it quickly became one of the most widely cited sources of information on quackery in the world, claiming over 100,000 hits a month by 1999. Barrett received so much notoriety from the site that he was interviewed by *Time* and *People*. Barrett was billed as "one of America's premier debunkers" of what he liked to call quackery. While his site was widely cited by doctors and medical writers, it had also made Barrett a "lightning rod for herbalists, homeopaths, and assorted true believers" who regularly vilified him as "dishonest, incompetent, a bully, and a Nazi." Barrett unflinchingly excoriated specific promoters, entire systems of alternative medical practice, and institutions that supported what he called the "quack menace."[54]

In July 1997, *Science* magazine reported that some big guns were taking aim at one of the institutions that Barrett targeted—the NIH's renamed Office of Alternative Medicine (OAM), a place the magazine referred to as the "home of far-out ideas on medical therapy." Amidst Senate hearings to discuss renewal of the OAM's $12.5 million budget, a number of top scientists had sent letters to members of the appropriations committee, recommending that funding be cut or eliminated. Nobel Prize–winning biologist Paul Berg called OAM "an embarrassment to serious scientists," adding that "quackery will always prey on the gullible and uninformed, but we certainly should not provide it cover from the NIH." Biologist Ursula Goodenough of Washington University in St. Louis wrote that "Nothing coming from OAM indicates that it is conducting or planning any studies that would put any alternative treatments to [a] scientific test." Former presidential science adviser D. Allan Bromley, meanwhile, warned that OAM had given prestige to "highly dubious practices, some of which clearly violate basic laws of physics and more clearly resemble witchcraft than medicine." He recommended terminating the office.[55]

Despite facing widespread opposition, the Office of Alternative Medicine was still upgraded to the National Center for Complementary and Alternative Medicine (NCCAM) in 1999, a change that expanded its budget to $50 million and granted the new NCCAM Director Stephen Straus an unprecedented opportunity. Straus quickly reassured critics and skeptics that he wanted to allay fears of NIH-sponsored quackery. In an article titled "Stephen Straus's Impossible Job," published in *Science* in 2000, Straus insisted he was not an advocate of alternative therapies, only an advocate of good science. In taking the NCCAM job, he was also cognizant of the fact that he was walking a tightrope—skeptical scientists and powerful supporters of alternative medicine would both be measuring his performance by their own criteria.[56]

The same year that Congress created NCCAM, a report from the Stanford Center for Research in Disease and Prevention offered an explanation for the appeal of a wide range of therapies that had been dismissed as quackery by skeptics. The study concluded that most users found a number of health-care alternatives to be "more congruent with their own values, beliefs, and philosophical orientations toward health and life." Given evidence that the vast majority of medical symptoms experienced by people were being self-diagnosed and self-treated, and the fact that a significant portion of alternative medicine use fell into the realm of self-care, it appeared that unconventional therapies offered consumers a greater amount of autonomy in therapeutic decision making.[57]

Meanwhile, as the twentieth century drew to a close, the critiques of NCCAM's work, and critical explanations for the appeal of complementary and alternative medicine, recapitulated many of the arguments that antiquackery crusaders had employed for at least a hundred years. They argued that studying complementary and alternative medicine (CAM) was a waste of effort and precious research money. They focused on what they called the "pseudoscientific" basis of many CAM practices. They identified a conspiracy to undermine the scientific basis of mainstream medicine. Critics attributed NCCAM's existence to political maneuvering and denied the value in studying medical modalities that had no clear basis in medical science. They assumed that people who chose complementary and alternative medicine made the same mistakes that victims of quackery had made all along.[58]

CONCLUSION

On the occasions when members of the remaining, fragmented antiquackery network addressed the more inscrutable reasons for the persistence of quackery as the twentieth century came to a close, they most often came to the same unsatisfying conclusion. The NCAHF's Jarvis, for example, identified what he called an unavoidable "cultural vulnerability" to health fraud that arose "chiefly from the fact that beliefs central to our views of ourselves and our place in the world, good ideas many of them, can be exaggerated and distorted." He admitted, like others, that it could therefore not be expected that efforts to combat medical quackery would ever eradicate it. "Rather, like any chronic disease, we will have to live with it while we do our best to fight it," Jarvis concluded. Jarvis and other leaders in the antiquackery crusade nevertheless held to the same hope that the father of the antiquackery network, Arthur J. Cramp, had expressed in the early twentieth century. In addition to increased regulatory authority, Cramp believed education and information would be the primary tools in future battles. Educational efforts and regulations ultimately nevertheless failed to have their intended effect. In fact, as the twentieth century drew to a close, complementary and alternative medicine became an increasingly popular choice for Americans. CAM advocates successfully argued that many therapeutic approaches long derided as quackery should be considered legitimate, mainstream complements to orthodox medical practice. This left antiquackery crusaders to preach the common early twentieth-century mantra of *caveat emptor*—let the buyer beware.[59]

Medical therapies judged to be quackery shared a common characteristic throughout the twentieth century. They appealed to patients' values, beliefs, and philosophical orientations toward health and life. While historians and quackbusters have occasionally acknowledged this appeal in offering an explanation for the proliferation of medical alternatives, more often than not they have primarily attributed the persistent buying and selling of alleged quack medicines to a shared delusion. Presuming a shared delusion, however, meant that antiquackery crusaders at the end of the twentieth century refused to believe that anything in the field of complementary and alternative medicine might actually work, despite evidence to the contrary. By categorically condemning dozens of popular therapeutic practices, the most ardent quackbusters even managed to alienate some of their former network allies. Strident skeptics failed to adequately address the shortcomings of their own crusade. Meanwhile, those pilloried as quacks reaped the benefits of their apparent successes. Quackery—defined by quackbusters so broadly that it included dozens of increasingly mainstream therapeutic practices—arguably remained as popular as ever.[60]

NOTES

INTRODUCTION

1. Arthur J. Cramp, *Nostrums and Quackery and Pseudo-Medicine* (Chicago: American Medical Association, 1936), vii.

2. Thomas Gieryn, *Cultural Boundaries of Science: Credibility on the Line* (Chicago: University of Chicago Press, 1999); Jackie Goode and David Greatbatch, "Boundary Work: The Production and Consumption of Health Information and Advice," *Journal of Consumer Culture* 5 (2005): 315–37; Gert H. Brieger, "Bodies and Borders: A New Cultural History of Medicine," *Perspectives in Biology and Medicine* 47 (Summer 2004): 402–21; Paul Starr, *The Social Transformation of American Medicine: The Rise of a Sovereign Profession and the Making of a Vast Industry* (New York: Basic Books, 1982).

3. Arthur J. Cramp to E. E. Valentini, 21 March 1929; Cramp to Clarence W. Brown, 8 April 1929; Box 290, Folder 1, Historical Health Fraud Collection (HFF), American Medical Association (Chicago, Illinois).

4. James Harvey Young, *The Medical Messiahs: A Social History of Health Quackery in Twentieth-Century America* (Princeton, NJ: Princeton University Press, 1992), 26.

CHAPTER ONE

1. Dan King, *Quackery Unmasked: A Consideration of the Most Prominent Empirical Schemes of the Present Time, with an Enumeration of Some of the Causes Which Contribute to Their Support* (Boston: David Clapp, 1858), 322.

2. King, *Quackery Unmasked*, 4–5; J. P. Epperson, *A Bomb in the Camp of the Enemy, or an Exposure of Quackery and "Patent Medicines"* (Columbia, TN: Rosboroughs & Kidd, 1845), 5–6.

3. Joseph F. Kett, *The Formation of the American Medical Profession: The Role of Institutions, 1780–1860* (New Haven, CT: Yale University Press, 1968); Paul Starr, *The Social Transformation of American Medicine: The Rise of a Sovereign Profession and the Making of a Vast Industry* (New York: Basic Books, 1982); James H. Cassedy, *Medicine in America: A Short History* (Baltimore: Johns Hopkins University Press, 1991); King, *Quackery Unmasked*, 295; "Character and Abuses of the Medical Profession: Rules and Regulations of the Boston Medical Association," *North American Review* 32 (April 1831): 368.

4. Lamar Riley Murphy, *Enter the Physician: The Transformation of Domestic Medicine, 1760–1860* (Tuscaloosa: University of Alabama Press, 1991); John S. Haller, *American Medicine in Transition, 1840–1910* (Urbana: University of Illinois Press, 1981), 65–83; George Rosen, *The Structure of American Medical Practice, 1875–1941* (Philadelphia: University of Pennsylvania Press, 1983); John C. Burnham, "American Medicine's Golden Age: What Happened to It," *Science* 215 (March 19, 1982): 1474–79. Burnham suggests that during the nineteenth century, physicians seeking to professionalize were "fair game for hostile comment, with quacks and sectarians on one side and the practitioners' actual therapeutic impotence on the other," 1474.

5. Arthur Wrobel, *Pseudo-Science and Society in Nineteenth Century America* (Lexington: University Press of Kentucky, 1987); Catherine L. Albanese, "Physic and Metaphysic in Nineteenth-Century America: Medical Sectarians and Religious Healing," *Church History* 55 (Dec. 1986): 489–502; Alanson Mosher, *Learned Quackery Exposed: Or the Difference Shown Between Poisons and Medicines* (Schoharie, NY: Gallup and Lawyer, 1846); "More 'Regular' Quackery," *Independent Botanic Advocate* 1 (Sept. 1839): 1–2.

6. For an overview of sectarianism in the nineteenth century, see William Rothstein, *American Physicians in the Nineteenth Century: From Sects to Science* (Baltimore: Johns Hopkins University Press, 1972); Norman Gevitz, ed., *Other Healers: Unorthodox Medicine in America* (Baltimore: Johns Hopkins University Press, 1988); James C. Whorton, *Nature Cures: The History of Alternative Medicine in America* (New York: Oxford University Press, 2002); Worthington Hooker, *The Treatment Due from the Profession to Physicians Who Become Homœopathic Practitioners* (Norwhich, CT: John G. Cooley, 1852). On therapeutics as a systematic approach, see Charles E. Rosenberg, "The Therapeutic Revolution: Medicine, Meaning, and Social Change in Nineteenth-Century America," in Morris J. Vogel and Charles E. Rosenberg, eds., *The Therapeutic Revolution: Essays in the Social History of American Medicine* (Philadelphia: University of Pennsylvania Press, 1979), 4–10; John Harley Warner, *The Therapeutic Perspective: Medical Practice, Knowledge, and Identity in America, 1820–1885* (Princeton, NJ: Princeton University Press, 1997), 13; Physician quoted in John

Harley Warner, "Medical Sectarianism, Therapeutic Conflict, and the Shaping of Orthodox Professional Identity in Antebellum American Medicine," in William F. Bynum and Roy Porter, eds., *Medical Fringe and Medical Orthodoxy* (London: Croom Helm, 1987) 246; Whorton's *Nature Cures* provides extensive coverage of each important nineteenth-century sectarian group.

7. These terms are drawn from sectarian medical journals (1838–1846) and are cited in Warner, "Medical Sectarianism," 256; "Some Things Explained," *American Journal of Homeopathy* 1 (1846): 13–14; Benjamin Colby, *A Guide to Health* (Nashua, NH: Gill, 1844), v.

8. Epperson, *A Bomb in the Camp of the Enemy*, 7–8; Philadelphia Medical Society, *First Report of the Committee of the Philadelphia Medical Society on Quack Medicines* (Philadelphia: Judah Dobson, 1828); Augustus Mason, *The Quackery of the Age: A Satire of the Times* (Boston: White, Lewis & Potter, 1845); John Parascandola, "Patent Medicines in Nineteenth-Century America," *Caduceus* 1 (1985): 1–39.

9. James Harvey Young, *The Toadstool Millionaires: A Social History of Patent Medicines in America Before Federal Regulation* (Princeton, NJ: Princeton University Press, 1961); John Parascandola, "Patent Medicines and the Public's Health," *Public Health Reports* 114 (Jul./Aug. 1999): 320; Edward H. Dixon, *A Treatise on Diseases of the Sexual Organs: Adapted to Popular and Professional Reading, and the Exposition of Quackery, Professional and Otherwise* (New York: Taylor, 1845); Frederick Fact, "Stop Thief!!! King Calomel Outlawed: Being an Hours Peep at the Mother of All Medical Mischief" (Boston, 1834), 2 (available at the New Hampshire Historical Society, Box 615, Folder 142).

10. William Porter, *Life and Its Forces: Health and Disease Correctly Defined: A Reliable Guide to Health without the Use of Mineral or Vegetable Poisons, or Irritants* (Hartford, CT: Case, Lockwood & Brainard Co., 1878), 73; John A. Brown, *Quackery Exposed, or a Few Remarks on the Thomsonian System of Medicine; Consisting of Testimonies and Extracts From Various Writers* (Boston: [s.n.], 1833), 22.

11. John Harley Warner, "Science in Medicine," *Osiris* 1 (1985): 37-58; Richard H. Shryock, "Empiricism versus Rationalism in American Medicine, 1650–1950," *Proceedings of the American Antiquarian Society* (April 1969): 99–150; Bernard Aschner, "Empiricism and Rationalism in Past and Present Medicine" *Bulletin of the History of Medicine* 17 (1945): 269–86; J. H. Nutting, *An Essay on Some of the Principles of Medical Delusion* (Boston: David Clapp, 1853), 5–17.

12. Epperson, *A Bomb in the Camp of the Enemy*, 10–12; King, *Quackery Unmasked*, 248–51 and 276–78; Henry Gibbons, *Illustrations of the Literature of Quackery* (San Francisco: [s.n.], 1874).

13. King, *Quackery Unmasked*, 265; Laurens Hull, *Annual Address Delivered before the Medical Society of the State of New York* (Albany: J. Munsell, 1839).

14. King, *Quackery Unmasked*, 265–71 and 301–06; "Character and Abuses of the Medical Profession," *North American Review* 32 (Apr. 1831): 367–86; James Jackson, "Currents and Counter-Currents in Medical Science," *North American Review* 93 (Jul. 1861): 195–211; John P. Harrison, *A Lecture on the Best Mode of Discouraging Empiricism* (Cincinnati, OH: R. P. Donogh, 1843); Othniel Hart Taylor, *Medical Reform and the Present System of Medical Instruction: An Address Delivered at the Semi-Annual Meeting of the New Jersey Medical Society* (Camden, NJ: Gray & Elliott, 1850).

15. Carl H. Horsch, *Facts Regarding the Medical Profession and Sanitary Science: The Pathies, Isms and Quackery* (Dover, NH: State Press Job Print, 1883), 19; Warner, "Medical Sectarianism," 240–41; Starr, *The Social Transformation of American Medicine*, 94–102; William Rothstein, *American Medical Schools and the Practice of Medicine: A History* (New York: Oxford University Press, 1987).

16. For a discussion of Holmes on homeopathy, see Martin Kaufman, *Homeopathy in America: The Rise and Fall of a Medical Heresy* (Baltimore: Johns Hopkins University Press, 1971), 35–43; Whorton, *Nature Cures*, 72–75; and for the broader context of the contemporary assault on homeopathy, see Harris L. Coulter, *Divided Legacy: A History of the Schism in Medical Thought* Vol. 3 (Washington, DC: McGrath, 1973), 158–219; Oliver Wendell Holmes, "Homeopathy and Its Kindred Delusions," in *Medical Essays: 1842–1882* (Boston: Houghton, Mifflin, 1899), 106–17.

17. Warner, "Medical Sectarianism," 246; Dr. Badger, *The Principles of Physiology and Medical Botany Illustrated: Fully Demonstrating the Great Principles of Life and Death* (Petersborough: K. C. Scott, 1859), 3.

18. Warner, *The Therapeutic Perspective*, 37–57; "Recent Advances in Medicine," *Science* 17 (Mar. 27, 1891): 170–71.

19. Whorton, *Nature Cures*, 3–16; Warner, *The Therapeutic Perspective*, 258–83; Epperson, *A Bomb in the Camp of the Enemy*, 19.

20. Louis Elsberg, "Lecture, Introductory to the Eighty-Seventh Course of Instruction in the Medical Department of Dartmouth College," 1883, New Hampshire Historical Society, Call no. 378.73 D227ma; Warner, *The Therapeutic Perspective*, 258–68.

21. George M. Sternberg, "Science and Pseudo-Science in Medicine," *Science* 5 (Feb. 5, 1897): 199–206; W. F. Bynum, *Science and the Practice of Medicine in the Nineteenth Century* (Cambridge: Cambridge University Press, 1994), 17; Alfred George Tebault, "Notes on Medical Lectures Taken at the University of Virginia: Alfred George Tebault Papers," cited in Warner, *The Therapeutic Perspective*, 341.

22. Guenter B. Risse, "The Road to Twentieth-Century Therapeutics: Shifting Perspectives and Approaches," in Gregory J. Higby and Elaine C. Stroud, eds., *The Inside Story of Medicines: A Symposium* (Madison, WI: American Institute of the History of Pharmacy, Publication No. 16, 1997), pp. 51–73.

23. James Harvey Young, *The Medical Messiahs: A Social History of Health Quackery in Twentieth-Century America* (Princeton, NJ: Princeton University Press, 1992), 25. Young uses data from the Bureau of the Census as the basis for these figures.

24. Sternberg, "Science and Pseudo-Science in Medicine," 202–06; "Aerated Oxygen," pamphlet from General Western Offices (Nashua, NH: AN Flinn, ca. 1890), New Hampshire Historical Society, Call no. 615.5 A254; Young, *The Medical Messiahs*, 27.

25. W. F. Bynum, *Science and Practice*, 165; Young, *The Medical Messiahs*, 27.

26. Nutting, *An Essay on Some of the Principles of Medical Delusion*, 20–29; Epperson, *A Bomb in the Camp of the Enemy*, 13–14.

27. Willis P. King, *Quacks and Quackery in Missouri* (St. Louis: [s.n.], 1882); Charles F. J. Lehlbach, *State Protection against Quackery* (Newark, NJ: [s.n.], 1888); Henry Gathmann and

John J. Seelman, *Medicine vs. Quackery* (Milwaukee, WI: Western Publishing, 1901); Epperson, *A Bomb in the Camp of the Enemy*, 13–14; King, *Quackery Unmasked*, 258.

28. "Code of Ethics of the American Medical Association," Chapter II, Article 1, Section 4. *New York Journal of Medicine* 9 (1847): 261; F. J. L. Blasingame, ed., *Digest of Official Actions, 1846–1958* Vol. 1 (Chicago: American Medical Association, 1959), 177–96.

29. Harry M. Marks, *The Progress of Experiment: Science and Therapeutic Reform in the United States, 1900–1990* (New York: Cambridge University Press, 1997), 23; Starr, *The Social Transformation of American Medicine*, 127–29; Martin Pernick, *A Calculus of Suffering: Pain, Professionalism and Anesthesia in Nineteenth-Century America* (New York: Columbia University Press, 1985), 21–31 and 93–124; Morris Fishbein, *A History of the American Medical Association, 1847 to 1947* (Philadelphia: W. B. Saunders, 1947); James G. Burrow, *AMA: Voice of American Medicine* (Baltimore: Johns Hopkins Press, 1963); William G. Rothstein, *American Physicians.*

30. Blasingame, *Digest of Official Actions*, 178–79; Fishbein, *A History of the American Medical Association*, 163–64. Fishbein notes that many *Journal* subscribers even cancelled their subscriptions in protest. The dilemma facing the board of trustees was how to adhere to standards and still pay the journal's publication. They took as their standard what other journals were doing; "Report of the Board of Trustees," *JAMA* 22 (Sept. 12, 1894): 804.

31. King, *Quackery Unmasked*, 301; "The Subject of Medical Legislation," *Science* 10 (Aug. 19, 1887): 85; William G. Eggleston, Austin Flint, and R. Ogden Doremus, "The Open Door of Quackery," *North American Review* 149 (Oct. 1889): 492.

32. William G. Eggleston, "The Closing Door of Quackery," *North American Review* 152 (May 1891): 633–35.

33. J. R. Jones, "Medical Education," *JAMA* 37 (1901): 743; Kenneth Ludmerer, *Learning to Heal: The Development of American Medical Education* (New York: Basic Books, 1985).

34. Ludmerer, *Learning to Heal*; Starr, *The Social Transformation of American Medicine*; Rosen, *The Structure of American Medical Practice*; Rothstein, *American Physicians*,; Ronald Numbers, ed. *The Education of American Physicians: Historical Essays* (Berkeley: University of California Press, 1980); Kett, *The Formation of the American Medical Profession*; Thomas Neville Bonner, *Becoming a Physician: Medical Education in Britain, France, Germany and the United States, 1750–1945* (New York: Oxford University Press, 1995).

35. Rothstein suggests that modern medicine emerged almost entirely because of scientific advances, in *American Physicians*. For an overview of changes in basic science instruction during this period, on subjects including anatomy, physiology, specialization, internal medicine, chemistry, pathology, public health, pharmacology, and surgery, see Ronald Numbers, ed., *The Education of American Physicians: Historical Essays* (Berkeley: University of California Press, 1980). On sectarian developments, see Coulter, *Divided Legacy*, 328–82; Kaufman, *Homeopathy in America*, 76–109; Haller, *The History of American Homeopathy*, 182–223; John S. Haller, *Medical Protestants: The Eclectics in American Medicine, 1825–1939* (Carbondale: Southern Illinois University Press, 1994), 198–219. On the impact of bacteriology specifically, see Nancy Tomes, *The Gospel of Germs: Men, Women, and the Microbe in American Life* (Cambridge, MA: Harvard University Press, 1998); Vogel and Rosenberg, eds.,

The Therapeutic Revolution, 3–108. For more information on related changes, see John Parascandola, *The Development of American Pharmacology: John J. Abel and the Shaping of a Discipline* (Baltimore: Johns Hopkins University Press, 1992); Charles Rosenberg, *The Care of Strangers: The Rise of America's Hospital System* (New York: Basic Books, 1987), 142–54 and 262–85; Starr, *The Social Transformation of American Medicine*, 99–103; Richard H. Shryock, *Medical Licensing in America, 1650–1965* (Baltimore: Johns Hopkins Press, 1967), 43–33.

36. J. R. Jones, "Medical Education," *JAMA* 35 (Sept. 21, 1901): 776.

37. King, *Quackery Unmasked*, 317; Eggleston, Flint, and Doremus, "The Open Door of Quackery," 492, 504.

CHAPTER TWO

1. A photocopy of this article from *Grocery World* (Dec. 6, 1915) was sent to the American Medical Association for their files on quackery by C. H. LaWall, Box 23, Folder 1, HHF.

2. "Dangers of the Use of Proprietary Remedies," *JAMA* 35 (July 21, 1900): 166; J. A. Witherspoon, "A Protest against Some of the Evils of the Profession of Medicine," *JAMA* 34 (June 23, 1900): 1589.

3. The value of drug products sold is taken from U.S. Census Office, *Report on Manufactures of the United States* (Washington, DC: Government Printing Office, 1882), 34, 63; and *Manufactures* (Washington, DC: Government Printing Office, 1902), 180–91, 340–41. On the role of the patent medicine industry in the rise of professional advertising, see Jackson Lears, *Fables of Abundance: A Cultural History of Advertising in America* (New York: Basic Books, 1994), 88–99; and Pamela Laird, *Advertising Progress: American Business and the Rise of Consumer Marketing* (Baltimore: Johns Hopkins University Press, 1998). On the state of the marketplace at the turn of the twentieth century, see Phillip J. Hilts, *Protecting America's Health: The FDA, Business, and One Hundred Years of Regulation* (New York: Alfred A. Knopf, 2003), 6–7; James Harvey Young, *American Health Quackery* (Princeton, NJ: Princeton University Press, 1992), 43; J. Worth Estes, "Public Pharmacology: Modes of Action of Nineteenth-Century 'Patent' Medicines," *Medical Heritage* 2 (1986): 218–28; Robert Hessler, "A Study of Reprints and Clinical Reports on Proprietary Medicines," *American Medicine* 9 (June 10, 1905): 951–54; James Harvey Young, *The Toadstool Millionaires: A Social History of Patent Medicines in America Before Federal Regulation* (Princeton, NJ: Princeton University Press, 1961), 67–75.

4. Morris J. Vogel and Charles E. Rosenberg, eds., *The Therapeutic Revolution: : Essays in the Social History of American Medicine* (Philadelphia: University of Pennsylvania Press, 1979); Roy Porter, "The Language of Quackery in England, 1660–1800," in Peter Burke and Roy Porter, eds., *The Social History of Language* (Cambridge: Cambridge University Press, 1987), 73–103; Harry M. Marks, *The Progress of Experiment: Science and Therapeutic Reform in the United States, 1900–1990* (New York: Cambridge University Press, 1997); Wallace Janssen, "Outline of the History of U.S. Drug Regulation and Labeling," *Food, Drug, Cosmetic Law Journal* 36 (1981): 420–41; Ann Anderson, *Snake Oil, Hustlers, and Hambones: The American Medicine Show* (Jefferson, NC, McFarland and Co., 2000).

5. Harry F. Dowling, *Medicines for Man: The Development, Regulation, and Use of Prescription Drug* (New York: Alfred A. Knopf, 1970); Peter Temin, *Taking Your Medicine:*

Drug Regulation in the United States (Cambridge, MA: Harvard University Press, 1980); Oscar E. Anderson, *Health of a Nation: Harvey W. Wiley and the Fight for Pure Food* (Chicago: University of Chicago Press, 1980).

6. "Pure Food and Drugs," *Pharmacist* 13 (March 1880): 109.

7. Marks, *The Progress of Experiment,* 19–23.

8. "Report of the Board of Trustees," *JAMA* 24 (Nov. 14, 1895): 760.

9. "The Organization of the Medical Profession," *JAMA* 36 (May 25, 1902): 113; William W. Keen, "The President's Address," *JAMA* 34 (June 9, 1900): 1445; on the political strategies of the AMA at this time, see Oliver Garceau, *The Political Life of the American Medical Association* (Hamden, CT: Archon Books, 1961); Elton Rayack, *Professional Power and American Medicine: The Economics of the American Medical Association* (New York: World Publishing, 1967); James G. Burrow, *Organized Medicine in the Progressive Era: The Move Toward Monopoly* (Baltimore: Johns Hopkins University Press, 1977). For statistics on AMA membership and *JAMA* revenues, see "Report of the Board of Trustees," *JAMA* 20 (Feb. 12, 1893): 686; 24 (Feb. 10, 1895): 760; 34 (Feb. 8, 1900): 1554; 34 (Feb. 7, 1900): 1635; 54 (Feb. 11, 1910): 1967.

10. "Relations of Pharmacy to the Medical Profession," Parts I through VIII, *JAMA* 34 (April 21, 1900): 986–88; (April 28, 1900): 1049–51; (May 5, 1900) 1114–16; (May 12, 1900); 1178–79; (May 26, 1900) 1327–29; (June 2, 1900) 1405–07; *JAMA* 35 (July 7, 1900): 27–29; (July 14, 1900): 89–91.; "Secret Nostrums and the Journal," *JAMA* 34 (June 2, 1900): 1420; "Dangers from the Use of Proprietary Remedies," *JAMA* 35 (July 14, 1900): 166.

11. On Simmons's career and role in the reorganization process, see Morris H. Fishbein, "George Henry Simmons, 1852–1937," *Proceedings of the Institute of Medicine of Chicago* 11 (Nov. 15, 1937): 397–401; "Obituary: George Henry Simmons," *JAMA* 109 (Dec. 23, 1937): 807. On the role of *JAMA* editors in relation to professional objectives, see Elizabeth Knoll, "The American Medical Association and Its Journal," in W. F. Bynum, Stephen Lock, and Roy Porter, eds., *Medical Journals and Medical Knowledge: Historical Essays* (New York: Routledge, 1992): 146–59.

12. "Secret Nostrums and the Journal," *JAMA* 34 (June 2, 1900): 1420; Foshay quoted in Morris Fishbein, *A History of the American Medical Association, 1847 to 1947* (Philadelphia: W.B. Saunders, 1947). 198; Robert Hessler, "A Study of Proprietary Advertisements," *JAMA* 44 (June 24, 1905): 1983.

13. *JAMA* 36 (July 7, 1900): 2–26.

14. James G. Burrow, "The Prescription-Drug Policies of the American Medical Association in the Progressive Era," in John B. Blake, ed., *Safeguarding the Public: Historical Aspects of Medicinal Drug Control* (Baltimore: Johns Hopkins University Press, 1968): 112–22; "The Secret Nostrum vs. the Ethical Proprietary Preparation," *JAMA* 44 (March 4, 1905): 718–19; "Proprietary Drug Trade," *JAMA* 46 (March 17, 1906): 718.

15. William J. Robinson, "The Composition of Some So-Called Ethical Synthetics and 'Ethical' Nostrums," *JAMA* 41 (April 16, 1904): 1016–17; E. L. Boothby, "Regarding the Lack of Progress in Scientific Therapeutics," *Wisconsin Medical Journal* 3 (1904): 270; N. S. Davis, "Effect of Proprietary Literature on Medical Men," *JAMA* 46 (May 5, 1906): 1339; Reid Hunt, "What Physicians Can Do to Improve Materia Medica," *JAMA* 53 (Aug. 14,

1909): 497–99. For earlier recommendations for a federal agency to do the same job as the council, see F. E. Stewart, "Proposed National Bureau of Materia Medica," *JAMA* 35 (April 21, 1901): 1175–78.

16. "The Secret Nostrum vs. the Ethical Proprietary Preparation," 718; American Medical Association, *New and Non-Official Remedies* (1st ed.) (Chicago: American Medical Association, 1907).

17. Robinson, "The Composition of Some So-Called Ethical Synthetics and 'Ethical' Nostrums," 1016; Simmons is quoted from "The Secret Nostrum vs. the Ethical Proprietary Preparation," 719.

18. "The Secret Nostrum vs. the Ethical Proprietary Preparation," 719; Marks, *The Progress of Experiment*, 21. On the movement for an experimentally based therapeutics, reinforced by achievements in laboratory science and the influence of German laboratory medicine in particular, see John Harley Warner, *Therapeutic Perspective*, 235–57; John Harley Warner, "Ideals of Science and Their Discontents in Late Nineteenth–Century American Medicine," *Isis* 82 (1991): 454–78.

19. This continued discussion of rational therapeutics employs the argument of Harry Marks in *The Progress of Experiment*, 20–22. While Marks identifies rational therapeutics as an objective of therapeutic reformers that was self-evidently positive, the discussion of the council in this chapter also seeks to analyze the critiques inspired by this approach. Marks is primarily concerned with how the council systematized rational therapeutics at the level of drug analysis and subsequently employed it in practice, whereas the focus in this chapter is on how rational therapeutics shaped public discourse about the boundaries of therapeutic orthodoxy. Solomon Solis-Cohen, "Progress in Therapeutics," *Proceedings of the Philadelphia County Medical Society* 21 (March 1900): 119–20. On "rational" symptomatic treatment, see also Joseph I. Miller, "The Value of Symptomatic Treatment," *Transactions of the Association of American Physicians* 30 (1915): 516–18; J. H. Means and A. L. Barach, "The Symptomatic Treatment of Pneumonia," *JAMA* 77 (Oct. 15, 1921): 1217. On the faith in the rational therapeutics approach and the need for reform in this direction, see N. S. Davis, "Need of Much More Accurate Knowledge Concerning Both the Immediate and Remote Effects of the Remedial Agents in General Use," *JAMA* 38 (May 31, 1902): 1415–16; A. Jacobi, "Phases in the Development of Therapy," *Yale Medical Journal* 41 (1905–1906): 490–92.

20. *New and Non-Official Remedies* (Chicago: American Medical Association, 1907), 3.

21. Young, *The Medical Messiahs*, 39; Paul Starr, *The Social Transformation of American Medicine: The Rise of a Sovereign Profession and the Making of a Vast Industry* (New York: Basic Books, 1982), 131–32; James G. Burrow, *AMA: Voice of American Medicine* (Baltimore: Johns Hopkins Press, 1963)108–09; "Report of the Board of Trustees," *JAMA* 20 (Feb. 12, 1893): 686; 24 (Feb. 10, 1895): 760; 34 (Feb. 8, 1900): 1554; 34 (Feb. 7, 1900): 1635; 54 (Feb. 11, 1910): 1967.

22. Torald Sollman, *The Broader Aims of the Council on Pharmacy of the American Medical Association* (Chicago: AMA, 1908), 21; George H. Simmons, "The Commercial Domination of Therapeutics and the Movement for Reform," *JAMA* 48 (May 18, 1907): 1645; George Blumer, "The Need of Reorganization in the Methods and Teaching of Therapeutics," *Boston Medical and Surgical Journal* 169 (1913): 261–66.

23. The text for each of the rules here and later in the chapter is drawn from "The Secret Nostrum vs. the Ethical Proprietary Preparation," 720–21. In his mention of rule 4 in *Divided Legacy: A History of the Schism in Medical Thought* Vol. 3 (Washington, DC: McGrath, 1973), Harris L. Coulter writes that it "came in like a lion and went out like a lamb," 423.

24. "The Secret Nostrum vs. the Ethical Proprietary Preparation," 720–21; W. A. Puckner, "The Nostrum from the Point of View of the Pharmacist," *JAMA* 46 (May 5, 1906): 1340. On recent problems in this area, see Jerry Avorn, "Drug Regulation and Drug Information:Who Should Do What to Whom?" *American Journal of the History of Pharmacy* 85 (Jan. 1995): 18; Temin, *Taking Your Medicine*. Temin argues that drug regulation epitomizes the liberal dilemma inherent in government operation because controls are warranted for the protection of the public, but there is no clear way to determine how much regulation is justified. Meanwhile, doctors may not get enough information about drugs, so it is difficult for them to make rational therapeutic choices in many cases.

25. "The Secret Nostrum vs. the Ethical Proprietary Preparation," 720–21.

26. "The Requirements of the Council on Pharmacy and Chemistry," *JAMA* 66 (March 18, 1916): 913.

27. For a case study of a drug neglected due to ambiguous standards, see James S. Goodwin and Jean M. Goodwin, "Failure to Recognize Efficacious Treatments: A History of Salicylate Therapy in Rheumatoid Arthritis," *Perspectives in Biology and Medicine* 25 (Autumn 1981): 78–92.

28. Marks, *The Progress of Experiment*, 32–33; Torald Sollman, "Yesterday, Today and Tomorrow: The Activities of the Council on Pharmacy and Chemistry," *JAMA* 61 (July 12, 1912): 5–6; Paul Nicholas Leech, "Chemistry in the Service of Pharmaceutical Medicine," *JAMA* 85 (July 11, 1925): 139–40.

29. Harvard Medical School's David Edsall noted that distinguishing between trustworthy and untrustworthy manufacturers was no simple task. Even "reputable" firms could hire disreputable individuals or decide to take advantage of the council's lack of scrutiny. See "Council on Pharmacy and Chemistry," *Bulletin* 7 (April, 2, 1908): 152–53; Torald Sollman, "Evaluation of Therapeutic Remedies in the Hospital," *JAMA* 94 (April 26, 1930): 1279–80. On distinguishing between motives of researchers, see also L. G. Rowntree, "The Role and Development of Drug Therapy," *JAMA* 77 (Oct. 1, 1921): 1061–65. For another example of how character was emphasized in evaluating science in other contexts, see Steven Shapin, *A Social History of Truth: Civility and Science in Seventeenth-Century England* (Chicago: University of Chicago Press, 1994).

30. John Harley Warner, "The Fall and Rise of Professional Mystery: Epistemology, Authority and the Emergence of Laboratory Medicine in Nineteenth-Century America," in Andrew Cunningham and Perry Williams, eds., *The Laboratory Revolution in Medicine* (Cambridge: Cambridge University Press, 1992), 110–41. Sollman quote comes from his article, "Experimental Therapeutics," *JAMA* 58 (Jan. 27, 1912): 244; "The Secret Nostrum vs. the Ethical Proprietary Preparation," 719.

31. Sollman, "Experimental Therapeutics," 234–244; see also Albion Walter Hewlitt, "The Cooperation between Pharmacology and Therapeutics," *JAMA* 59 (Oct. 6, 1917): 1123. According to Marks, the term "weakest link," to some degree, reflects the beliefs of

pharmacologists on the council in a hierarchy of evidence, with laboratory studies being the most secure and clinical investigations the least reliable (34). This discussion of the challenges of clinical investigations employs the analysis of the Council on Pharmacy and Chemistry's minutes in a series of *Bulletins* cited by Marks in *The Progress of Experiment*, 34–36. For an explicit discussion of this hierarchy of evidence, and the problem of inconsistencies in the criterion used to judge therapeutic claims, see *Bulletin of the Council of Pharmacy and Chemistry* 49 (March 20, 1929), 237. "The Therapeutic Research Committee of the Council on Pharmacy and Chemistry of the American Medical Association," *JAMA* 67 (Nov. 11, 1916): 1440.

32. Council on Pharmacy and Chemistry, "Preliminary Announcement," *JAMA* 44 (March 4, 1905): 720–21; "Expressions on the Announcement: Comments on the Plan of Work as Temporarily Outlined by the Council on Pharmacy and Chemistry," *JAMA* 46 (March 25, 1905): 971; "Cleveland Society Endorses Plan," *JAMA* 16 (April 28, 1905): 1380; "Some Comments on the Creation of the Council of Pharmacy and Chemistry," *JAMA* 46 (March 18, 1905): 893; "Further Comments Quoted," *JAMA* 46 (April 28, 1905): 1381–82.

33. "Some Comments on the Creation of the Council of Pharmacy and Chemistry," 893–94; "Further Comments Quoted," *JAMA* 46 (April 28, 1905): 1395.

34. "Symposium: 'The Propaganda for Reform,'" *The Medical Council* (Aug. 1913): 308–10; Gerald Geison, "Divided We Stand: Physiologists and Clinicians in the American Context," in Vogel and Rosenberg, eds., *The Therapeutic Revolution*, 67–90; Russell Maulitz, "'Physician Versus Bacteriologist': The Ideology of Science in Clinical Medicine," in Ibid., 91–107; John Parascandola, "The Search for the Active Oxytocic Principal of Ergot: Laboratory Science and Clinical Medicine in Conflict," in *Neue Beitrage zur Arzneimittelgeschichte*, E. Hickel and G. Schroder, eds. (Stuttgart, Germany: Wissenschaftliche Verlagsgesellschaft, 1982), 205–27 (reprinted in John Parascandola, *Studies in the History of Modern Pharmacology and Drug Therapy* [Farnham, UK: Ashgate, 2012]).

35. For thumbnail biographical sketches on early members of the council, see August Smith, "The Council on Pharmacy and Chemistry and the Chemical Laboratory," in Fishbein, ed., *A History of the American Medical Association*, 866–68; Marks, *The Progress of Experiment*, 24.

36. "Symposium: The Propaganda for Reform," 309.

37. Arthur J. Cramp to Col. E. Bright, 3 May 1916, Box 174, Folder 11, Health Fraud Collection (HFC), American Medical Association (Chicago, IL); Arthur J. Cramp to F. J. Schlink, 30 Nov. 1926, Box 174, Folder 11, HFC.

38. "A Neglected Field for the Council of Chemistry and Pharmacy," *Medical Standard* 32 (December 1909): 626–27.

39. "Shall the Physician Be Compelled to Inform His Patients as to the Identity of Medicines Dispensed?" *American Journal of Clinical Medicine* (Feb. 1915): 173–80.

40. "The Legislative Schemes of the American Medical Association: A Conspiracy to Establish a Physicians' Trust," reprint from *National Druggist*, 1906, Folder A4(d)I; "Giving the Doctors a Dose of Their Own Medicine," reprint from *National Druggist*, 1906, Folder A4(d)1, Kremers Reference Files, American Institute of the History of Pharmacy (Madison, WI).

41. "The Legislative Schemes of the American Medical Association," 6.

42. Samuel Hopkins Adams, "The Great American Fraud," *Collier's* (Oct. 7, 1905): 15–16.

43. For a history of the early efforts toward the 1906 act and the predecessor agency of the Food and Drug Administration, see Oscar E. Anderson, *Health of a Nation: Harvey W. Wiley and the Fight for Pure Food* (Chicago: University of Chicago Press, 1980); Harvey W. Wiley, *An Autobiography* (Indianapolis: Bobbs-Merrill, 1930); Young, *The Medical Messiahs*, 3–65; Lorine Swainston Goodwin, *The Pure Food, Drink, and Drug Crusaders, 1879–1914* (New York: McFarlan & Co., 1999); Burrow, "The Prescription-Drug Policies of the American Medical Association in the Progressive Era," 116–20. For a shorter overview of the government's role in regulating the practice of pharmacy, see John P. Swann, "FDA and the Practice of Pharmacy: The History of Prescription Drug Regulation before the Durham-Humphrey Amendment of 1951," *Pharmacy in History* 36 (1994): 55–70.

44. For the broadest look at the various interest groups involved in this coalition, see James Harvey Young, *Pure Food: Securing the Federal Food and Drugs Act of 1906* (Princeton, NJ: Princeton University Press, 1989). On the reform process and collaborative relationships, see Hilts, *Protecting America's Health*; W. Steven Pray, *A History of Nonprescription Product Regulation* (Binghamton, NY: Pharmaceutical Products Press, 2003); Marks, *The Progress of Experiment*, 27; Smith, "The Council on Pharmacy and Chemistry," 868–70; Ramunas Kondratas, "The Biologics Control Act of 1902," in James Harvey Young, ed., *The Early Years of Federal Food and Drug Control* (Madison, WI: American Institute of the History of Pharmacy, 1982), 8–27; Young, *The Medical Messiahs*, 41–65; John Parascandola, *The Development of American Pharmacology: John H. Abel and the Shaping of a Discipline* (Baltimore: Johns Hopkins University Press, 1992), 91–100. Parascandola argues that American pharmacology grew as a discipline primarily as a result of government bureau work and that regulatory work was key in bringing pharmacologists into the pharmaceutical industry via efforts at standardization and the accelerated quest for new medicines.

45. Samuel Hopkins Adams, "Patent Medicines, the Law and the Public," "The Fraud above the Law," and "Patent Medicines under the Pure Food Law," in *The Great American Fraud* (Chicago: American Medical Association, 1913), reprinted from *Collier's* (June 8, 1907), 122–32, 133–45, and 177.

46. Editorial, *JAMA* 47 (July 7, 1906): 41; Burrow, "The Prescription Drug Policies of the American Medical Association in the Progressive Era," 115–17; Editorial, *JAMA* 47 (July 14, 1906): 116; Young, *Pure Food*, 265.

47. Editorial, *JAMA* 47 (Aug. 4, 1906): 365; Young, *Pure Food*, 265–70.

48. James C. Munch and James C. Munch, Jr., "The First Thousand," presentation at Historical Pharmacy Section, American Pharmaceutical Association, Boston: August 26, 1954. Munch and Munch analyzed the first 10,000 of the 31,157 Notices of Judgment published by the federal government under the 1906 act and authored by the Board of Food and Drug Inspection. Upon request, these Notices of Judgment were made available to the public. Of the first 1,000 Notices of Judgment, only 221 had drug, pharmaceutical, or pharmacological aspects. Of the 124 preparations distinctly designated as drug products in the first 1,000 Notices of Judgment, 76 pled guilty and most paid a fine of less than $100. In some cases, a shipment seized by the authorities was merely destroyed.

49. Burrow, *AMA: Voice of American Medicine*, 89; "Decision in Johnson Case," *JAMA* 56 (June 17, 1911): 1832–35; Young, *American Health Quackery*, 94–96 and *The Medial Messiahs*, 48–51; John G. Kuniholm, "Constitutional Limitations on the Regulation of Therapeutic Claims under 1938 Federal, Food, Drug, and Cosmetic Act," *Food, Drug and Cosmetic Law Journal* 9 (Nov. 1954): 636–41.

50. Editorial, *JAMA* 56 (June 17, 1911): 1819; Burrow, *AMA: Voice of American Medicine*, 90; "Petition to Amend the Pure Food and Drugs Act," *JAMA* 57 (July 8, 1911): 133.

51. Young, *The Medical Messiahs*, 49–65 and 88–112; Michael S. Torbeson and Jonathan Erlen, "A Case Study of the Lash's Bitters Company: Advertising Changes after the Federal Food and Drugs Act of 1906 and the Sherley Amendment of 1912," *Pharmacy in History* 45 (2003): 139–49.

52. Sollman, *Broader Aims of the Council*, 3.

53. Marks, *The Progress of Experiment*, 40; Victor Robinson, "A Symposium on Drugs," *Review of Reviews* 22 (1916): 15–26.

CHAPTER THREE

1. J. H. Salisbury, "The Subordination of Medical Journals to Proprietary Interests," *JAMA* 46 (June 2, 1906): 1337–38.

2. F. J. L. Blasingame, ed., *Digest of Official Actions, 1846–1958* Vol. 1 (Chicago: American Medical Association, 1959), 184; James G. Burrow, *AMA: Voice of American Medicine* (Baltimore: Johns Hopkins Press, 1963), 111.

3. "Patent Medicine Advertising," *JAMA* 58 (April 13, 1912): 1118–19; Burrow, *AMA*, 111–14.

4. Adriance & Adriance to the AMA, Feb. 9, 1914, Box 23, Folder 1, HHF; *JAMA* to Adriance, Feb. 10, 1914, Box 23, Folder 1, HHF; AMA to Theo W. Singer, March 12, 1914, Box 23, Folder 1, HHF.

5. "Current Comment," *JAMA* 48 (Feb. 2, 1907): 422; 64 (Jan. 2, 1915): 61; 64 (April 24, 1915): 1430.

6. "And Still They Come: Another Daily Paper Rejects All Patent Medicine Advertisements," Box 23, Folder 1, HHF; "New Standard of Newspaper Decency," *Republican* (Dec. 14, 1913), Box 23, Folder 1, HHF; "Decency Pays: The Phoenix Republican Proves It," Box 23, Folder 11, HHF; Anonymous to AMA Manager, Feb. 7, 1914, Box 23, Folder 1, HHF.

7. "Why Vigilance Committees?" pamphlet by Associated Advertising Clubs of America, ca. 1918, Box 61, Folder 8, HHF; "Advertising Reform Successful," *JAMA* 58 (May 3, 1912): 36; Samuel Hopkins Adams, "The Patent-Medicine Conspiracy against the Freedom of the Press," in *The Great American Fraud* (Chicago: American Medical Association, 1912), pp. 146–65; Frank Armstrong of the Associated Vigilance Committee of Iowa to AMA, Sept. 18, 1917; AMA to Armstrong, 20 Sept. 1917; A. R. Henthorn of the Vigilance Bureau of the Minneapolis Advertising Forum to Arthur J. Cramp, Sept. 25, 1918; Cramp to Henthorn, Sept. 27, 1918; "Help Enforce the New Ohio Advertising Law," pamphlet from the Cleveland Advertising Clubs, 1913; Special Bulletin of the Advertisers Protective Bureau,

Inc. of the Kansas City Advertising Club, May 20, 1922; Third Annual Report of the Vigilance Bureau of the Minneapolis Advertising Forum, 1916–1917; Box 61, Folder 8, HHF; Jacob A. Goldberg, "The Advertising Physician," *Hygeia* 1 (Aug. 1923): 308–11.

    8. "The Year's Fight," *Kentucky Medical Journal* (Nov. 1907): 3.

    9. Burrow, *AMA*, 112; "The Big Six: Six Reasons for the Perpetuation of the Proprietary Evil," *JAMA* 63 (Oct. 31, 1914): 1594–95; "Representative Medical Publications," advertisement in Box 84, Folder 13, HHF; "The Big Six," July 9, 1914, Box 84, Folder 13, HHF; "The Big Six: Six Reasons for the Perpetuation of the Proprietary Evil," 1595. The Big Six were the *American Journal of Clinical Practice* (Chicago), *American Journal of Surgery* (New York), *American Medicine* (Burlington, VT), *Interstate Medical Journal* (St. Louis), the *Therapeutic Gazette* (Detroit), and *Medical Council* (Philadelphia).

    10. This quote and other material cited from *Medical Council* in this paragraph come from an unsigned and undated internal AMA memorandum titled "This Is an Honest Market-Place." Other items in the folder suggest the author of the material from the AMA is *Journal* editor George H. Simmons. Circulars from the business manager of the *Medical Council* corroborate the contents of the memo, Feb. 21, 1912 and Feb. 15, 1914, Box 50, Folder 1, HHF; "This is an Honest Market-Place," 1914, Box 50, Folder 1, HHF.

    11. AMA House of Delegates, *Proceedings* (66th Annual Session, 1915): 3; *JAMA* 76 (Nov. 22, 1921): 1658; *JAMA* 48 (June 12, 1917): 1714; Burrow, *AMA*, 130–31; *Nostrums and Quackery* (Chicago: American Medical Association, 1912), 7; *The Propaganda for Reform in Proprietary Medicines* Vol. I (Chicago: American Medical Association, 1922). Newspaper clippings from Box 61, Folder 8, HHF, include the following headlines regarding advertising reform: "Advertising Fakes Checked," 1913; "Square Deal Advertising," 1913; "Papers Reject Fraudulent Ads," 1925; "Menace to Health Removed," 1926; "Council Wars on Worthless Drugs: American Medical Association Subjects All Remedies to Analysis," Aug. 20, 1927, Box 174, Folder 10, HHF; Paul Nicholas Leech, "Drug Reform: Medical and Dental," *Journal of the American Dental Association* 18 (Jan. 1931): 79.

    12. "The Secret Nostrum vs. the Ethical Proprietary Preparation," *JAMA* 44 (March 4, 1905): 718; Milton Silverman and Philip R. Lee, *Pills, Profits, and Politics* (Berkeley: University of California Press, 1974), 49.

    13. "A Study of the Scientific Action and Therapeutic Value of Antiphlogistine," pamphlet by Denver Chemical Manufacturing Company, 1903, Box 23, Folder 1, Medical Trade Ephemera Collection, College of Physicians of Philadelphia (CPP); "Infected Wound Therapy," pamphlet by Denver Chemical Manufacturing Company, ca. 1939, in Box 56, Folder 6, HHF; Cramp to A. E. Holmes, Nov. 22, 1932, Box 56, Folder 6, HHF; Cramp to C. D. Giauque, 24 Feb. 1936, Box 56, Folder 6, HHF; "Antiphlogistine," report from the Bureau of Chemistry, reprinted from *Journal of the American Dental Association* (Aug. 1929), 2; Federal Trade Commission Release, 31 March 1950, Complaint No. 5755; copy in Box 56, Folder 6, HHF.

    14. "Vanadium," pamphlet by Vanadium Chemical Company, 1912, Box 91, Folder 1, CPP.

    15. "Vanadium as a Therapeutic Agent," *JAMA* 49 (May 9, 1908): 1548.

    16. "Vanadium in Tuberculosis," "Vanadiol Preparations," pamphlets by Vanadium Chemical Co., 1911, in Box 877, Folder 7, HHF; "Vanadiol Preparations," monograph sent

to by Turner to Samuel C. Stanton, Nov. 23, 1911, Box 877, Folder 6, HHF; "Proprietary Vanadium Preparations: Report of the Council on Pharmacy and Chemistry," (Chicago: AMA, 1913), 3; "Experience with Vanadium in Tuberculosis," *Journal of the American Institute of Homeopathy* (Sept. 1912): 26–32.

17. The AMA learned about Turner's involvement with the Dr. Turner Company responsible for the obesity cure scheme via correspondence with a Pittsburgh doctor who knew Turner. Following the publication of the article exposing Turner in the *Journal*, he contacted inquiring physicians and refuted the claims in the article. Dr. Grayson, along with other doctors, also secretly sent their correspondence with Turner to the AMA. T. W. Grayson to Cramp, May 4, 1912; Cramp to Grayson, May 9, 1912; Richard M. Riley to AMA, July 11, 1912; Turner to Riley, July 9, 1912; Cramp to Riley, July 13, 1912; Box 877, Folder 8, HHF. The article in question was "Another Fraudulent Fat–Reducing Concern," *JAMA* (June 22, 1912): 714.

18. Editorial, *JAMA* (Jan. 18, 1913): 226.

19. "Refreshing Sleep, Restored Energy," 1905; "A Dramatic Event in the History of a Distressful Disease," 1920; pamphlets by Winthrop Chemical Company, Box 96, Folder 4, CPP; "Luminal," *JAMA* 60 (May 17, 1913): 1541; John Phillips, "Phenobarbital Luminal Poisoning: Report of Case," *JAMA* 78 (April 22, 1922): 1199–1201.

20. Julius Grinker, "Experiences with Luminal in Epilepsy," *JAMA* 75 (Aug. 28, 1920): 588–92; Cecil E. Reynolds, "Experiences with Luminal in Epilepsy," *JAMA* 75 (Sept. 18, 1920): 829–30; L. F. Kebler to Cramp, Sept. 22, 1929, Box 482, Folder 3, HHF; Cramp to Kebler, 24 Jan. 1929, Box 482, Folder 3, HHF. Luminal also provides an early example of what came to be known as the therapeutic cycle: when a new drug is promoted to doctors and covered excitedly by the media, which increases patient interest and demand for the drug, the drug begins to be overprescribed for ailments it cannot cure. As more people use it over a longer period of time, problems with adverse side effects and questions regarding therapeutic effectiveness increase dramatically. For a later example of this, see Mickey Smith, *Small Comfort: A History of Minor Tranquilizers* (New York: Praeger Press, 1985), 4–7.

21. "Our Scientific Chemicals," pamphlet by Liberty Chemical Company, ca. 1910, Box 52, Folder 1, MFEC-CPP.

22. "Syllabus of Bacteriology: A Compact Treatise Designed to Aid the Physician in the Scientific Diagnosis of Disease," handbook by Palisade Manufacturing Company, ca. 1901, Box 72, Folder 4, CPP.

23. "An Outline of Some of the Uses and Advantages of Petrolagar," pamphlet by Deshell Laboratories Inc., 1928, Box 23, Folder 1, CPP; "Report in the Matter of the Chemical, Bacteriological, and Biological Investigation of Zonite to Determine Its Value as a Germicide and Local Antiseptic," report by Pease Laboratories, successors to Lederle Laboratories, 1911, Box 48, Folder 1, CPP; "Organic Chemical Mfg. Company: Its Products," Organic Chemical Manufacturing Company, 1905, Box 71, Folder 1, CPP; James Whorton, *Inner Hygiene: Constipation and the Pursuit of Health in Modern Society* (New York: Oxford University Press, 2000).

24. *Homeopathic Medical Index: A Guide to Homeopathic Treatment of Common Ailments* (Philadelphia: Boericke & Tafel, 1907); *Boericke & Tafel's Physician's Price Current*

(Philadelphia: Boericke & Tafel, 1907), 3; AMA to Eugene E. Thomas, Feb. 8, 1934, Box 359, Folder 4, HHF; Paul C. Barton to Homer Calver, Feb. 14, 1940, Box 359, Folder 4, HHF.

25. "The Pennsylvania Orthopaedic Institute and School of Mechanotherapy," pamphlet by the Pennsylvania Orthopaedic Institute and School of Mechanotherapy, 1905, in Box 75, Folder 2, CPP; Max J. Walter, "Mechano–Therapy of To-Day," reprint from *The Trained Nurse and Hospital Review* (March 1905), 1; in Box 9, Folder 7, CPP.

26. Christopher Toumey, *Conjuring Science: Scientific Symbols and Cultural Meanings in American Life* (New Brunswick, NJ: Rutgers University Press, 1996), 151.

27. Frederick Humphreys, *Humphreys' Mentor: Medical Advisor in the Use of Humphrey's Remedies* (New York: Humphrey's Homeopathic Medicine Co., 1926), 2; AMA to E. A. McLaughlin, Jan. 14, 1936, Box 359, Folder 6, HHF; S. Adolphus Knopf to Frank J. Clancy, Aug. 17, 1937, Box 359, Folder 6, HHF. Knopf quipped: "I need not discuss with you the value of similia similibus curantur. Its principle is to the best of my knowledge violated by all progressive homeopathic physicians."

28. E. L. Shope, "Word to My Fellow Practitioners: The Road to Success I Have Followed: Others Have Tried it Successfully: Will You?" advertisement for Frank S. Betz Company, 1912, in Box 9, Folder 1, CPP.

29. "The Importance of Aquatone Pure Spring Water," pamphlet by Keasbey and Mattison Company, ca. 1895, in Box 43, Folder 4, CPP.

30. For an extended analysis of a variety of neo-Hippocratic incarnations, see David Cantor, ed., *Reinventing Hippocrates* (Aldershot, England: Ashgate, 2002); James C. Whorton, *Nature Cures: The History of Alternative Medicine in America* (Oxford: Oxford University Press, 2002), xii; John Harley Warner, "The 'Nature-Trusting Heresy': American Physicians and the Concept of the Healing Power of Nature," *Perspectives in American History* 11 (1977–1978): 291–324; Catherine L. Albanese, *Nature Religion in America: From the Algonkian Indians to the New Age* (Chicago: University of Chicago Press, 1990).

31. Kickapoo Indian Medicine Co., "Souvenir of the Kickapoo Indian Medicine Co.'s Demonstration and Indian Exhibition," Clintonville, CT: 1909, Connecticut Historical Society, Folio 615.88.6 K46k; Kickapoo Indian Medicine Co., "Kickapoo Indian Dream Book," Clintonville, CT: ca. 1907, Connecticut Historical Society, Call no. 615.866 K46k; "Kickapoo Cough Cure," *JAMA* 52 (June 24, 1911): 275; Arthur J. Cramp to Edward M. Burke, June 1, 1935, Box 413, Folder 10, HHF.

32. "Fraser's Tablets," pamphlet by The Fraser Tablet Company, 1906, in Box 31, Folder 7, CPP; "Biogen and Dermogen: Portable Oxygen Products, As Considered by Leading Medical and Pharmaceutical Journals," pamphlet by Biogen Company, ca. 1907, in Box 12, Folder 1, CPP; article quoted in "A Realization: 'Biogen' Magnesium Dioxide," *International Journal of Surgery* (May 1903: 15; William J. Robinson, "The Composition of Some So-Called Synthetics and 'Ethical' Nostrums," *JAMA* 42 (June 16, 1904): 1017.

33. George H. Sherman, "The Steady Progress toward Efficient Therapeutic Immunization in the Treatment of Acute Infections," pamphlet by G. H. Sherman Bacteriological Laboratories, 1920, in Box 83, Folder 2, CPP; Untitled Circular, Standard Emulsion Company, 1923, in Box 87, Folder 1, CPP; "Health, Beauty and Perpetual Youth by Using the Niagara Vapor Bath Cabinet," pamphlet by Jones & Co.; *Cleanliness Is Next to Godliness:*

Health, Beauty and Perpetual Youth by Using the Niagara Vapor Bath Cabinet, ca. 1910, Box 42, Folder 1, CPP.

34. "Safety in Administering Sedatives," pamphlet by Dios Chemical Company, 1929, in Box 24, Folder 2, CPP; "Materia Medica Bayer," catalogue by Bayer Pharmaceutical Company, 1915: 14, Box 10, Folder 1, CPP; "Neurosine: The Safe Soporific," pamphlet by Dios Chemical Company, 1934, Box 213, Folder 22, HHF; "The Dangers of Empiricism in the Use of Sedatives," pamphlet by Dios Chemical Company, 1940, Box 213, Folder 22, HHF.

35. BOH to M. T. Jarvis, Nov. 6, 1936, Box 213, Folder 22, HHF; BOH to Philip Reichert, July 19, 1937, Box 213, Folder 22, HHF; "Neurosine and the Original Package Evil," *JAMA* (April 27, 1918): 1251; "Neurosine Poisoning," *JAMA* (April 11, 1931): 1225. BOH to Marion E. Console, May 11, 1939, Box 213, Folder 22, HHF; AMA to Fred D. L. Squires, Dec. 20, 1939, Box 213, Folder 22, HHF; "An Extraordinary Large Dose of Neurosine with no Bad After Effects," ca. 1915, Box 213, Folder 22, HHF.

36. "Will it Be Asking Too Much to Beg Permission to Save Your Life?" pamphlet by Stafford Mineral Springs & Hotel Co., ca. 1905, Box 87, Folder 1, CPP; "From the President of the United States to our Former Washington, D.C. Agents," pamphlet by Stafford Mineral Springs & Hotel Co., ca. 1898, Box 87, Folder 1, CPP.

37. "New Remedies," catalog by Boericke & Tafel, 1907, Box 13, Folder 1, CPP; "Prescription Blanks and Some Practical Points on Hydrotherapy," pamphlet by Pennsylvania Orthopaedic Institute of Mechano-therapy, ca. 1915, Box 75, Folder 1, CPP.

38. Charles A. Tyrrell, Circular, ca. 1920, in Box 90, Folder 1, CPP; "Why Man of To-Day is Only 50 Per Cent Efficient," pamphlet by Tyrrell's Hygienic Institute, 1904, Box 867, Folder 9, HHF; "The What, The Why, The Way of Internal Baths," pamphlet by Tyrrell's Hygienic Institute, 1916, in Box 90, Folder 1, CPP; Casey A. Wood to George H. Simmons, Jan. 13, 1911, Box 868, Folder 4, HHF.

39. "The What, The Why, The Way of Internal Baths"; Simmons to Wood, Jan. 17, 1911, Box 868, Folder 4, HHF; Arthur J. Cramp to Dr. E. Dreifus, July 6, 1911, Box 868, Folder 4, HHF; Edmund F. Healey to *JAMA*, May 5, 1913, Box 868, Folder 4, HHF; *JAMA* to Healey, 11 March 1913, Box 868, Folder 4, HHF.

40. "The What, The Why, The Way of Internal Baths," 3.

41. "Testimonials," ca. 1913, Box 301, Folder 4, HHF.

CHAPTER FOUR

1. "Teach the Public That Medical Practice Is More Than Drug-Giving," *JAMA* 48 (May 11, 1907): 1617.

2. Oliver Garceau, *The Political Life of the American Medical Association* (Hamden, CT: Archon Books, 1961); Elton Rayack, *Professional Power and American Medicine: The Economics of the American Medical Association* (New York: World Publishing, 1967); James G. Burrow, *Organized Medicine in the Progressive Era: The Move Toward Monopoly* (Baltimore: Johns Hopkins University Press, 1977).

3. Arthur J. Cramp (AJC), "What is the Bureau of Investigation?" Mar. 25, 1932, Box 187, Folder 1, HHF.

4. F. L. Smith, Jr., "The Archfoe of the Quacks," 1928, Box 175, Folder 10, HHF; Obituary (Arthur J. Cramp), *JAMA* 147 (1951): 1773; Oliver Field, "The A.M.A. Bureau of Investigation," *A.M.A. Woman's Auxiliary Bulletin* 17 (1956): 244; William W. Alderdyce, "Dr. Cramp of the A.M.A.," *Toledo Academy of Medicine Bulletin* (March 1927): 7–8; James Harvey Young, *The Medical Messiahs: A Social History of Health Quackery in Twentieth-Century America* (Princeton, NJ: Princeton University Press, 1992), 129.

5. Austin Smith, "The Council on Pharmacy and Chemistry," in Morris Fishbein, ed., *A History of the American Medical Association, 1847 to 1947* (Philadelphia: W. B. Saunders, 1957), 866–77; Bliss O. Harding, "The Bureau of Investigation," in Ibid., 1034; AJC to Dr. Robert S. Lynd, Secretary of the Social Sciences Research Council, April 10, 1931, Box 292, Folder 1, HHF.

6. "Great American Fraud, Correspondence," 1906–1961, Box 301, Folder 5, HHF; "The Great American Fraud," *JAMA* 48 (May 11, 1907): 1617; Editorial, *JAMA* 54 (March 5, 1910): 237.

7. AJC, *Nostrums and Quackery*, Vol. I (Chicago: American Medical Association, 1911), 8–11; AJC, *Nostrums and Quackery*, Vol. II (Chicago: American Medical Association, 1921), 6.

8. AJC *Nostrums and Quackery*, Vol. I, 11–13; AJC, "The Bureau of Investigation of the American Medical Association," *American Journal of Police Science* 2 (July–Aug. 1931): 288.

9. AJC to George Simmons, Oct. 23, 1928, Box 929, Folder 1, HHF; "A Great Paper Attempts the Impossible," *JAMA* 58 (April 13, 1912): 1118.

10. AMA House of Delegates, *Proceedings* (67th Annual Session, 1916): 7.

11. AJC to William F. Herren, Jan. 26, 1931, Box 929, Folder 6, HHF.

12. AMA House of Delegates, *Proceedings* (68th Annual Session, 1917): 12; AMA House of Delegates, *Proceedings* (65th Annual Session, 1914): 6; AMA House of Delegates, *Proceedings* (66th Annual Session, 1915): 4; AJC to Samuel A. Visanska, Jul. 7, 1922, Box 929, F6, HHF.

13. "The Bureau of Investigation," *AMA Report of Board of Trustees* (1929): 68; Frederick R. Green to Simon Flexner, Jul. 6, 1912, Series 1, "American Medical Association," Folder 1, Simon Flexner Papers, American Philosophical Society (Philadelphia).

14. House of Delegates, *Proceedings* (69th Annual Session, 1918): 7; AJC "The Bureau of Investigation of the American Medical Association," 286; House of Delegates, *Proceedings* (73rd Annual Session, 1922): 10; Marion Plovak to AJC, Dec. 1, 1935, Box 929, Folder 7, HHF; BOH to Richard M. Hewitt of the Mayo Clinic, April 20, 1936; W. W. Bauer to Joseph DeBrum of Sequoia Union High School in California, Aug. 6, 1956; and W. W. Bauer to W. H. Frisker, Head of the Home Economics Department at State Teachers College in Wisconsin, Feb. 25, 1937, Box 929, Folder 2, HHF.

15. "The Bureau of Investigation," *AMA Report of Board of Trustees* (1929): 68–69. A complete set of all 28 posters could be purchased for $5.00.

16. "Propaganda Department Exhibit," June 10, 1918, Box 187, Folder 1, HHF; Cramp, "The Bureau of Investigation of the American Medical Association," 288.

17. A few of Cramp's articles include "Modern Advertising and the Nostrum," *American Journal of Public Health* 8 (1918): 756–58; "Therapeutic Thaumaturgy," *American Mercury* 3 (1924): 423–30; "The Nostrum and the Public Health," *New England Journal of Medicine*

201 (1929): 1297–1300; "The Bureau of Investigation of the American Medical Association," *American Journal of Police Science* 2 (July–Aug. 1931): 285–89; "The Work of the Bureau of Investigation," *Law and Contemporary Problems* 1 (Dec. 1933): 51–54.

18. AJC to William D. Cutter, May 15, 1933, Box 929, Folder 2, HHF.

19. AJC to Samuel A. Visanska, July 7, 1922, Box 929, Folder 6, HHF.

20. AJC to Robert S. Lynd, April 10, 1931, Box 929, Folder 1, HHF; House of Delegates, *Proceedings* (76th Annual Session, 1925): 12; F. A. Conrad to AJC, May 2, 1927, Box 929, Folder 1, HHF; Cramp to Conrad, May 6, 1927, Box 929, Folder 6, HHF.

21. "Reports of Officers: Bureau of Investigation," *JAMA* 96 (May 2, 1932): 1490–91.

22. Young, *The Medical Messiahs*, 131.

23. Memoranda, Aug. 6, 1937, Box 256, F5; Dozens of case memoranda and extensive correspondence can be found in the HHF files, Box 667, Folders 1–15.

24. "The Federal Trade Commission: How This Governmental Agency Is Protecting the Public in the Medical Field," *JAMA* (April 30, 1932): 1584–85; Memoranda, Aug. 6, 1937, Box 256, Folder 5, HHF.

25. AJC to William L. Taggart, May 31, 1938, Box 256, Folder 5; Otis B. Johnson to AJC, Feb. 24, 1933, Box 256, Folder 5; Trial Attorney DeWitt T. Puckett to Frank J. Clancy, Feb. 20, 1937; Trial Attorney William L. Taggart to AJC, March 20, 1937; Commissioner Ewin L. Davis to Olin West, June 30, 1938, Box 256, Folder 5; AJC to William E. Humphrey, April 25, 1932, Box 256, Folder 5, HHF; "The Federal Trade Commission: Further Good Work in Protecting the Public," *JAMA* (Jan. 28, 1933): 275; "The Federal Trade Commission: More Nostrum Exploiters Brought to Time," *JAMA* (Sept. 30, 1933): 1093.

26. AJC, "Let the Seller Beware! How the Federal Trade Commission Protects the Public," *Hygeia* (April 1933): 336–39.

27. AJC to A. E. Backman, Nov. 24, 1929, Box 929, Folder 1, HHF.

28. M. D. Moore to Roland H. Langelier, Oct. 1, 1931, Box 174, Folder 11, HHF; R. S. Hadsell to the AMA Jan. 30, 1937, Box 929, Folder 2, HHF; AJC, Memorandum, June 10, 1918, Box 187, Folder 1, HHF.

29. "Reports of Officers: Bureau of Investigation," *JAMA* 96 (May 2, 1932): 1490–91; J. G. Crownhart to AJC, Jan. 8, 1926, Box 502, Folder 2, HHF; AJC to J. C. Crownhart, Jan. 12, 1926, Box 502, Folder 2, HHF.

30. Sara E. Morse to AJC, Aug. 8, 1918, Box 929, Folder 8, HHF.

31. House of Delegates, *Proceedings* (76th Annual Meeting, 1925): 12; Kenneth B. Backman to AJC, Feb. 15, 1932, Box 929, Folder 7, HHF; "The Bureau of Investigation," *AMA Report of Board of Trustees* (1929): 67–68; "Reports of Officers: Bureau of Investigation," *JAMA* 96 (May 2, 1932): 1490.

32. House of Delegates, *Proceedings* (65th Annual Session, 1914): 5; "The Bureau of Investigation," *AMA Report of the Board of Trustees* (1929): 66; AJC to Dr. Robert S. Lynd, April 10, 1931, Box 292, Folder 1, HHF.

33. Eric W. Boyle, "Beyond Mirage and Magic Bullets: Redefining Therapeutic Orthodoxy in An Age of Reform," see Chapter 5, "Widening the Educational Divide" (PhD diss., University of California Santa Barbara, 2007); William Rothstein, *American Medical Schools and the Practice of Medicine: A History* (New York: Oxford University Press, 1987); Ronald

Numbers, ed. *The Education of American Physicians: Historical Essays* (Berkeley: University of California Press, 1980); John S. Haller, *The History of American Homeopathy: The Academic Years, 1820–1935* (New York: Haworth, 2005); Ludmerer, *Learning to Heal: The Development of American Medical Education*; James G. Burrow, *AMA: Voice of American Medicine* (Baltimore: Johns Hopkins Press, 1963) George Rosen, *The Structure of American Medical Practice, 1875–1941* (Philadelphia: University of Pennsylvania Press, 1983).

34. "The Bureau of Investigation," *AMA Report of Board of Trustees* (1929): 70.

35. Young, *Medical Messiahs*, 131–32. Figures are based on information in AMA files and reports by the Bureau of Investigation on the period 1910–1913; AJC to Yan Y. Caldwell, April 17, 1931, Box 929, Folder 1, HHF; AJC, "Bureau of Investigation: For *JAMA*," March 1937, Box 187, Folder 1, HHF.

36. Young, *The Medical Messiahs*, 133. As part of his research, Young conducted interviews with Cramp's colleagues, and this habit was reported by W. W. Bynum; Cramp, *Nostrums and Quackery* Vol. II, 3.

37. AJC to Harry F. Ferguson, Nov. 22, 1932, Box 929, Folder 7, HHF; "Some Comments Made by University of Chicago Students," 1915, Box 929, Folder 6, HHF; John O. Holliwell to *JAMA* Editor, July 16, 1915, Box 929, Folder 6, HHF; Elbert J. Mandeville to the AMA, Nov. 16, 1918, Box 929, Folder 6, HHF; W. C. Rodgers to *JAMA* Editor, May 7, 1937, Box 929, Folder 6, HHF; M. J. Donnelly to AMA, June 1, 1932, Box 929, Folder 7, HHF; W. M. Shurr to AMA, Jan. 6, 1937, Box 929, Folder 7, HHF; Dr. John A. Haynis to AJC, Dec. 4, 1916, Box 929, Folder 6, HHF; Joseph B. Webber to *JAMA* Editor, Dec. 15, 1920, Box 929, Folder 6, HHF; T. J. Williams to Olin West, July 20, 1932, Box 929, Folder 7, HHF; Alda George to AMA, Jan. 5, 1918, Box 929, Folder 6; dozens of similar letters are available in Box 929, Folders 6 and 7, HHF.

38. C. Ward Crampton of the Medical Society of the State of New York to AJC, May 19, 1931; "Investigation and Advertising Censorship," *Weekly Roster and Medical Digest* 26 (July 4, 1931): 19; R. B. Baer of the New York Tribune to AJC, Feb. 8, 1918; Margaret C. Munna of the National Woman's Christian Temperance Union and *Union Signal* to AJC, Jan. 14, 1918; Rose Young of *Woman Citizen* to AJC, Jan. 20, 1919; Box 929, Folder 6, HHF.

39. Oscar Dowling, "Charlatan Tactics," *Bunkie, Louisiana Record* (March 4, 1927): A1.

40. F. J. Schlink to AJC, July 18, 1932, Box 929, Folder 7, HHF; Cramp to Schlink, July 22, 1932, Box 929, Folder 7; Schlink to Cramp, July 29, 1932, Box 929, Folder 7, HHF.

41. Editorial, *National Eclectic Medical Association Quarterly* (Dec. 1916): 181; Samuel A. Visanska to *JAMA* Editor, July 3, 1922, Box 929, Folder 6, HHF.

42. "The 'Journal of the American Medical Association' Begs the Question," *Medical Brief* 38 (April 1910): 195. This argument was repeated by Charles J. Whalen, "The American Medical Association Becomes an Autocracy," *American Medical Press* (Jan. 1923): 5–20; "The Blind Infatuation of the A.M.A. Leaders," *Medical Brief* 38 (Oct. 1910): 567; "A Critical Laboratory," *Medical Standard* 34 (Feb. 1911): 42.

43. Martin Kaufman, *Homeopathy in America: The Rise and Fall of a Medical Heresy* (Baltimore: Johns Hopkins University Press, 1971), 125–40; Harris L. Coulter, *Divided Legacy: A History of the Schism in Medical Thought* Vol. 3 (Washington, DC: McGrath, 1973), 402–10; Ronald L. Numbers, "Do-It Yourself the Sectarian Way," in Guenter Risse,

Ronald Numbers, and Judith Leavitt, eds., *Medicine without Doctors* (New York: Science History, 1977), 59; Frederick Humphreys, *Manual of Specific Homœopathy* (New York: Humphreys' Specific Homœopathic Medicine Company, 1869); *Humphreys' Homeopathic Mentor of Family Adviser* (New York: Humphreys' Homeopathic Medicine Company, 1876). Homeopathic colleaque quoted in Numbers, 61; J. S. Douglas, *Practical Homeopathy for the People* (15th ed.) (Milwaukee: Lewis Sherman, 1894), p. iii.

44. "Editorial Comment," *California Journal of Medicine* (Oct. 1917): 389, Box 359, Folder 6, HHF; "Ad-Mirror," *Detroit Times* (Feb. 5, 1918), in Box 359, Folder 6; J. F. Norton to Cramp, July 16, 1923, Box 358, Folder 6, HHF; M. Tierney to Cramp, June 10, 1926, Box 359, Folder 6, HHF; E. A. McLaughlin to AMA, Jan. 11, 1936, Box 359, Folder 6, HHF; Frank Stratton to AMA Chemical Laboratory, July 29, 1936, Box 359, Folder 6, HHF; S. Adolphus Knopf to Frank J. Clancy, Aug. 17, 1937, Box 359, Folder 6, HHF; Gordon J. McCurdy to AMA, Jan. 26, 1944, Box 359, Folder 6, HHF; John J. Burke of the National Better Business Bureau to AMA, Dec. 22, 1948, Box 359, Folder 6, HHF.

45. Bureau of Investigation to Jean Y. Gratz, Jan. 17, 1938, Box 358, Folder 6, HHF; Gratz to AMA, Jan. 8, 1938, Box 358, Folder 6, HHF; Gratz to AMA, Jan. 9, 1938, Box 358, Folder 6, HHF. A subsequent reply to an inquiry from the *Chicago Tribune* also reported that FDA chemists in 1931 had identified the presence of aconite, an ingredient on which the Council on Pharmacy and Chemistry had issued a warning due to its effect on heart rate; see Bureau of Investigation to M. Tierney, Nov. 29, 1939, Box 358, Folder 6, HHF.

46. Cramp, *Nostrums and Quackery,* Vol. II, 31; Natalie Robins, *Copeland's Cure: Homeopathy and the War Between Conventional and Alternative Medicine* (New York: Alfred A. Knopf, 2005), 137–39; James C. Whorton, *Nature Cures: The History of Alternative Medicine in America* (New York: Oxford University Press, 2002), 194–214.

47. AMA Propaganda Department to Irwin B. Thompson, May 20, 1919, Box 542, Folder 4, HHF.

48. Cramp to Hugh Smith, Nov. 10, 1920, Box 542, Folder 4, HHF; Cramp to A. J. Reiter, March 19, 1924, Box 524, Folder 4, HHF; Cramp to A. J. Grenstein, May 19, 1924, Box 524, Folder 4, HHF.

49. Cramp to J. E. Britton, Nov. 22, 1923, Box 524, Folder 4, HHF; Cramp to Helen Huber, Feb. 2, 1933, Box 174, Folder 11, HHF.

50. "Chiropractors and Others Prosecuted," 91 *JAMA* (July 14, 1928): 416; "Illegal Practice by Medical Cult Practitioners," *JAMA* (July 7, 1920): 24; "Chiropractors Refuse to Comply with the Law," 91 *JAMA* (Oct. 6, 1928): 1044; "Chiropractor Fined," *JAMA* (July 21, 1920): 324; "Chiropractic Pathology" and "Michigan Turns Down Chiropractors," clippings of articles, 1921, Box 126, Folder 14; "Leslie's on Chiropractic," "Physicians Organize to Fight Chiropractor Bill," and "Fair Play to the Public," 1921–22, Box 126, Folder 14, HHF.

51. "Medical Testimonials for Chiropractic: Opinions of Some Alleged Well-Known Medical Men on Chiropractic," 79 *JAMA* (July 1, 1922) 57–59. "Lo, the Poor Chiropractor," 82 *JAMA* (May 17, 1924): 1613.

52. "An Estimate of Chiropractic by the Journal of the A.M.A.," clipping from the *Echo Enterprise* (Nov. 5, 1914), Box 624, Folder 5, HHF.

53. C. O. Wamscott to *JAMA*, Nov. 11, 1914, Box 624, Folder 5, HHF; Cramp to Wamscott, Nov. 14, 1914, Box 624, Folder 5, HHF; Hobart P. Shattuck to Cramp, Oct. 29, 1909, Box 624, Folder 5, HHF; Cramp to Shattuck, 3 Nov. 1909, Box 624, Folder 5; Cramp to H. B. Vallette, Jan. 11, 1910, Box 624, Folder 5, HHF.

54. AJC to Smith Ely Jelliffe, April 25, 1918, Box 174, Folder 11, HHF; Jelliffe to Cramp, April 17, 1918, Box 174, Folder 11, HHF; Cramp to Jelliffe, April 25, 1918, Box 174, Folder 11, HHF; *JAMA* to Hamilton, Aug. 3, 1912, Box 624, Folder 5, HHF. The quotations in the remainder of this paragraph are attributed to theletter from Smith Ely Jelliffe to AJC, April 27, 1918, Box 174, Folder 11, HHF.

CHAPTER FIVE

1. Barbara Bridgman Perkins, "Economic Organization of Medicine and the Committee on the Costs of Medical Care," *American Journal of Public Health* 88 (1998): 1721–26; Joseph S. Ross, "The Committee on the Costs of Medical Care and the History of Health Insurance in the United States," *Einstein Quarterly Journal of Biological Medicine* 19 (2002): 129–34. Ross places the formation of the committee in the context of debates over health insurance inspired by rising costs and poor health-care coverage for many Americans.

2. "The Committee on the Costs of Medical Care," *JAMA* 99 (Dec. 3, 1932): 1950–51.

3. Lee Anderson and Gregory J. Higby, *The Spirit of Voluntarism: A Legacy of Commitment and Contribution: The United States Pharmacopeia, 1820–1995* (Rockville, MD: United States Pharmacopeia Convention, 1995); Gregory J. Higby, ed., *One Hundred Years of the National Formulary: A Symposium* (Madison, WI: American Institute of the History of Pharmacy, 1989).

4. C. Rufus Rorem and Robert P. Fischelis, *The Costs of Medicine: The Manufacture and Distribution of Drugs and Medicines in the United States and the Services of Pharmacy in Medical Care* (Chicago: University of Chicago Press, 1932), v–20; Committee on the Costs of Medical Care, *Medical Care for the American People*, 28–29.

5. Rorem and Fischelis, *The Costs of Medicines*, 114–15, 135–36, and 196–97.

6. Surveys were initially conducted in Birmingham, New York City, Chicago, Dallas, New Orleans, and Washington, DC "Quackery and Drug Store Treatments in Birmingham, Alabama," 1932–33, Box 98, Folder 1, Social Welfare History Archives, American Social Hygiene Association, University of Minnesota (SWHA), Minneapolis, MN; "Quackery in Relation to Syphilis and Gonorrhea in Chicago," 1931, Box 99, Folder 3, SWHA; "Quackery and Drug Store Treatment in Relation to Venereal Disease in North Harlem," 1931, Box 100, Folder 14, SWHA; "Report on Extent of Sale of Nostrums and Prescribing for and Treatment of Venereal Disease by Druggists," 1927, Box 101, Folder 11, SWHA; "Quackery and Drug Store Treatment in Relation to Syphilis and Gonorrhea in Dallas, Texas," 1932, Box 102, Folder 4, SWHA; "The Medical Charlatan: Exploiter of the Sick, Well, Ignorant, Credulous," pamphlet ca. 1935, Box 173, Folder 15, SWHA; "Jerry Learns a Lesson: Keep Away from Quacks," pamphlet ca. 1933, Box 173, Folder 15,SWHA .

7. "Replies to Dr. McCormack: Frank J. Cheney, President of the Proprietary Association, Shows the Falsity of the Position of the Representative of the American Medical Association

Regarding 'Patent' Medicines," 1908, Box 678, Folder 11; Arthur J. Cramp to S. H. Landrum, March 31, 1910, Box 678, Folder 11, HHF.

8. Louis S. Reed, *The Healing Cults: A Study of Sectarian Medical Practice: Its Extent, Causes, and Control* (Chicago: University of Chicago Press, 1932), 11.

9. For a characterization of the "healing cults" or sects similar to Reed's, see Morris Fishbein, *The Medical Follies: An Analysis of the Foibles of Some Healing Cults, Including Osteopathy, Homeopathy, Chiropractic, and the Electronic Reactions of Abrams, with Essays on the Antivivisectionists, Health Legislation, Physical Culture, and Rejuvenation* (New York: Bonsi & Liveright, 1925).

10. Reed, *The Healing Cults*, 110–11; John C. Burnham, *How Superstition Won and Science Lost: Popularizing Science and Health in the United States* (New Brunswick, NJ: Rutgers University Press, 1987), 45–84.

11. Edward Bok, "My 'Attack' On Doctors," *JAMA* 50 (March 21, 1908): 961.

12. Reed, *The Healing Cults*, 110–15.

13. Charles W. Warner, *Quacks* (Jackson, MI: 1930), 20–28. Warner's book underwent seven printings between 1930 and 1934. It is unclear where he obtained the numbers of sufferers of the various ailments he identified.

14. Stuart Chase, *The Tragedy of Waste* (New York: MacMillan, 1937); AJC to William D. Cutter, 15 May 1933, Box 929, Folder 2, HHF; Young, *The Medical Messiahs*, 123.

15. Charles O. Jackson, "Muckraking and Consumer Protection: The Case of the 1938 Food, Drug and Cosmetic Act," *Pharmacy in History* 13 (1971): 103–10; C. B. Larrabee, "Guinea Pig Books," *Printer's Ink* 175 (April 16, 1936): 72; Stuart High, "Guinea Pigs, Left March," *Forum* 102 (October 1939): 153.

16. Jackson, "Muckraking and Consumer Protection," 105; James Harvey Young, *The Medical Messiahs: A Social History of Health Quackery in Twentieth-Century America* (Princeton: Princeton University Press, 1992), 152; James Corbett, "The Activities of Consumers' Organizations," *Law and Contemporary Problems* 1 (Dec. 19, 1933): 61–62; David F. Cavers, "The Food, Drug, and Cosmetic Act of 1938: Its Legislative History and Its Substantive Provisions," *Law and Contemporary Problems* 6 (Winter 1939): 2–42.

17. Young, *Medical Messiahs*, 153–54; Phillip J. Hilts, *Protecting America's Health: The FDA, Business, and One Hundred Years of Regulation* (New York: Alfred A. Knopf, 2003), 83–84.

18. Young, *Medical Messiahs*, 154; Arthur Kallet and F. J. Schlink, *100,000,000 Guinea Pigs: Dangers in Everyday Food, Drugs and Cosmetics* (New York: Vanguard, 1933), 6, 10, 16, 178, 181–83.

19. Kallet and Schlink, 116–17.

20. "The Consumer's Protection under the Federal Pure Food and Drugs Act," *Columbia Law Review* 32 (April 1932): 720–36.

21. E. Pendleton Herring, "The Balance of Social Forces in the Administration of the Pure Food and Drug Act," *Social Forces* 13 (March 1935): 358–66; Lauffer T. Hayes and Frank J. Ruff, "The Administration of the Federal Food and Drugs Act," *Law and Contemporary Problems* 1 (December 1933): 16–35.

22. Hilts, *Protecting America's Health*, 73–77; Charles Wesley Dunn, *The Federal Food, Drug, and Cosmetic Act: A Statement of Its Legislative Record* (New York: G. E. Stechert and Co., 1938), 24–30.

23. Charles O. Jackson, *Food and Drug Legislation in the New Deal* (Princeton, NJ: Princeton University Press, 1970). For information on the problems faced by the FTC, see "The Federal Trade Commission Act of 1938," *Columbia Law Review* 39 (February 1939): 259–73; Milton Handler, "The Control of False Advertising under the Wheeler-Lea Act," *Law and Contemporary Problems* 6 (Winter 1939): 91–110.

24. Kallet and Schlink, *100,000,000 Guinea Pigs*, 189–93; T. Swann Harding, *Fads, Frauds and Physicians: Diagnosis and Treatment of the Doctor's Dilemma* (New York: The Dial Press, 1930), 152.

25. Kallet and Schlink, 159, 190–93, 213.

26. Young, *Medical Messiahs*, 156.

27. As Young notes, Wiley expressed his views in testifying before a House Committee in 1912 in *The Pure Food and Drugs Act: Hearings before the Committee on Interstate and Foreign Commerce, House of Representatives* (62nd Congress, 2nd Session). Carl Alsberg, chief of the Bureau of Chemistry, described "serious limitations" of the law in his *1917 Report of Bureau of Chemistry* in *Food Law Institute, Federal Food, Drug and Cosmetic Law Administrative Reports, 1907–49* (Washington, DC: U.S. Government Printing Office, 1951): 355, 366–76; cited in Young, *Medical Messiahs*, 159. For more on Wiley's critique of the act, see Harvey W. Wiley, *An Autobiography* (Indianapolis: The Bobbs-Merrill Co., 1930); Wiley, *History of a Crime against the Food Law* (Washington: Arno Press, 1929); Wiley, "A Criticism of Some Drug Law Regulations," *American Druggist* 80 (October 1929): 60. Lamb, *American Chamber of Horrors: The Truth About Food and Drugs* (New York: Farrar & Rinehart, 1936).

28. Paul B. Dunbar, "Memories of Early Days of Federal Food and Drug Law Enforcement," *Food, Drug, Cosmetic Law Journal* 14 (February 1959): 134–35; Jackson, *Food and Drug Legislation in the New Deal*, 3–24; *The Journal of Quackery* (New York: The Olof Company, 1912).

29. Lamb, *American Chamber of Horrors*, 278–80; Hilts, *Protecting America's Health*, 76–78.

30. The five-year struggle to pass what became known as the Federal Food, Drug and Cosmetic Act of 1938 is covered in the greatest detail by Jackson, *Food and Drug Legislation in the New Deal*. In *Medical Messiahs*, Young also devotes a chapter to this subject. In *Federal Food, Drug, and Cosmetic Act: A Statement of Its Legislative Record* (New York: G. E. Stechert & Co., 1938), Charles W. Dunn has reprinted all the pertinent portions of the *Congressional Record* relating to the efforts to secure the law as well as portions of congressional hearings citing testimony from the FDA and FTC, consumer groups, and industry representatives. For an interpretation focused on the FDA, see Hilts, *Protecting America's Health*, 72–94. For a perspective from someone involved in the process of securing the new law, see Lamb, *America Chamber of Horrors*, 278–327. On Tugwell's involvement, see Bernard Sternsher, *Rexford Tugwell and the New Deal* (New Brunswick, NJ: Rutgers University Press, 1964).

31. Dunn, *Federal Food, Drug and Cosmetic Act*, 37–50; Lamb, *Chamber of Horrors*, 287–88; Young, *Medical Messiahs*, 165–66; Cavers, "The Food, Drug, and Cosmetic Act of 1938," 7–8.

32. Opposition to Copeland and Tugwell is addressed in Young, *Medical Messiahs*, 164–68; Hilts, *Protecting America's Health*, 81–82; Jackson, *Food and Drug Legislation in the New Deal*, 32–36; Lamb, *American Chamber of Horrors*, 290–92; and Raymond Joseph Potter, *Royal Samuel Copeland 1868-1938: A Physician in Politics*, (University of Cleveland, unpublished Ph.D. dissertation, 1967), 448–52. The preceding characterizations are also drawn from articles that can be found in FDA Scrapbooks, Vol. 1, Records of the Office of the Commissioners of FDA, RG 88, Accession No. 52–A86, National Archives. Specifically, see G. A. Nichols, "Beat the Tugwell Bill," *Printer's Ink* 165 (November 2, 1933): 6ff; Frank Blair, "Effects of Proposed Legislative Changes upon Industry," *Standard Remedies* 20 (November 1933): 6; Stephen Wilson, *Food and Drug Regulation* (Washington, DC: American Council on Public Affairs, 1942), 93.

33. *Food, Drugs, and Cosmetics Hearings before a Subcommittee of the Committee of Commerce* (U.S. Senate, 73rd Congress, 2nd Sess. On S. 1944 held December 7 and 8, 1933): 101, 104, 132, 192–94, 405. Hereafter these hearings are cited as *Senate Hearings on S. 1944* (December 1933).

34. Young, *Medical Messiahs*, 166; Jackson, *Food and Drug Legislation in the New Deal*, 31–33; *Senate Hearings on S. 1944* (December 1933): 104; "The Case against the Tugwell Bill," *Advertising and Selling* 22 (November 9, 1933): 13–14; "Food and Drug Bill Pending," *Standard Remedies* 20 (September 1933): 5; Charles LaWall, "Fads and Frauds in Foods and Drugs," *American Journal of Pharmacy* 109 (March 1937): 119.

35. *Senate Hearings on S. 1944* (December 1933): 336–37, 109; *Standard Remedies* 20 (August 1933): 1; Nichols, "Beat the Tugwell Bill," 6.

36. Jackson, *Food and Drug Legislation in the New Deal*, 37–38; Cavers, "The Food, Drug, and Cosmetic Act of 1938," 9–10; E. E. Calkins, "Another Look at the Pure Food Bill," *Good Housekeeping* 97 (December 1933): 90.

37. Jackson, *Food and Drug Legislation in the New Deal*, 38–39.

38. Jackson, *Food and Drug Legislation in the New Deal*, 39–42; Jackson, "Muckraking and Consumer Protection," 105–6; Cavers, "The Food, Drug, and Cosmetic Act of 1938," 3; George Seldes, *Lords of the Press* (New York: 1938), 300; C. C. Regier, "The Struggle for Federal Food and Drugs Legislation," *Law and Contemporary Problems* 1 (December 1933): 3–15.

39. FDA information officer Ruth deForest Lamb covered each of these cases in detail in her book *American Chamber of Horrors*, which included reproductions of a number of posters used in the exhibit. For coverage of the Chamber of Horrors, see Young, *Medical Messiahs*, 169–71; Jackson, *Food and Drug Legislation in the New Deal*, 43–45; Hilts, *Protecting America's Health*, 85–88. Contemporary press coverage is exemplified by John Mitchell, "Pink Pills for Dead People," *New Republic* 77 (Dec. 13, 1933): 119–21.

40. Arthur Kallet, "A Consumer Looks at the Food and Drugs Bill," *Law and Contemporary Problems* 1 (Dec. 1933): 127; *Senate Hearings on S. 1944* (Dec. 1933): 355–57; "Tugwell Bill Tension," *Business Week* (Dec. 16, 1933): 8; Young, *Medical Messiahs*, 169–70; Jackson, *Food and Drug Legislation in the New Deal*, 45–47.

41. For the most extensive coverage of the period from 1933 to 1947, see Jackson, *Food and Drug Legislation in the New Deal*, 47–200; and Young, *The Medical Messiahs*, 170–90.

42. This account of the Elixir Sulfanilamide crisis is drawn from James Harvey Young, "The 'Elixir Sulfanilamide' Disaster," *Emory University Quarterly* 14 (1958): 230–47; Young, *Medical Messiahs*, 184–87; Jackson, *Food and Drug Legislation in the New Deal*, 175–88; and Hilts, *Protecting America's Health*, 89–92.

43. Ibid.

44. Jackson, *Food and Drug Legislation in the New Deal*, 175–200; Young, *The Medical Messiahs*, 187–190; Hilts, *Protecting America's Health*, 92–93.

45. John P. Swann, *Academic Scientists and the Pharmaceutical Industry: Cooperative Research in Twentieth Century America* (Baltimore: Johns Hopkins University Press, 1988).

46. Many of these weaknesses, and the benefits outlined in subsequent paragraphs, are identified and discussed in the following sources: Jackson, *Food and Drug Legislation in the New Deal*, 192–200; Young, *The Medical Messiahs*, 189–90; Hilts, *Protecting America's Health*, 93–94; Cavers, "The Food, Drug, and Cosmetic Act of 1938," 31–40.

CHAPTER SIX

1. Peter Temin, "The Origin of Compulsory Drug Prescriptions," *Journal of Law and Economics* 22 (April 1979): 91–105; Harry M. Marks, "Revisiting 'The Origins of Compulsory Drug Prescriptions,'" *American Journal of Public Health* 85 (Jan. 1995): 109–15; Arthur Daemmrich, *Pharmacopolitics: Drug Regulation in the United States and Germany* (Chapel Hill: University of North Carolina Press, 2004); Jonathan Liebenau, *The Formation of the American Pharmaceutical Industry* (Baltimore: Johns Hopkins University Press, 1987).

2. "To Distributors of Sulfanilamide and Related Drugs," FDA Trade Correspondence, reprinted in Vincent Kleinfeld and Charles Wesley Dunn, *Federal Food, Drug and Cosmetic Act: Judicial and Administrative Record, 1938–1949* (Chicago: Commerce Clearing House, 1949), 561; Edward J. Matson, "Some Historical Notes on the Refilling of Prescriptions," *Food, Drug, and Cosmetic Law Quarterly* (*FDCLQ*) 4 (Dec. 1949): 575–85; Harrry M. Marks, *The Progress of Experiment: Science and Therapeutic Reform in the United States, 1900–1990* (New York: Cambridge University Press, 1997), 80.

3. Marks, *The Progress of Experiment*, 80–81; Marks, "Revisiting 'The Origin of Compulsory Drug Prescriptions,'" 109–15; Temin, "The Origin of Compulsory Drug Prescriptions," 97–98.

4. H. E. Moskey, "The Drug Manufacturer's Duties," *Food, Drug and Cosmetic Law Journal* (*FDCLJ*) 6 (March 1951): 374–82; Carl M. Anderson, "The 'New Drug' Section," *FDCLQ* 1 (March 1946), 84; Robert T. Stormont, "Application of the Federal Act to New Drugs," *FDCLQ* 2 (December 1947): 490–97; Erwin E. Nelson, "New Drug Requirements of the Federal Food, Drug, and Cosmetic Act," *FDCLQ* 4 (June 1949): 227–32; Nelson, "Development of New Drugs," *FDCLJ* 5 (March 1950): 238–50; Frederic P. Lee, "The Basic Philosophy of Federal Food and Drug Legislation," *FDCLQ* 3 (March 1948): 44–48; Marks, *The Progress of Experiment*, 85–93.

5. Marks, *The Progress of Experiment*, 80–82, 92–95; Theodore G. Klumpp to John P. Peters, Dec. 29, 1939, 88-58A-277, Box 38, Folder 511.07-512, Washington National

Record Center, Suitland, MD; J. J. Durrett, "Some of the Implications of Section 505(b) (I) of the Food, Drug and Cosmetic Act," American Drug Manufacturers Association, *Proceedings*, 28th Annual Meeting (1939): 98–104.

6. William A. Quinlan, "The Sullivan Case," *FDCLQ* 3 (Dec. 1948): 532–51. For an extended discussion of the Sullivan Case, see James Harvey Young, *The Medical Messiahs: A Social History of Health Quackery in Twentieth-Century America* (Princeton: Princeton University Press, 1992), 269–71. Case-related documents are reprinted in Kleinfeld and Dunn, *Federal Food, Drug, and Cosmetic Act* 319–58. The *FDCLQ* published the text of the Supreme Court justices' opinions in their entirety under the title, "The Sullivan Case" (March 1948): 131–44.

7. Robert L Swain, "The Impact of the Sullivan Case upon the Local Sale and Distribution of Drugs and Medicine," *FDCLQ* 4 (March 1949): 79–84; Young, *The Medical Messiahs*, 271; Temin, "The Origin of Compulsory Drug Prescriptions," 100–01; *1948 Report of the Food and Drug Administration*, 26 (All annual reports from the FDA here cited and in the remainder of the chapter are reprinted in *Federal Food, Drug and Cosmetic Law: Administrative Reports, 1907–1949* (Chicago: Commerce Clearing House, 1951) and *Food and Drug Administration, Annual Reports, 1950–1974* (Washington: Government Printing Office, 1974); *1949 Report of the Food and Drug Administration*, 25–26; George P. Larrick, "Indiscriminate Sale of Dangerous and Habit-Forming Drugs," *FDCLJ* 5 (May 1950), 251–57.

8. Leonard P. Prusak, "Barbiturate Control by Legislation," *FDCLJ* 5 (September 1950), 598–603; H. J. Anslinger, "Barbiturate Legislation," *FDCLJ* 7 (March 1952): 211–14; R. T. Stormont, "Barbiturate Drug Legislation," *FDCLJ* 7 (1952): 215–21; "1951 Food and Drug Administration Annual Report of the Federal Security Agency," *FDCLJ* 7 (May 1952): 322–37; Young, *The Medical Messiahs*, 272–73; *1949 Report of the Food and Drug Administration*, 25–26; *1948 Report of the Food and Drug Administration*, 8–9.

9. "Drugs Dispensed on Physician's Prescription," and "Dangerous Drugs," FDA Trade Correspondence, reprinted in Kleinfeld and Dunn, *Federal Food, Drug, and Cosmetic Act*, 699, 708; Charles W. Crawford, "The Federal Law and the Druggist," *FDCLJ* 5 (Dec. 1950), 812–22; Walton M. Wheeler, Jr., "Prescription Refills," *FDCLJ* 5 (Dec. 1950), 746–54; John P. Swann, "FDA and the Practice of Pharmacy: Drug Regulation Before the Durham-Humphrey Amendment of 1951," *Pharmacy in History* 36, (1994), 55–70; Young, *The Medical Messiahs*, 274; Temin, "The Origin of Compulsory Drug Prescriptions," 102.

10. Oscar R. Ewing, "The Durham Bill Hearings," *FDCLJ* 5 (June 1951): 407–30; Richard Joseph Hopkins, "Medical Prescriptions and the Law: A Study of the Enactment of the Durham-Humphrey Amendment to the Federal Food, Drug and Cosmetic Act," (master's thesis, Emory University, 1965), 33–38; Young, *The Medical Messiahs*, 274–77.

11. James F. Hoge, "The Durham-Humphrey Bill," *FDCLJ* 6 (February 1951): 135–41 (quote on 139); "Testimony by Charles Wesley Dunn," from *Hearings on H.R. 298*, reprinted in *FDCLJ* 6 (June 1951): 430; Hopkins, "Medical Prescriptions and the Law," 175–88; Peter Temin, *Taking Your Medicine: Drug Regulation in the United States*. Cambridge, Mass.: Harvard University Press, 1980, 51–63; Marks, "Revisiting 'The Origins of Compulsory Drug Prescriptions,'" 112–13.

12. Charles Wesley Dunn, "The New Prescription Drug Law," *FDCLJ* 6 (December 1951): 951–69.

13. Temin, "The Origins of Compulsory Drug Prescriptions," 103–04; Temin, *Taking Your Medicine*, 63–67; Marks, "Revisiting 'The Origins of Compulsory Drug Prescriptions,' " 112–13.

14. This judgment of the chemotherapeutic revolution and related advances is recounted in Young, *The Medical Messiahs*, 260–63; *1956 Annual Report: Food and Drug Administration, Department of Health, Education and Welfare*, 172.

15. *1953 Report of the Food and Drug Administration, U.S. Department of Health, Education, and Welfare*, 200; Julius Stieglitz, ed., *Chemistry in Medicine* (New York: Chemical Foundation, 1929), 496; R. T. Stormont, "From Alchemy to Antibiotics," *FDCLJ* 11 (February 1956): 98–99; Frank H. Wiley, "The Analysis of Drugs," *FDCLJ* 16 (December 1961): 733–34; George Larrick, testimony before a House Committee, reprinted in *FDCLJ* 13 (April 1958): 230; Young, *The Medical Messiahs*, 263–65.

16. *1956 Report of the Food and Drug Administration, U.S. Department of Health, Education, and Welfare*, 36–37; Editorial, *Drug Trade News* 33 (March 10, 1958): 30; Young, *The Medical Messiahs*, 266–67.

17. Young, *The Medical Messiahs*, 262–65. Young cites the following sources for these trends: James F. Hoge, "Government Interest in the Drug Trade," mimeographed address distributed with the Proprietary Association *Executive News-Letter* 482 (June 7, 1959);; Bureau of the Census, *United States Census of Manufacturers: 1954*, II, *Industry Statistics*, Part I, *General Survey and Major Groups 20 to 28* (Washington, DC, 1957): 28C-10 through 28C-12.

18. James F. Hoge, "An Appraisal of the New Drug and Cosmetic Legislation from the Viewpoint of Those Industries," *Law and Contemporary Problems* 6 (1939): 111–28; Charles Crawford, "Problems of Compliance and Enforcement under the Drug Law," *FDCLQ* 2 (1947): 445.

19. *1941 Annual Report of Food and Drug Administration*, 15–22.

20. Ibid.

21. Charles W. Crawford, "Legislative and Administrative Progress under the Federal Food, Drug, and Cosmetic Act," *FDCLJ* 5 (March 1950): 17; Crawford, "Problems of Compliance and Enforcement under the Drug Law," 445; Young, *The Medical Messiahs*, 191–93.

22. Rayburn D. Tousley, "The Federal Food, Drug, and Cosmetic Act of 1938," *Journal of Marketing* 5 (Jan. 1941): 259–69; Edward B. Williams, "Exemption from the Requirement of Adequate Directions for Use in the Labeling of Drugs," *FDCLQ* 2 (June 1947): 155–72; U.S. Department of Agriculture, Food and Drug Administration, "Federal Food, Drug, and Cosmetic Act and General Regulations for Its Enforcement" (Washington, DC: Government Printing Office, Aug. 1939): 4; "Directions for Use," "Warning Statements for Drug Preparations," FDA Trade Correspondence, in Kleinfeld and Dunn, *Federal Food, Drug, and Cosmetic Act, 1938–1949*, 745, 574–78.

23. For an extended discussion of the Colgrove case, see Young, *The Medical Messiahs*, 197–200. The case records involving Colgrove and Colusa Natural Oil are reprinted in Kleinfeld and Dunn, *Federal Food, Drug, and Cosmetic Act, 1938–1949*, 218–21; Kleinfeld

and Dunn, *Federal Food, Drug, and Cosmetic Act, 1949–50*, 114–20, 237–41. The account of Colgrove's litigious career is also evidenced in FDA Drugs and Devices Notices of Judgment numbers 380, 381, 1040, 1384, 2087, 2131, 2782, 2833, 3009, 3045, 3061, and 3989. Figures are taken from *1949 Report of Food and Drug Administration*, 27.

24. Ibid. See also Daniel P. Willis and William W. Goodrich, "Enforcement and Judicial Processes of the Federal Food, Drug, and Cosmetic Act," *FDCLJ* 5 (March 1950): 27–35.

25. Young, *The Medical Messiahs*, 198–200; *1949 Report of Food and Drug Administration*, 27.

26. Vincent A. Kleinfeld, "Applicability of the Federal Food, Drug, and Cosmetic Act to Drug Advertising," *FDCLJ* 5 (March 1950): 45–53; William W. Goodrich, "Enforcement and Judicial Progress in 1951 Under the Federal Food, Drug, and Cosmetic Act," *FDCLJ* 7 (March 1952): 197–209.

27. George Link, Jr., "Judicial Interpretation of the Words 'Accompanying Such Article,' Contained in the Federal Food, Drug and Cosmetic Law," *FDCLQ* 2 (June 1947): 207–15; Arthur D. Herrick, "Some Implications of the Kordel Decision," *FDCLQ* 4 (March 1949): 94–104; Thomas W. Christopher, "The Attitude of the Supreme Court," *FDCLJ* 7 (1952): 365–72. The Kordel and Urbeteit case reports are reprinted in Kleinfeld and Dunn, *Federal Food, Drug, and Cosmetic Act, 1938–1949*, 328–30, 343–48, 382–86, 212–15, 249–51, 521, 560.

28. Campbell, "Legislative and Administrative Progress under the Federal Food, Drug, and Cosmetic Act," 18–19; Campbell, *1942–43 Report of Food and Drug Administration*, in *Federal Food, Drug and Cosmetic Law Administrative Reports*, 1026–38; W. R. M. Wharton, "Wartime and Postwar Food and Drug Adulteration," *FDCLQ* 1 (February 1946): 465; C. W. Crawford, "Legislative and Administrative Progress Under the Federal Food, Drug, and Cosmetic Act," *FDCLJ* 5 (March 1950): 16–24.

29. Kleinfeld and Dunn, *Federal Food, Drug, and Cosmetic Act, 1938–1949*, Introduction, xv–xvi; Paul Dunbar, "The Enforcement of the Federal Food, Drug, and Cosmetic Act," *FDCLQ* 3 (June 1948): 154–65.

30. George P. Larrick, "Some Current Problems of Enforcement," *FDCLQ* 3 (June 1948): 261–69; James W. Cassedy, "Progress of Federal Law against False Advertisement of Food, Drugs, and Cosmetics," *FDCLQ* 4 (June 1949): 353–62.

31. Francis E. McKay and Benjamin Frauwirth, "The Penalty Provisions of the Federal Food, Drug, and Cosmetic Act," *FDCLJ* 6 (1951): 575–92; William W. Goodrich, "Judicial Highlights of 50 Years' Enforcement," *FDCLJ* 11 (February 1956): 70–76; George P. Larrick, "Administrative Progress of the Federal Food, Drug, and Cosmetic Act in 1951," *FDCLJ* 7 (February 1952): 153–60; Wallace F. Janssen, *Annual Reports, 1950–1974, on the Administration of the Federal Food, Drug, and Cosmetic Act and Related Laws* (Rockville, MD: Dept. of Health, Education and Welfare, 1975), xi.

CHAPTER SEVEN

1. George P. Larrick, "1956 Annual Report, Food and Drug Administration," from the *1956 Annual Report of the U.S. Department of Health, Education, and Welfare*, 201. All FDA reports cited in this chapter are collected in *Annual Reports 1950–1974 on the Administration*

of the Federal Food, Drug, and Cosmetic Act and Related Laws (Washington, DC: U.S. Government Printing Office, 1976).

2. George Larrick, "Fifty Years of Federal Food, Drug and Cosmetic Law," *Food, Drug and Cosmetic Law Journal (FDCLJ)* 11 (April 1956): 212–19; *1957 Annual Report, Food and Drug Administration,* 192–95. [All annual reports from the FDA cited below are published in *Food and Drug Administration, Annual Reports, 1950-1974* (Washington: Government Printing Office, 1974).]

3. Larrick, "The Achievements of 50 Years," *FDCLJ* 11 (June 1956): 36; *1956 Annual Report, Food and Drug Administration,* 209–13; *Report of the Citizens' Advisory Committee on the U.S. Food and Drug Administration to the Secretary of Health, Education and Welfare* (Washington, DC: HEW, 1955), typescript copy in "Special Data, 1955," Box 272, Folder 08, HHF; Daniel Carpenter, *Reputation and Power: Organizational Image and Pharmaceutical Regulation at the FDA* (Princeton, NJ: Princeton University Press, 2010), 132–33.

4. *1954 Annual Report, Food and Drug Administration,* 187–91; *1955 Annual Report, Food and Drug Administration,* 196–97; *1956 Annual Report, Food and Drug Administration,* 212.

5. James C. Munch, "A Half-Century of Drug Control," *FDCLJ* 11 (June 1956): 305–35; William W. Goodrich, "Searching for Medical Truths in the Courtroom," *FDCLJ* 11 (September 1956): 482–83.

6. Ronald W. Lamont-Havers, "Arthritis Quackery," *American Journal of Nursing* 63 (March 1963): 94; "FDA Wins Long Battles; Hoxsey, Tri-Wonda Hit," *AMA News* (Oct. 3, 1960): 3; "Government Wins Battle against Arthritis Remedy," *JAMA* 174 (Nov. 19, 1960): 1642; Goodrich, "Searching for Medical Truths," 483–84.

7. For extensive coverage of the Hoxsey saga, see James Harvey Young, *The Medical Messiahs: A Social History of Health Quackery in Twentieth-Century America* (Princeton: Princeton University Press, 1992), 360–89; Kenny Ausubel, *When Healing Becomes a Crime: The Amazing Story of the Hoxsey Cancer Clinics and the Return of Alternative Therapies* (Rochester, VT: Healing Arts Press, 2000); and Eric S. Juhnke, *Quacks and Crusaders: The Fabulous Careers of John Brinkley, Norman Baker, and Harry Hoxsey* (Lawrence: University of Kansas Press, 2002). The AMA HHF Archives also include extensive coverage on Hoxsey, especially in Boxes 366–377 as well as S01–09, S03–08, S03–09, and S04–01. Details of the trial are taken from Young, *The Medical Messiahs,* 375–80; Alan H. Kaplan, "Therapeutic Claims and the Federal Government," *FDCLJ* 11 (April 1956): 231–36; Goodrich, "Searching for Medical Truths in the Courtroom," 484–85.

8. Ibid.

9. "Public Warning against Hoxsey Cancer Treatment," FDA press release (Apr. 4, 1956); Wallace F. Janssen, "Quackery in the News," *Public Health Reports* 74 (July 1959): 635–38; Young, *The Medical Messiahs,* 387.

10. David Cantor, "Cancer Quackery and the Vernacular Meanings of Hope in 1950s America," *Journal of the History of Medicine* 61 (July 2006): 335–36, 345–49.

11. Ibid., 354–59.

12. Goodrich, "Searching for Medical Truth in the Courtroom," 483–85; Albert H. Holland, "The Medical Work of the Food and Drug Administration," *FDCLJ* 11 (April 1956): 181–84; Holland, "Current Problems under the Federal Food, Drug, and

Cosmetic Act," *FDCLJ* 11 (Sept. 1956): 486–92; David H. Vernon, "Labyrinthine Ways: The Handling of Food, Drug, Device and Cosmetic Cases by the Federal Trade Commission Since 1938," *FDCLJ* 8 (June 1953): 389–91.

13. James Cook, "The Nation's Nostrum Bill," *New York Post* (May 20, 1957): 2; Cook, *Remedies and Rackets: The Truth About Patent Medicines* (New York: W. W. Norton, 1958); Louis M. Orr, "Public Beware, Quackery Ahead!" address delivered before the Commonwealth Club, San Francisco, CA (June 27, 1958), 2–3; " 'Quack Boom,' Doctor Says," *San Francisco Examiner* (June 23, 1958): 3; "Quacks Still Flourish in Age of Science, MD Tells Club," *San Francisco News* (June 27, 1958): 1; "The Big Boom in Quackery," *Newsweek* (July 7, 1958): 60; Janssen, "Quackery in the News," 635–38.

14. Jaqueline Larkin, "Quack Nostrums Only Help Quacks: Their Bank Accounts Grow at Expense of Hopeful Patients," *Minneapolis Tribune* (February 23, 1958): 2; Norma Lee Browning, "Quackery: $500,000,000 Racket: The Snake Oil Salesman Was a Piker Compared with Grafters Fleecing the Gullible Today," *Chicago Sun Times Magazine* (June 14, 1959): 35–36; "Billion-Dollar Business Bared by Quack Hunt," *Medical Economics* (May 9, 1960): 44; Ralph Lee Smith, "America's Most Flourishing Fraud," *American Legion Magazine* (October 1959): 24–25, 50–55; "Medical Quacks' Take Hits Record Mark," *Rocky Mountain News* (August 13, 1960): A3; "A Revival of Quackery," *Time* (June 29, 1959): 60.

15. "Medical Frauds at New High: FDA Official Calls for More Aggressive Fight on Quacks," *Medical News* (March 1, 1958): 47; Eric W. Martin, "Murder by Mail," a copy of the editorial and an accompanying news release were sent to the AMA's Bureau of Investigation in March 1958, Box 711, File 10, HHF.

16. Jonathan Spivak, "Crusade on Quacks: Federal, State, Private Agencies Step Up Fight against False 'Cures'," *Wall Street Journal* (June 22, 1960): 1; Roald N. Grant et al., "Progress against Cancer Quacks," *JAMA* 175 (Feb. 4, 1961): 401–02; L. Henry Garlan, "Investigation of Cancer Remedies," *National Academy of Sciences, National Research Council News Report* 7 (Sept.–Oct. 1957): 73–77; Charles S. Cameron, *The Cancer Quacks* (Washington, DC: National Cancer Institute, 1963), reprinted with permission from U.S. Public Health Service, *The Truth About Cancer* (New York: Prentice-Hall, 1956); Kenneth N. Anderson, "What You Should Know about Phony Arthritis Remedies," *Today's Health* 39 (July 1961): 32–33; Ruth Walrad, *The Misrepresentation of Arthritis Drugs and Devices in the United States* (New York: The Arthritis and Rheumatism Foundation, 1961).

17. George Larrick, "Report from the Food and Drug Administration," *FDCLJ* 13 (March 1958): 151–52; Wallace F. Janssen, "Public Information under the Federal Food, Drug, and Cosmetic Act," *FDCLJ* 12 (Jan. 1957): 57–61; Young, *The Medical Messiahs*, 393–94.

18. U.S. Food and Drug Administration (FDA), *Your Money and Your Life: An FDA Catalog of Fakes and Swindles in the Health Field* (Washington, DC: U.S. Department of Health, Education, and Welfare, 1965); HEW Press Release, Nov. 18, 1958; Young, *Medical Messiahs*, 394.

19. Spivak, "Crusade on Quacks," 1; "New AMA Campaign," *AMA News* 3 (Oct. 3, 1960): 4; "What Does 'Quack' Mean to You?" *Today's Health* 33 (April 1955): 56–57; Jack Kytle, "Don't Help the Quacks," *Today's Health* 36 (Nov. 1956): 13. More than a million

copies of the pamphlet "Merchants of Menace" (Chicago: AMA, 1960) were distributed by the AMA by 1963.

20. Young, *Medical Messiahs*, 402–03; Don Blair, Associate Executive Secretary of the Oklahoma State Medical Association to Oliver Field, 3 Aug. 1961, and Field's reply to Blair, 8 August 1961, Box 524, Folder 13, HHF.

21. "First National Congress on Medical Quackery to Be Held in October," AMA press release (Chicago: July 31, 1961); J. W. Davis, "Nation's Big Guns Called Up for War on Medical Quackery," *Chicago Sun-Times* (Oct. 1, 1961): 9; "For Release in A.M. Papers," FDA press release (Washington, DC: Oct. 3, 1961).

22. Young provides a personal account of his attendance at the congress in *The Medical Messiahs*, 403.

23. C. Joseph Stetler and Abraham Ribicoff, "Introduction," *Proceedings, National Congress on Medical Quackery* (Chicago: American Medical Association, 1961), 1–6.

24. *Proceedings: National Congress on Medical Quackery*, 6, 47–48, 17–19; "Washington News: First National Quackery Congress: A Report," *JAMA* 178 (Oct. 21, 1961): 33.

25. *Proceedings: National Congress on Medical Quackery*, 35–40; "Quick Action Urged to Stamp Our Quacks," AMA press release (Chicago: Oct. 6, 1961).

26. *Proceedings: National Congress on Medical Quackery*,40–41, 6; "The Month in Washington," AMA memorandum (Chicago: Oct. 6, 1961); John Troan, "Quackery Is Near to Murder: End It," *S.F. News–Call Bulletin* (Oct. 6, 1961): 3.

27. "Publicity Highlights from the National Congress on Medical Quackery, October 6–7, 1961," Box, Folder, HHF "Quick-Buck Quacks Are Prospering More Than Ever, Conference Told," *Washington Post* (Oct. 7, 1961); Leonard W. Larson, "Join the New War against Quacks," *This Week* (Oct. 6, 1961): 4–10; "FDA and AMA Sponsor National Congress on Medical Quackery," *Journal of the American Pharmaceutical Association* (Nov. 1961): 692–93; Letter from Oliver Field to James Harvey Young, 21 Nov. 1961, Box 524, Folder 14, HHF. Field mentions the Congress got "round-the-world coverage," from Germany to New Zealand.

28. *Proceedings: National Congress on Medical Quackery*, 17–19; "AMA and FDA Unite on Urging New Crackdown but Split on Question of Federal Authority," *Medical World News* (Oct. 27, 1961): 26–28; "Physicians and Government Will Work Together at Protecting the Public from Medical Quackery," *Journal of the Iowa Medical Society* (Nov. 1961): 271–74.

29. *Proceedings: National Congress on Medical Quackery*, 2–3; Morris Fishbein, "Medical Quackery: A National Menace," *Medical World News* (Oct. 27, 1961): 72.

30. Carpenter, *Reputation and Power*, 204–09.

31. George Larrick, "Our Unfinished Business," address to Eastern Section of the American Pharmaceutical Manufacturers' Association, Waldorf-Astoria Hotel, New York, Dec. 8, 1954, Box 272, Folder 7, "Special Data, 1953–54," AMA; Larrick, "Fifty Years of Federal Food, Drug and Cosmetic Laws," 216–17; Carpenter, *Reputation and Power*, 195.

32. Larrick, "The Achievement of 50 Years," 38; Larrick, "Fifty Years of Federal Food, Drug and Cosmetic Laws," 216; Holland, "The Medical Work of the Food and Drug Administration," 184.

33. For an extended discussion of NDAs during this period, see Carpenter, *Reputation and Power*, 157–82. Carpenter cites Holland's statement in "Before the House Subcommittee on

Legal and Monetary Affairs of the House Committee on Government Operations," Feb. 18, 1958; DF 505, RG 88, National Archives. On considerations of the efficacy question before 1960, see John Swann, "Sure Cure: Public Policy on Drug Efficacy before 1962," in Gregory J. Higby and Elaine C. Stroud, eds., *The Inside Story of Medicines: A Symposium* (Madison, WI: American Institute for the History of Pharmacy, 1997), 223–62; Marks, *The Progress of Experiment*, 78–97.

34. Carpenter, *Reputation and Power*, 164. Prosecution and enforcement data, and related unpublished material detailing the increased activity in these areas, are available in "FDA, USDHEW, Larrick's Statement Before Kefauver Committee, 1960," Box 273, Folder 1 and "FDA, USDHEW, Special Data, 1959–69," Box 273, Folder 2, AMA.

35. This account of Kefauver, the Kefauver hearings, and the subsequent legislation that resulted is taken from Carpenter, *Reputation and Power*, 230–45, 260–80. For more information on Kefauver and his involvement with the pharmaceutical industry, see Richard Harris, *The Real Voice: The Kefauver Drug Hearings* (New York: McMillan, 1964); Richard E. McFadyen, *Estes Kefauver and the Drug Industry* (Ph.D. diss., History, Emory University, 1973); Morton Mintz, *By Prescription Only* [originally published as *The Therapeutic Nightmare*] (Boston: Houghton Mifflin, 1967); Hilts, *Protecting America's Health*, 129–65; Young, *The Medical Messiahs*, 413–22.

36. Carpenter, *Reputation and Power*, 190–94, 234.

37. Carpenter, *Reputation and Power*, 235–36; Hilts, *Protecting America's Health*, 132–43; McFadyen, *Estes Kefauver and the Drug Industry*, 214–50.

38. Morton Mintz, "Heroine of FDA Keeps Bad Drug Off Markets: Linked to Malformed Babies," *Washington Post* (July 15, 1962): A1; Carpenter, *Reputation and Power*, 238–45; Rock Brynner and Trent Stephens, *A Dark Remedy: The Impact of Thalidomide and Its Revival as a Vital Medicine* (New York: Basic Books, 2001), Chapter 2; Hilts, *Protecting America's Health*, 144–65; Harris, *The Real Voice*, 161; Richard E. McFadyen, "Thalidomide in America: A Brush with Tragedy," *Clio Medica* 11 (1976): 79–93; Max Sherman and Steven Strauss, "Thalidomide: A Twenty-Five Year Perspective," *FDCLJ* 41 (1986): 458–66.

39. Campbell, *Reputation and Power*, 260–63. The standard of "well-controlled investigations" was set in law by the "Drug Amendments of 1962," section 102, 2, Public Law 87–871, Oct. 10, 1962. In *The Progress of Experiment*, Harry Marks notes that the FDA did not define the standards for such "well-controlled" studies until 1970, when it designated that such studies must (ideally) incorporate a contemporaneous control group assigned at random, sufficient quantitative evaluation, and the use of appropriate statistical methods (129).

40. C. L. Wilbar, "Summary," *Proceedings of First Pennsylvania Congress To Combat Health Quackery* (Philadelphia: Pennsylvania Department of Health, 1962), 81–84.

41. Irving Ladimer, "Quackery and the Consumer: Responsibility of the Medical Profession," speech delivered before the Connecticut State Congress on Medical Quackery (Berlin, CT: Sept. 26, 1962): 1–4.

42. Ladimer, "Quackery and the Consumer," 13–14; K. L. Milstead, "The Food and Drug Administration's Program against Quackery," speech delivered before the Yonkers Academy of Medicine (Yonkers, NY: May 16, 1962): 1–14.

43. Martha Dudley, "Why People Fall for Quackery," *RN* (Jan. 1963): 48–54; S. William Kalb, "Fads, Fallacies and Fakery," *Essex County (N.J.) Medical Society Bulletin* (April 1963): 165–67; K. L. Milstead, "Enforcement of Antiquackery Laws" and Warren Braren, "Broadcasting Code against Quackery," *Journal of the American Pharmaceutical Association* NS3 (Sept. 1963): 458–60, 464–67.

44. Morris Fishebein, "Quackery in American Medicine," *Medical Bulletin of Los Angeles* 92 (Aug. 16, 1962): 16, 32–38; John C. Keene and C. Grove McCown, "Medical Quackery and the Law," *Philadelphia Medicine* (Feb. 22, 1963): 219–22; Karl L. Kaufman, "Haven for Hucksters?" *Torch* (Jan. 1963): 25–28, 47–50; "Medical Quackery," *Industrial News Review* (Dec. 1963): 22–24.

45. *Proceedings: Second National Congress on Medical Quackery* (Chicago: AMA, 1963)—on the limitations and challenges faced by regulatory agencies, see Sidney W. Bishop, "Report from the Post Office Department," 17; on the challenges of educational efforts, see W. W. Bauer, "Education: A Weapon against Quackery?" 50–51; on the difficulties faced in unifying efforts in the media, see Donald Dunham, "Newspapers," 78–79; Kenneth Ward, "The Role of Advertising Agencies in Combating Medical Quackery," 85–88.

46. Charles L. Hudson, "Address of Welcome," *Proceedings: Third National Congress on Medical Quackery* (Chicago: AMA, 1966): 4–6.

47. John W. Knutson, "Address of Welcome," *Proceedings: Third National Congress on Medical Quackery*, 1–3.

48. James Harvey Young, "Combating Health Quackery: The Weapons: Enforcement and Education," in *Proceedings: Fourth Congress on Medical Quackery*, 5–6.

49. Wilbur, "Health Quackery: Costly in More Ways Than One," *Proceedings: Fourth Congress on Medical Quackery*, 2–4.

CHAPTER EIGHT

1. James Harvey Young, "Why Quackery Persists: Quacks Never Sleep," in Stephen Barrett and William T. Jarvis, eds., *The Health Robbers: How to Protect Your Money and Your Life* (Philadelphia: George F. Stickley, 1976), 317.

2. "Fight against Fraud Tracks 'Miracle Cure,'" *JAMA* 254 (Oct. 25, 1985): 2201–02; *Quackery: A $10 Billion Scandal*, Hearing before the Subcommittee on Health and Long-Term Care, 98th Congress, 2nd Session, May 31, 1984, Comm. Pub. No. 98-463 (Washington, DC: U.S. Government Printing Office, 1984), 1–4.

3. *Quackery: A $10 Billion Scandal*, 2–3, 7–8, 142–44.

4. U.S. Senate Special Committee on Aging, Frauds and Misrepresentations Affecting the Elderly, Hearings before Sub-Committee, 88th Congress, 2nd Session, Part I (Washington, DC: U.S. Government Printing Office, 1964); *A Study of Health Practices and Opinions* was conducted by National Analysts, Inc. and published by the National Technical Information Service of Springfield, VA, in June 1972; J. W. Buchan, "America's Health: Fallacies, Beliefs, Practices," *FDA Consumer* 6 (Oct. 1972): 4–10; "A Study of Health Practices and Opinions," *(Health Education and Welfare) HEW News* press release (Oct. 9, 1972): 1–4.

5. "A Study of Health Practices and Opinions," x–xii; "U.S. Overmedicated, FDA Warns," *Chicago Today* (Oct. 15, 1972): 2; Marilynn Preston, "Stay Healthy and Avoid the Swindle," *Family Today–Chicago Today* (Oct. 1, 1970): 42; Raymond O. West, "The Menace of Common Quackery," *These Times* (Feb. 1971): 28–32.

6. "A Study of Health Practices and Opinions," xii–xv; "Food, Pill Fads Gyp Millions, Report Says," *Washington Post* (Oct. 16, 1972): C1; J. A. Sabatier, "Quackery," *Journal of the Louisiana State Medical Society* 123 (May 1971): 185; Thierry Sagnier, "Medical Quackery in the U.S.," *Des Moines Tribune* (Jan. 11, 1971): 13.

7. Richard D. Lyons, "Patent Remedies Abused, FDA Says: Ads, Ignorance and Bias Are Found to Cause Overuse" *New York Times* (Oct. 9, 1972): D1; "Quackery Persists," *JAMA* 221 (Aug. 21, 1972): 217.

8. Nicholas von Hoffman, "Medicine's Unhealthy Outlook," *Chicago Tribune* (Oct. 23, 1972): 20; "Health and Hucksterism," *Time* (Oct. 23, 1972): 27–28.

9. Julian B. Roebuck and Bruce Hunter, "The Awareness of Health-Care Quackery as Deviant Behavior," *Journal of Health & Social Behavior* 18 (June 1972): 162–66; Roebuck and Hunter, "Medical Quackery as Deviant Behavior," *Criminology* 8 (May 1970): 48–62.

10. David K. Gast, "Consumer Education and the Madison Avenue Morality," *Phi Delta Kappan* 48 (June 1967): 485; "And now a word about commercials," *Time* 92 (July 12, 1968): 56; Robert E. Kime, *Health: A Consumer's Dilemma* (Belmont, CA: Wadsworth, 1970), 1–3.

11. "Feature Story," University of Wisconsin–Madison press release (Feb. 7, 1973), in "Nostrums and Quackery," Box 588, Folder 9, HHF Warren E. Schaller and Charles R. Carroll, *Health, Quackery & the Consumer* (Philadelphia: W. B. Saunders, 1976), 172.

12. William T. Jarvis, "Quackery and the Media," *FDA Consumer* (Dec. 1977): 5; Stephen Barrett, "Health Frauds and Quackery," *FDA Consumer* (Nov. 1977): 12–16; Alfred Soffer, "Consumers' Rights in Medicine," *Archives of Internal Medicine* 138 (June 1978): 905; Lawrence Cohen and Henry Rothschild, "The Bandwagons of Medicine," *Perspectives in Biology and Medicine* (Summer 1979): 531–52.

13. "A Study of Health Practices and Opinions," ii–vi; James Harvey Young, *American Self-Dosage Medicines: An Historical Perspective* (Lawrence, KA: Coronado Press, 1974), 46–52; James Harvey Young, "The Regulation of Health Quackery," *Pharmacy in History* 26 (1984): 3–12; Daniel Taktkon, *The Great Vitamin Hoax* (New York: MacMillan, 1968); Victor Herbert and Stephen Barrett, *The Vitamin Pushers: How the 'Health Food' Industry Is Selling America a Bill of Goods* (Amherst, NY: Prometheus, 1994).

14. James Harvey Young, *The Medical Messiahs: A Social History of Health Quackery in Twentieth-Century America* (Princeton: Princeton University Press, 1992), 446–48; "Vitamin and Mineral Preparations," FDA news release (Aug. 1, 1973); H.R. 643, S. 2801, *Congressional Record*, 93rd Congress, 1st Session (1976); Thomas H. Jukes, "Megavitamin Therapy," *JAMA* 233 (Aug. 11, 1975): 550–51.

15. Young, *The Medical Messiahs*, 447–48; Harold Hopkins, "Regulating Vitamins and Minerals," *FDA Consumer* 10 (July–August 1976): 10–11; Jarvis, "Quackery and the Media," 5; Philip L. White, "Megavitamin This, Megavitamin That," *JAMA* 233 (Aug. 11, 1975): 538–39.

16. James Harvey Young, "Business Booming for Medical Quacks, History Professor Warns," *American Medical News* 20 (Oct. 3, 1977): 17–18; Ray Hyman, "Occult Healing," in Stephen Barret, ed., *The Health Robbers* (2nd ed.) (Philadelphia: George F. Stickley, 1980), 34; John C. Burnham, *How Superstition Won and Science Lost: Popularizing Science and Health in the United States* (New Brunswick, NJ: Rutgers University Press, 1987).

17. Myra Heims, "Medical Quacks: Peddlers of Hope," *Medical Record News* (April 1976): 63–69; Young, *The Medical Messiahs*, 441–42; Marilynn Preston, "Stay Healthy and Avoid the Swindle," *Chicago Today* (Oct. 1, 1970): 42; Edward Finch Cox, Robert C. Fellmeth, and John E. Schulz, *The Nader Report on the Federal Trade Commission* (New York: R. W. Baron, 1969).

18. Young, *The Medical Messiahs*, 449.

19. James Harvey Young, "Combating Health Quackery: The Weapons: Enforcement and Education," in *Proceedins of the Fourth National Congress on Quackery* (Chicago: American Medical Association, 1968), 3; Brian Inglis, "Fringe Medicine," *Journal of the Royal College of Physicians* 9 (July 1975): 347–62.

20. Kime, *Health: A Consumer's Dilemma*, 3–4; Wilbur J. Cohen, *Health, Education, and Welfare: Accomplishments, 1963–1968, Problems and Challenges, and a Look to the Future* (Washington, DC: U.S. Government Printing Office, 1968); Kenneth L. Jones, Louis M. Shainberg, and Curtis O. Byer, *Consumer Health* (San Francisco: Canfield Press, 1975); Inglis, "Fringe Medicine," 347–48; E. K. Lederman, *Philosophy and Medicine* (Brookfield, VT: Gower, 1970), 26–27; George L. Engel, "The Need for a New Medical Model: A Challenge for Biomedicine," in *Concepts of Health and Disease: Interdisciplinary Perspectives*, Arthur L. Caplan, H. Tristram Engelhardt, Jr., and James J. McCartney, eds. (Reading, MA: Addison-Wesley Pub. Co, 1981), 591.

21. Stephen Barrett, "The Health Quack: Supersaleman of the Seventies," *Archives of Internal Medicine* 138 (July 1978): 1065–66.

22. Barrett, "Health Frauds and Quackery," 13–14; West, "The Menace of Common Quackery," 31; A. J. de Craen, T. J. Kaptchuk, J. G. Tijssen, and J. Kleijnen, "Placebos and Placebo Effects in Medicine: Historical Overview," *Journal of the Royal Society of Medicine* 92 (Oct. 1999): 511–15; Anne Harrington, ed., *The Placebo Effect: An Interdisciplinary Exploration* (Cambridge, MA: Harvard University Press, 1997); Arthur K. Shapiro and Elaine Shapiro, *The Powerful Placebo: From Ancient Priest to Modern Physician* (Baltimore: Johns Hopkins University Press, 1997).

23. "A Study of Health Practices and Opinions," iii–v; Young, *American Self-Dosage Medicines*, 33–61; *Advertising of Proprietary Medicines: Hearings Before the Subcommittee on Monopoly of the Select Committee on Small Business*, United States Senate, 92nd Congress, 1st Session, May 25, 1971 (Washington, DC: U.S. Government Printing Office, 1971); John D. Cooper, ed., *The Efficacy of Self-Medication*, Philosophy and Technology of Drug Assessment, Vol. IV (Washington, DC: Interdisciplinary Communication Associates, Inc., for Interdisciplinary Communications Program, Smithsonian Institution, 1973), 216–18; Charles E. Edwards, Nelson Senate Subcommittee Hearings, part 1, 1–25, 177–91; Office of Technology Assessment, *Assessing the Efficacy and Safety of Medical Technologies* (Washington, DC: U.S. Government Printing Office, 1978).

24. Leonard Tushnet, *The Medicine Men: The Myth of Quality Care in America Today* (New York: St. Martin's Press, 1971); Harry F. Dowling, *Medicines for Man: The Development, Regulation, and Use of Prescription Drugs* (New York: Alfred A. Knopf, 1970); Young, *American Self-Dosage Medicines*, 34–35; Schaller and Carroll, *Health, Quackery & the Consumer*, 174–75; Milton Silverman and Philip R. Lee, *Pills, Profits and Politics* (Berkeley: University of California Press, 1974), 262–71; *Congressional Quarterly Weekly Report*, Vol. 29, July 11, 1971, p. 4; Morton Mintz, *The Therapeutic Nightmare: A Report on Prescription Drugs, the Men Who Make Them and the Agency That Controls Them* (Boston: Houghton Mifflin, 1965).

25. Anne Harrington, *The Cure Within: A History of Mind–Body Medicine* (New York: W.W. Norton & Co., 2008), 124; Ivan Illich, *Medical Nemesis: The Expropriation of Health* (New York: Penguin, 1977); Lawrence Foss, *The End of Modern Medicine: Biomedical Science Under a Microscope* (New York: State University of New York Press, 1992); John Dupre, *The Disorder of Things: Metaphysical Foundations of the Disunity of Science* (Harvard: University of Harvard Press, 1995); Schaller and Carroll, *Health, Quackery & the Consumer*, 174–75.

26. "Commission Challenges AMA's Ethical Ban on Advertising," *FTC News Summary* (Dec. 16, 1975): 1; "Mail Law Violations Are Charged to A.M.A.: Postal Service Accuses Association of Underpaying $1,048,967 for Delivery of Medical Journal," *New York Times* (April 23, 1977): D1.

27. Frank D. Campion, *The AMA and U.S. Health Policy Since 1940* (Chicago: Chicago Review Press, 1984).

28. Marguerite Michaels, "Medicine: Sore Throat Attacks," *Time* (Aug. 18, 1975): 28; David Burnham, "4 A.M.A. Employees Quizzed on Leak," *New York Times* (Aug. 6, 1975): D1.

29. David Burnham, "A.M.A. Criticized on Chiropractic: House Unit Poses Question of Antitrust Aspects," *New York Times* (Oct. 29, 1975) D4; Susan Getzendanner, "Permanent Injunction Order against AMA," *JAMA* 259 (Jan. 1, 1988): 81–82; Norman N. Gevitz, "The Chiropractors and the AMA: Reflections on the History of the Consultation Clause," *Perspectives in Biology and Medicine* 32 (1989): 281–99.

30. "Nation: A Battle over Cancer," *Time* (Feb. 12, 1979): A1; Thomas H. Jukes, "Laetrile for Cancer," *JAMA* 236 (Sept. 13, 1976): 1284–86; Stuart Nightingale, "Laetrile: The Regulatory Challenge of an Unproven Remedy," *Public Health Reports* 99 (July–Aug. 1984): 333–38; James Harvey Young, "Laetrile in Historical Perspective," in Gerald E. Markle and James C. Petersen, eds., *Politics, Science, and Cancer: The Laetrile Phenomenon*, (Boulder, CO: Westview Press, 1981), 60; "Medicine: Debate over Laetrile," *Time* (Aug. 12, 1971): 23; Food and Drug Administration, "Laetrile: The Commissioner's Decision," HEW Publication No. 77-3056 (Washington, DC: U.S. Government Printing Office, 1977).

31. Nightingale, "Laetrile: The Regulatory Challenge of an Unproven Remedy," 333–34; Richard D. Lyons, "Backers of Laetrile Charge a Plot Is Preventing the Cure of Cancer," *New York Times* (July 13, 1977): A8; "Medicine: Victories for Laetrile's Lobby," *Time* (May 21, 1977): 12; Frederic Golden, "*Time* Essay: Freedom of Choice and Apricot Pits," *Time* (June 20, 1977): 3; "Laetrile: The Political Success of a Scientific Failure," *Consumer Reports* 42 (Aug. 1977): 444–47.

32. Nightingale, "Laetrile: The Regulatory Challenge of an Unproven Method," 336; Lawrence K. Altman, "Four Year Test of Laetrile Finds No Evidence It Can Cure Cancer," *New York Times* (June 16, 1977): 18; Mark J. Rubno and Frank Davidoff, "Cyanide Poisoning from Apricot Seeds," *JAMA* 241 (Jan. 26, 1979): 359; N. M. Ellison, D. P. Bayer, and G. R. Newell, "Special Report on Laetrile: The NCI Laetrile Review: Results of the National Cancer Institute's Retrospective Laetrile Analysis," *New England Journal of Medicine* 299 (Sept. 7, 1978): 549–52; Thomas H. Jukes, "Laetrile on Trial," *JAMA* 242 (Feb. 16, 1979): 719–20.

33. "National Cancer Institute begins Laetrile Clinical Trial," *JAMA* 244 (Feb. 8, 1980): 538; C. G. Mortel et al., "A Clinical Trail of Amygdalin (Laetrile) in the Treatment of Human Cancer," *New England Journal of Medicine* 306 (Jan. 28, 1982): 201–06; "Update on Laetrile," *FDA Drug Bulletin* 7 (Jan.–April 1977): 1; "Medicine: Laetrile Flunks," *Time* (May 11, 1981): 24; Margot Slade and Eva Hoffman, "Laetrile Verdict: It's the Pits," *New York Times* (Jan. 31, 1982): C1; Barrie Cassileth, "Laetrile by Any Other Name Is Still Bogus," *Los Angeles Times* (Jan. 1, 2001): D1.

34. "Fight against Fraud Tracks 'Miracle Cures,' " 2201–02; *Quackery: A $10 Billion Scandal*, 141–45.

35. "NCAHF's History," http://www.ncahf.org/about/history.html; Rex Dalton, "Quackbusters Inc.: Hot on the Heels of Medical Hucksters," *Scientist* 2 (May 16, 1988): 1; "National Council against Health Fraud: What is Their Agenda?" *Dynamic Chiropractic* 8 (Oct. 10, 1990): 1–5; "An Invitation to Join in Combating Health Fraud, Misinformation, and Quackery," National Council Against Health Fraud (NCAHF) Pamphlet (Loma Linda, CA: NCAHF, 1988).

36. "NCAHF's History"; "An Invitation to Join in Combating Health Fraud, Misinformation, and Quackery"; "Available Resource Materials: Sixth Edition," pamphlets (Loma Linda, CA: NACHF, n.d.).

37. Eliot Marshall, "OTA Peers into Cancer Therapy Fog," *Science* 35 (1990): 67–68; Office of Technology Assessment, *Unconventional Cancer Treatments. OTA-H-405* (Washington, DC: U.S. Government Printing Office, 1990), 3–7; Michael Lerner, "The Role of Autonomous Cancer Self-Help Groups as a 'Third Force' in the Development of New Perspectives on Health Promotion, Conventional Cancer Treatments and Complementary Systems of Cancer Therapy and Self-Care," paper presented at the World Health Organization Conference on Health Promotion and Chronic Illness, Bad Honeff, Germany, June 1987.

38. Wallace Sampson, "The Rise of Alternative Medicine: Anti-Science and Propaganda," *Profacto Newsletter* 2 (Spring 1996): 1–3.

39. *Quackery: A $10 Billion Scandal*, 141; William T. Jarvis, "How Quackery Is Promoted," in Stephen Barrett and Barrie R. Cassileth, eds., *Dubious Cancer Treatments* (Tampa, FL: American Cancer Society, 1991), 7–9.

40. Tim Gorski, "William Jarvis Speaks at Dallas–Fort Worth Council against Health Fraud Annual Meeting," *The Skeptic: The Newsletter of the North Texas Skeptics* 3 (Nov.–Dec. 1989): 1–3; William T. Jarvis, "Quackery: A National Scandal," *Clinical Chemistry* 38 (Aug. 1992): 1574–86; *Quackery: A $10 Billion Scandal*, 2.

41. "NACHF Manifesto," http://www.ncahf.org/about/manifesto.html.

42. "OAM Legislative History," 16–17 Sept. 1996, Rec. No. 443-03-4110, Box 1, Folder 10, Office of Alternative Medicine Collection (OAMC), Office of NIH History, Bethesda, MD; Eric W. Boyle, "The Politics of Alternative Medicine at the National Institutes of Health," *Federal History Journal* 3 (January 2011): 16–32.

43. Daniel Glick, "New Age Meets Hippocrates: Medicine Gets Serious about Unconventional Therapy," *Newsweek* (July 13, 1992): 32–33.

44. Natalie Angier, "U.S. Opens the Door Just a Crack to Alternative Medicine," *New York Times* (Jan. 10, 1993): 1.

45. Stephen Barrett and William T. Jarvis, eds., *The Health Robbers: A Close Look at Quackery in America* (New York: Prometheus, 1993); James Gorman, "Take a Little Deadly Nightshade and You'll Feel Better," *New York Times* (Aug. 30, 1992): A2; Arnold E. Bender, *Health or Hoax: The Truth about Health Foods and Diets* (Buffalo: Prometheus, 1986); Wallis, Horowitz, and Lafferty, "Why New Age Medicine Is Catching On," 54.

46. David M. Eisenberg, Ronald C. Kessler, et al., "Unconventional Medicine in the United States: Prevalence, Costs, and Patterns of Use," *New England Journal of Medicine* 328 (January 28, 1993): 246–52.

47. R. H. Murray and A. J. Rubel, "Physicians and Healers: Unwitting Partners in Health Care," *New England Journal of Medicine* 326 (1992): 61–64; Eisenberg, "Unconventional Medicine in the United States," 247–49; Edward W. Campion, "Why Unconventional Medicine," *New England Journal of Medicine* 328 (January 28, 1993): 282–83.

48. Trisha L. Beckstead, "Buyer Beware: Deregulation of Dietary Supplements Upon Enactment of the Dietary Supplement Health and Education Act of 1994," *San Joaquin Annual Law Review* 11 (2001): 121–54; Anthony L. Young and I. Scott Bass, "The Dietary Supplement Health and Education Act," *Food, Drug and Law Journal* 50 (1995): 285–307; Mike Mitka, "The FDA Never Promised an Herb Garden: But Buyers and Sellers Eager to See One Grow," *JAMA* 280 (1998): 1544–46; Oren G. Hatch, "Congress versus the Food and Drug Administration: How One Government Health Agency Harms the Public Health," *Journal of Public Policy and Marketing* 13 (Spring 1994): 150–52.

49. Peter Barton Hutt, "FDA Statutory Authority to Regulate the Safety of Dietary Supplements," *American Journal of Law and Medicine* 31 (2005): 155–76; Suzan Onel, "Dietary Supplements: A Definition That Is Black, White, and Gray," *American Journal of Law and Medicine* 31 (2005): 177–94; Bruce Silverglade, "The Vitamin Wars: Marketing, Lobbying and the Consumer," *Journal of Public Policy and Marketing* 13 (Spring 1994) 154–56; Stephen Barrett, "How the Dietary Supplement Health and Education Act of 1994 Weakened the FDA," http://www.quackwatch.org/02ConsumerProtection/dshea.html.

50. Lauren J. Sloane, "Herbal Garden of Good and Evil: The Ongoing Struggles of Dietary Supplement Regulation," *Administrative Law Review* 51 (Winter 1999): 135–57; Joshua H. Beisler, "Dietary Supplements and Their Discontents: FDA Regulation and the Dietary Supplement Health and Education Act of 1994," *Rutgers Law Journal* 31 (Winter 2000): 111–31; Marlys J. Mason, "Drugs or Dietary Supplements: FDA's Enforcement of DSHEA," *Journal of Public Policy and Marketing* 17 (Fall 1998): 296–302; Laura A. W. Khatcheressian, "Regulation of Dietary Supplements: Five Years of DSHEA," *Food, Drug and Law Journal* 54 (1999): 693–703.

51. Gina Kolata, "Ideas and Trends: The Unwholesome Tale of the Herb Market," *New York Times* (April 12, 1996): 1B.

52. Stephen Barrett et al., *Health Schemes, Scams, and Frauds* (Mount Vernon, NY: Consumers Union, 1990), 8–11; John H. Renner, *Health Smarts: How to Spot the Quacks, Avoid the Nonsense, and Get the Facts That Affect Your Health* (Kansas City, MO: HealthFacts Publishing, 1990); P. Joseph Lisa, *The Assault on Medical Freedom* (Norfolk, VA: Hampton Roads Publishing, 1994), 52–55, 67–91; *AMA Policy Compendium: Current Policies of the AMA House of Delegates* (Chicago: AMA, 1990).

53. Kurt Butler, *A Consumer's Guide to Alternative Medicine* (Buffalo: Prometheus, 1992); Frederick Stare, Virginia Aronson, and Stephen Barrett, *Your Guide to Good Nutrition* (Amherst, NY: Prometheus Books, 1991); Peter Skrabanek and James McCormick, *Follies and Fallacies in Medicine*; James Randi, *The Faith Healers*; Arnold Bender, *Health or Hoax? The Truth about Health Foods and Diets*; George Magner, *Chiropractic: The Victim's Perspective*; Dalton, "Quackbusters Inc.: Hot on the Heels of Medical Hucksters," 2–3.

54. Quackwatch Mission Statement," http://quackwatch.org/00AboutQuackwatch/ mission.html, updated Jan. 13, 2012; "Awards Received by Quackwatch," http://quackwatch .org/00AboutQuackwatch/Awards/awards.html, updated July 11, 2004; Leon Jaroff, "The Man Who Loves to Bust Quacks," *Time* (Apr. 22, 2001): 52; Thomas Fields-Meyer, "Doctor No: Considering Treatments That Sound Too Good to Be True? Quackbuster Stephen Barrett Has a Word for You: Don't," *People* 51 (Jan. 25, 1999): 8–9.

55. "ScienceScope," *Science* 277 (July 11, 1997): 169.

56. "NIAID's Stephen Straus to Direct NCCAM," *NIH Record* LI (Nov. 2, 1999): 3; Erik Stokstad, "Stephen Straus' Impossible Job," *Science* 288 (June 2, 2000): 1568–70; William R. Harlan, "New Opportunities and Proven Approaches in Complementary and Alternative Medicine Research at the National Institutes of Health," *Journal of Alternative and Complementary Medicine* 7 (2001): S53–59; Stephen E. Straus, "Complementary and Alternative Medicine: Challenges and Opportunities for American Medicine," *Academic Medicine* 75 (June 2000): 572–73; Richard L. Nahin and Stephen E. Straus, "Research into Complementary and Alternative Medicine: Problems and Potential," *British Medical Journal* 322 (Jan. 20, 2001): 161–63.

57. John A. Astin, "Why Patients Use Alternative Medicine: Results of a National Survey," *JAMA* 279 (May 20, 1998): 1548–1553; Ivan Barofsky, "Compliance, Adherence and the Therapeutic Alliance: Steps in the development of Self-care," *Social Science and Medicine* 12A (1978): 369–76; Kathryn Dean, "Conceptual, Theoretical, and Methodological Issues in Self-Care Research," *Social Science and Medicine* 12 (1989): 117–23.

58. Jarvis, "Quackery: A National Scandal," 1576.

59. Gorski, "William Jarvis Speaks at D/FW Council against Health Fraud Annual Meeting," 3.

60. James Harvey Young, "Patent Medicines and the Self-Help Syndrome," in Guenter B. Risse, Ronald Numbers and Judith Leavitt, eds., *Medicine without Doctors* (New York: Science History, 1977), 95.

SELECTED BIBLIOGRAPHY

ARCHIVES AND SPECIAL COLLECTIONS

Kremers Reference Files and Cowen Reference Files, American Institute of the History of Pharmacy, University of Wisconsin–Madison, Madison (AIHP).

American Medical Association Archives, Historical Health Fraud Collection, Chicago (HHF).

American Philosophical Society Library, Simon Flexner Papers, Philadelphia (APS).

Bakken Library and Museum, Manuscripts, Rare Books, and Pamphlets, Minneapolis.

College of Physicians of Philadelphia Library, Historical Collections and Manuscripts, Medical Trade Ephemera Collection Philadelphia (CPP).

Connecticut Historical Society, Manuscripts, Broadsides, and Ephemera Collections, Rare Books, Hartford.

Francis A. Countway Library of Medicine, Harvard University, Professional Manuscripts, Rare Books, Boston.

Harvard Law School Library, Rare Books, Professional Manuscripts, Boston.

Massachusetts Historical Society, Manuscripts, Rare Books, and Pamphlets, Boston.

National Archives and Record Administration, FDA Records, College Park, MD (NA).

National Library of Medicine, History of Medicine Division, Rare Books and Pamphlet Collection, Bethesda, MD.

New Hampshire Historical Society, Special Collections, Rare Books, Concord.

Social Welfare History Archives, University of Minnesota, American Social Health Association Archives, National Health Council Records, Minneapolis (SWHA).

BOOKS

Adams, Samuel Hopkins. *The Great American Fraud* (Chicago: AMA, 1913).

Albanese, Catherine L. *Nature Religion in America: From the Algonkian Indians to the New Age* (Chicago: University of Chicago Press, 1990).

Anderson, Ann. *Snake Oil, Hustlers, and Hambones: The American Medicine Show* (Jefferson, NC, McFarland and Co., 2000).

Anderson, Lee and Gregory J. Higby, eds. *The Spirit of Voluntarism: A Legacy of Commitment and Contribution: The United States Pharmacopeia, 1820–1995* (Rockville, MD: United States Pharmacopeia Convention, 1995).

Anderson, Oscar E. *Health of a Nation: Harvey W. Wiley and the Fight for Pure Food* (Chicago: University of Chicago Press, 1980).

Annual Reports 1950–1974 on the Administration of the Federal Food, Drug, and Cosmetic Act and Related Laws (Washington, DC: Department of Health, Education and Welfare, 1976).

Armstrong, David and Elizabeth Metzger Armstrong. *The Great American Medicine Show: Being an Illustrated History of Hucksters, Healers, Health Evangelists, and Heroes From Plymouth Rock to the Present* (New York: Prentice Hall, 1991).

Ausubel, Kenny. *When Healing Becomes a Crime: The Amazing Story of the Hoxsey Cancer Clinics and the Return of Alternative Therapies* (Rochester, VT: Healing Arts Press, 2000).

Baker, Robert B., Arthur L. Caplan, Linda L. Emanuel, and Stephen R. Latham, eds. *The American Medical Ethics Revolution: How the AMA's Code of Ethics Has Transformed Physicians' Relationships to Patients, Professionals, and Society* (Baltimore: Johns Hopkins University Press, 1999).

Barrett, Stephen and Gilda Knight, eds. *The Health Robbers: How to Protect Your Money and Your Life* (Philadelphia: George F. Stickley, 1976).

Barrett, Stephen and Barrie R. Cassileth, eds. *Dubious Cancer Treatments* (Tampa, FL: American Cancer Society, 1991).

Barrett, Stephen et al. *Health Schemes, Scams, and Frauds* (Mount Vernon, NY: Consumers Union, 1990).

Bender, Arnold E. *Health or Hoax: The Truth About Health Foods and Diets* (Buffalo: Prometheus, 1986).

Blake, John, ed. *Safeguarding the Public: Historical Aspects of Medicinal Drug Control* (Baltimore: Johns Hopkins University Press, 1970).

Blasingame, F. J. L., ed. *Digest of Official Actions, 1846–1958* (Chicago: AMA, 1959).

Bonner, Thomas Neville. *Becoming a Physician: Medical Education in Britain, France, Germany and the United States, 1750–1945* (New York: Oxford University Press, 1995).

Brock, Pope. *Charlatan: America's Most Dangerous Huckster, the Man Who Pursued Him, and the Age of Flimflam* (New York: Crown, 2008).

Brown, John A. *Quackery Exposed, or a Few Remarks on the Thomsonian System of Medicine; Consisting of Testimonies and Extracts From Various Writers* (Boston: 1833).

Brynner, Rock and Trent Stephens. *A Dark Remedy: The Impact of Thalidomide and Its Revival as a Vital Medicine* (New York: Basic Books, 2001).

Burnham, John C. *How Superstition Won and Science Lost: Popularizing Science and Health in the United States* (New Brunswick, NJ: Rutgers University Press, 1987).

Burrow, James G. *AMA: Voice of American Medicine* (Baltimore: Johns Hopkins Press, 1963).

Burrow, James G. *Organized Medicine in the Progressive Era: The Move Toward Monopoly* (Baltimore: Johns Hopkins University Press, 1977).

Butler, Kurt. *A Consumer's Guide to Alternative Medicine* (Buffalo: Prometheus, 1992).

Bynum, W. F. *Science and the Practice of Medicine in the Nineteenth Century* (Cambridge: Cambridge University Press, 1994).

Bynum W. F., and Roy Porter, eds. *Medical Fringe and Medical Orthodoxy, 1750–1850* (London: Croom Helm, 1987).

Campion, Frank D. *The AMA and U.S. Health Policy Since 1940* (Chicago: Chicago Review Press, 1984).

Carpenter, Daniel. *Reputation and Power: Organizational Image and Pharmaceutical Regulation at the FDA* (Princeton, NJ: Princeton University Press, 2010).

Cassedy, James H. *Medicine in America: A Short History* (Baltimore: Johns Hopkins University Press, 1991).

Collins, Selwyn D., ed. *The Incidence of Illness and the Volume of Medical Services Among 9,000 Canvassed Families* (Washington, DC: U.S. Public Health Service, 1944).

Committee on the Costs of Medical Care. *Medical Care for the American People* (Chicago: University of Chicago Press, 1932).

Cook, James. *Remedies and Rackets: The Truth About Patent Medicines* (New York: W. W. Norton, 1958).

Coulter, Harris. *Divided Legacy: A History of the Schism in Medical Thought*, Vol. 3 (Washington, DC: McGrath, 1973).

Cramp, Arthur J. *Nostrums and Quackery: Articles on the Nostrum Evil and Quackery Reprinted from the Journal of the American Medical Association* (2nd ed.) (Chicago: AMA, 1913).

Cramp, Arthur J. *Nostrums and Quackery and Pseudo-Medicine* (Chicago: AMA, 1936).

Cramp, Arthur J. *The Propaganda for Reform in Proprietary Medicines*, Vol. I (Chicago: AMA, 1922).

Cunningham, Andrew, and Perry Williams, eds. *The Laboratory Revolution in Medicine* (Cambridge: Cambridge University Press, 1992).

Daemmrich, Arthur. *Pharmacopolitics: Drug Regulation in the United States and Germany* (Chapel Hill: University of North Carolina Press, 2004).

Dixon, Edward H. *A Treatise on Diseases of the Sexual Organs: Adapted to Popular and Professional Reading, and the Exposition of Quackery, Professional and Otherwise* (New York: Taylor, 1845).

Dowling, Harry F. *Medicines for Man: The Development, Regulation, and Use of Prescription Drug* (New York: Alfred A. Knopf, 1970).

Dunn, Charles Wesley. *The Federal Food, Drug, and Cosmetic Act: A Statement of Its Legislative Record* (New York: G. E. Stechert and Co., 1938).

Dupre, John. *The Disorder of Things: Metaphysical Foundations of the Disunity of Science* (Cambridge, MA: Harvard University Press, 1995).

Epperson, J. P. *A Bomb in the Camp of the Enemy, or an Exposure of Quackery and 'Patent Medicines'* (Columbia, TN: Rosboroughs & Kidd, 1845).

Fishbein, Morris. *The Medical Follies: An Analysis of the Foibles of Some Healing Cults, Including Osteopathy, Homeopathy, Chiropractic, and the Electronic Reactions of Abrams, with Essays on The Antivivisectionists, Health Legislation, Physical Culture, Birth Control, and Rejuvenation* (New York: Boni and Liveright, 1925).

Fishbein, Morris. *A History of the American Medical Association, 1847 to 1947* (Philadelphia: W. B. Saunders, 1947).

Flexner, Abraham. *Medical Education in the United States and Canada: A Report to the Carnegie Foundation for the Advancement of Teaching* (New York: Carnegie Foundation, 1910).

Foss, Lawrence. *The End of Modern Medicine: Biomedical Science under a Microscope* (New York: State University of New York Press, 1992).

Freidson, Eliot. *Professional Dominance: The Social Structure of Medicine* (New York: Atherton, 1970).

Freidson, Eliot. *Profession of Medicine* (New York, Dodd, Mead, 1970).

Garceau, Oliver. *The Political Life of the American Medical Association* (Hamden, CT: Archon Books, 1961).

Gevitz, Norman. *Other Healers: Unorthodox Medicine in America* (Baltimore: Johns Hopkins University Press, 1988).

Gevitz, Norman. *The D.O.'s: Osteopathic Medicine in America* (Baltimore: Johns Hopkins University Press, 1991).

Gieryn, Thomas. *Cultural Boundaries of Science: Credibility on the Line* (Chicago: University of Chicago Press, 1999).

Goodwin, Lorine Swainston. *The Pure Food, Drink, and Drug Crusaders, 1879–1914* (New York: McFarlan & Co., 1999).

Haller, John S. *The History of Homeopathy: The Academic Years, 1820–1910* (Binghamton, NY: Haworth Press, 2005).

Haller, John S. *Medical Protestants: The Eclectics in American Medicine, 1825–1939* (Carbondale: Southern Illinois University Press, 1994).

Haller, John S. *American Medicine in Transition, 1840–1910* (Urbana: University of Illinois Press, 1981).

Harding, T. Swann. *Fads, Frauds and Physicians: Diagnosis and Treatment of the Doctor's Dilemma* (New York: Dial Press, 1930).

Harrington, Anne. *The Cure Within: A History of Mind-Body Medicine* (New York: W. W. Norton & Co., 2008).

Harrington, Anne, ed. *The Placebo Effect: An Interdisciplinary Exploration* (Cambridge, MA: Harvard University Press, 1997).

Harrison, John P. *A Lecture on the Best Mode of Discouraging Empiricism* (Cincinnati: R. P. Donogh, 1843).

Hawthorne, Fran. *Inside the FDA: The Business and Politics behind the Drugs We Take and the Food We Eat* (Hoboken, NJ: John Wiley & Sons, 2005).

Herbert, Victor and Stephen Barrett. *The Vitamin Pushers: How the "Health Food" Industry is Selling America a Bill of Goods* (Amherst, NY: Prometheus, 1994).

Higby, Gregory J. and Elaine C. Stroud, eds. *The Inside Story of Medicines: A Symposium* (Madison, WI: American Institute of the History of Pharmacy, 1997).

Higby, Gregory J. ed., *One Hundred Years of the National Formulary: A Symposium* (Madison, WI: American Institute of the History of Pharmacy, 1989).

Hilts, Phillip J. *Protecting America's Health: The FDA, Business, and One Hundred Years of Regulation* (New York: Alfred A. Knopf, 2003).

Holbrook, Steward H. *The Golden Age of Quackery* (New York: MacMillan, 1959).

Hooker, Worthington. *The Treatment Due from the Profession to Physicians Who Become Homœopathic Practitioners* (Norwhich, CT: John G. Cooley, 1852).

Horsch, Carl H. *Facts Regarding the Medical Profession and Sanitary Science: The Pathies, Isms and Quackery* (Dover, NH: State Press Job Print, 1883).

Illich, Ivan. *Medical Nemesis: The Expropriation of Health* (New York: Penguin, 1977).

Jackson, Charles O. *Food and Drug Legislation in the New Deal* (Princeton, NJ: Princeton University Press, 1970).

Johnston, Robert, ed. *The Politics of Healing: Histories of Alternative Medicine in Twentieth-Century North America* (New York: Routledge, 2004).

Juhnke, Eric S. *Quacks and Crusaders: The Fabulous Careers of John Brinkley, Norman Baker, and Harry Hoxsey* (Lawrence: University of Kansas Press, 2002).

Kallet, Arthur and F. J. Schlink. *100,000,000 Guinea Pigs* (New York: Vanguard Press, 1933).

Kaufman, Martin. *Homeopathy in America: The Rise and Fall of a Medical Heresy* (Baltimore: Johns Hopkins University Press, 1971).

Kett, Joseph. *The Formation of the American Medical Profession: The Role of Institutions, 1780–1860* (New Haven, CT: Yale University Press, 1968).

King, Dan. *Quackery Unmasked: A Consideration of the Most Prominent Empirical Schemes of the Present Time, with an Enumeration of Some of the Causes Which Contribute to Their Support* (Boston: David Clapp, 1858).

Kleinfeld, Vincent and Charles Wesley Dunn. *Federal Food, Drug and Cosmetic Act, Judicial and Administrative Record* (New York: Commerce Clearing House, 1949).

Laird, Pamela. *Advertising Progress: American Business and the Rise of Consumer Marketing* (Baltimore: Johns Hopkins University Press, 1998).

Lamb, Ruth Deforest. *American Chamber of Horrors: The Truth about Food and Drugs* (New York: Farrar & Rinehart, 1936).

Lears, Jackson. *Fables of Abundance: A Cultural History of Advertising in America* (New York: Basic Books, 1994).

Leavitt Judith Walzer and Ronald L. Numbers, eds. *Sickness and Health in America: Reading in the History of Medicine and Public Health* (Madison: University of Wisconsin Press, 1985).

Liebenau, Jonathan. *The Formation of the American Pharmaceutical Industry* (Baltimore: Johns Hopkins University Press, 1987).

Lisa, P. Joseph. *The Assault on Medical Freedom* (Norfolk, VA: Hampton Roads Publishing, 1994).

Ludmerer, Kenneth. *Learning to Heal: The Development of American Medical Education* (New York: Basic Books, 1985).

Ludmerer, Kenneth. *A Time to Heal: American Medical Education from the Turn of the Century to the Era of Managed Care* (New York: Oxford University Press, 1999).

Markle, Gerald E. and James C. Petersen, eds. *Politics, Science, and Cancer: The Laetrile Phenomenon* (Boulder, CO: Westview Press, 1981).

Marks, Harry M. *The Progress of Experiment: Science and Therapeutic Reform in the United States, 1900–1990* (New York: Cambridge University Press, 1997).

Mason, Augustus. *The Quackery of the Age: A Satire of the Times* (Boston: White, Lewis & Potter, 1845).

McNamara, Brooks. *Step Right Up* (Jackson: University of Mississippi Press, 1995).

Mintz, Morton. *The Therapeutic Nightmare: A Report on Prescription Drugs, the Men Who Make Them and the Agency That Controls Them* (Boston: Houghton Mifflin, 1965).

Moore, J. Stuart. *Chiropractic in America: The History of a Medical Alternative* (Baltimore: Johns Hopkins University Press, 1993).

Mosher, Alanson. *Learned Quackery Exposed: Or the Difference Shown Between Poisons and Medicines* (Schoharie: Gallup and Lawyer, 1846).

Murphy, Lamar Riley. *Enter the Physician: The Transformation of Domestic Medicine, 1760– 1860* (Tuscaloosa: University of Alabama Press, 1991).

National Analysts. *A Study of Health Practices and Opinions* (Springfield, VA: 1972).

New and Non-Official Remedies (1st ed.) (Chicago: American Medical Association, 1907).

Numbers, Ronald L., ed. *The Education of American Physicians: Historical Essays* (Berkeley: University of California Press, 1980).

Office of Technology Assessment, *Unconventional Cancer Treatments. OTA-H-405* (Washington, DC: U.S. Government Printing Office, 1990).

Parascandola, John. *The Development of American Pharmacology: John H. Abel and the Shaping of a Discipline* (Baltimore: Johns Hopkins University Press, 1992).

Parascandola, John. *Studies in the History of Modern Pharmacology and Drug Therapy* (Farnham, UK: Ashgate, 2012).

Pellegrino, Edmund and David C. Thomasma. *A Philosophical Basis of Medical Practice* (New York: Oxford University Press, 1981).

Pernick, Martin. *A Calculus of Suffering: Pain, Professionalism and Anesthesia in Nineteenth-Century America* (New York: Columbia University Press, 1985).

Porter, Roy. *Quacks: Fakers and Charlatans in Medicine* (Gloucestershire, UK: Tempus, 2003, revised edition).

Porter, William. *Life and Its Forces: Health and Disease Correctly Defined. A Reliable Guide to Health without the Use of Mineral or Vegetable Poisons, or Irritants* (Hartford, CT: Case, Lockwood & Brainard Co., 1878).

Pray, W. Steven. *A History of Nonprescription Product Regulation* (Binghamton, NY: Pharmaceutical Products Press, 2003).

Rayack, Elton. *Professional Power and American Medicine: The Economics of the American Medical Association* (New York: World Publishing, 1967).

Reed, Louis S. *The Healing Cults: A Study of Sectarian Medical Practice: Its Extent, Causes, and Control* (Chicago: University of Chicago Press, 1932).

Renner, John H. *Health Smarts: How to Spot the Quacks, Avoid the Nonsense, and Get the Facts That Affect Your Health* (Kansas City, MO: HealthFacts Publishing, 1990).

Risse, Guenter B., Ronald L. Numbers, and Judith Walzer Leavitt, eds. *Medicine Without Doctors: Home Health Care in American History* (New York: Science History, 1977).

Robins, Natali. *Copeland's Cure: Homeopathy and the War Between Conventional and Alternative Medicine* (New York: Alfred A. Knopf, 2005).

Rogers, Naomi. *An Alternative Path: The Making and Remaking of Hahnemann Medical College and Hospital of Philadelphia* (New Brunswick, NJ: Rutgers University Press, 1998).

Rorem, C. Rufus and Robert P. Fischelis. *The Costs of Medicine: The Manufacture and Distribution of Drugs and Medicines in the United States and the Services of Pharmacy in Medical Care* (Chicago: University of Chicago Press, 1932).

Rosen, George. *The Structure of American Medical Practice, 1875–1941* (Philadelphia: University of Pennsylvania Press, 1983).

Rosenberg, Charles. *The Care of Strangers: The Rise of America's Hospital System* (New York: Basic Books, 1987).

Rothstein, William. *American Medical Schools and the Practice of Medicine: A History* (New York: Oxford University Press, 1987).

Rothstein, William. *American Physicians in the 19th Century: From Sects to Science* (Baltimore: Johns Hopkins University Press, 1972).

Salmon, J. Warren, ed. *Alternative Medicine: Popular and Policy Perspectives* (New York: Tavistock, 1984).

Schaller, Warren E. and Charles R. Carroll. *Health, Quackery & the Consumer* (Philadelphia: W. B. Saunders, 1976).

Shapin, Steven. *A Social History of Truth: Civility and Science in Seventeenth-Century England* (Chicago: University of Chicago Press, 1994).

Shapiro, Arthur K. and Elaine Shapiro. *The Powerful Placebo: From Ancient Priest to Modern Physician* (Baltimore: Johns Hopkins University Press, 1997).

Silverman, Milton and Philip R. Lee. *Pills, Profits, and Politics* (Berkeley: University of California Press, 1974).

Sivulka, Juliann. *Stronger Than Dirt: A Cultural History of Advertising Personal Hygiene in America, 1875 to 1940* (New York: Humanity Books, 2001).

Smith, Elmer L. *Patent Medicine: The Golden Days of Quackery* (Lebanon, PA: Applied Arts, 1979).

Smith, Mickey. *Small Comfort: A History of Minor Tranquilizers* (New York: Praeger, 1985).

Sollmann, Torald. *The Broader Aims of the Council on Pharmacy of the American Medical Association* (Chicago: American Medical Association, 1908).

Starr, Paul. *The Social Transformation of American Medicine: The Rise of a Sovereign Profession and the Making of a Vast Industry* (New York: Basic Books, 1982).

Swann, John P. *Academic Scientists and the Pharmaceutical Industry: Cooperative Research in Twentieth-Century America* (Baltimore: Johns Hopkins University Press, 1988).

Taktkon, Daniel. *The Great Vitamin Hoax* (New York: MacMillan, 1968).

Taylor, Othniel Hart. *Medical Reform and the Present System of Medical Instruction: An Address Delivered at the Semi-Annual Meeting of the New Jersey Medical Society* (Camden, NJ: Gray & Elliott, 1850).

Temin, Peter. *Taking Your Medicine: Drug Regulation in the United States* (Cambridge, MA: Harvard University Press, 1980).

Tomes, Nancy. *The Gospel of Germs: Men, Women, and the Microbe in American Life* (Cambridge, MA: Harvard University Press, 1998).

Toumey, Christopher. *Conjuring Science: Scientific Symbols and Cultural Meanings in American Life* (New Brunswick, NJ: Rutgers University Press, 1996).

Tushnet, Leonard. *The Medicine Men: The Myth of Quality Care in America Today* (New York: St. Martin's Press, 1971).

Vogel, Morris J. and Charles E. Rosenberg, eds. *The Therapeutic Revolution: Essays in the Social History of American Medicine* (Philadelphia: University of Pennsylvania Press, 1979).

Warner, Charles W. *Quacks* (Jackson, MI: 1930).

Warner, John Harley. *The Therapeutic Perspective: Medical Practice, Knowledge, and Identity in America, 1820–1885* (Princeton, NJ: Princeton University Press, 1997).

Whorton, James C. *Nature Cures: The History of Alternative Medicine in America* (New York: Oxford University Press, 2002).

Whorton, James C. *Inner Hygiene: Constipation and the Pursuit of Health in Modern Society* (New York: Oxford University Press, 2000).

Wiley, Harvey W. *An Autobiography* (Indianapolis: Bobbs-Merrill, 1930).

Wrobel, Arthur. *Pseudo-Science and Society in Nineteenth Century America* (Lexington: University Press of Kentucky, 1987).

Young, James Harvey. *The Toadstool Millionaires: A Social History of Patent Medicines in America before Federal Regulation* (Princeton: Princeton University Press, 1961).

Young, James Harvey. *American Self-Dosage Medicines: An Historical Perspective* (Lawrence, KN: Coronado, 1974).

Young, James Harvey. *Pure Food: Securing the Federal Food and Drugs Act of 1906* (Princeton, NJ: Princeton University Press, 1989).

Young, James Harvey. *The Medical Messiahs: A Social History of Health Quackery in Twentieth-Century America* (Princeton, NJ: Princeton University Press, 1992).

Young, James Harvey, ed., *The Early Years of Federal Food and Drug Control* (Madison, WI: American Institute of the History of Pharmacy, 1982).

ARTICLES

Albanese, Catherine L. "Physic and Metaphysic in Nineteenth-Century America: Medical Sectarians and Religious Healing." *Church History* 55 (Dec. 1986): 489–502.

Arthur, Irvin. "The Medical Profession and the People." *Journal of the Indiana State Medical Association* 16 (Nov. 1923): 369.

Astin, John A. "Why Patients Use Alternative Medicine: Results of a National Survey." *JAMA* 279 (May 20, 1998): 1548–1553.

Barrett, Stephen. "Health Frauds and Quackery." *FDA Consumer* (Nov. 1977): 12–16.

Billings, Frank. "The Medical Profession and the Medical Journals in Relation to Nostrums." *JAMA* 46 (March 10, 1906): 715–19.

Boyle, Eric W. "The Politics of Alternative Medicine at the National Institutes of Health." *Federal History Journal* 3 (January 2011): 16–32.

Brieger, Gert H. "Bodies and Borders: A New Cultural History of Medicine." *Perspectives in Biology and Medicine* 47 (Summer 2004): 402–21.

Burnham, John C. "American Medicine's Golden Age: What Happened to It?" *Science* 215 (March 19, 1982): 1474–79.

Cantor, David. "Cancer Quackery and the Vernacular Meanings of Hope in 1950s America." *Journal of the History of Medicine and Allied Sciences* 61 (July 2006): 324–68.

Cohen, Lawrence and Henry Rothschild. "The Bandwagons of Medicine." *Perspectives in Biology and Medicine* (Summer 1979): 531–52.

Cramp, Arthur J. "Modern Advertising and the Nostrum." *American Journal of Public Health* 8 (1918): 756–58.

Cramp, Arthur J. "Therapeutic Thaumaturgy." *American Mercury* 3 (1924): 423–30.

Cramp, Arthur J. "The Nostrum and the Public Health." *New England Journal of Medicine* 201 (1929): 1297–1300.

Cramp, Arthur J. "The Bureau of Investigation of the American Medical Association." *American Journal of Police Science* 2 (July–Aug. 1931): 285–89.

Cramp, Arthur J. "The Work of the Bureau of Investigation." *Law and Contemporary Problems* 1 (Dec. 1933): 51–54.

de Craen, A. J., T. J. Kaptchuk, J. G. Tijssen, and J. Kleijnen. "Placebos and Placebo Effects in Medicine: Historical Overview." *Journal of the Royal Society of Medicine* 92 (Oct. 1999): 511–15.

Eisenberg, David M., Ronald C. Kessler, et al. "Unconventional Medicine in the United States: Prevalence, Costs, and Patterns of Use." *The New England Journal of Medicine* 328 (Jan. 28, 1993): 246–252.

Eisenberg, David M., Roger B. Davis, et al. "Trends in Alternative Medicine Use in the United States, 1990–1997: Results of a Follow–up National Survey." *JAMA* 280 (Nov. 11, 1998): 1569–75.

Estes, J. Worth. "Public Pharmacology: Modes of Action of Nineteenth-Century 'Patent' Medicines." *Medical Heritage* 2 (1986): 218–28

Fontanarosa, Phil B., and George D. Lundberg. "Alternative Medicine Meets Science." *JAMA* 280 (1998): 1618–19.

Gieryn, Thomas. "Boundary-Work and the Demarcation of Science from Non-Science: Strains and Interests in Professional Ideologies of Scientists." *American Sociological Review* 48 (Dec. 1983): 781–95.

Goldstein, Michael S. "The Persistence and Resurgence of Medical Pluralism." *Journal of Health Politics, Policy and Law* 29 (Aug.–Oct. 2004): 926–45.

Goode, Jackie and David Greatbatch. "Boundary Work: The Production and consumption of Health Information and Advice." *Journal of Consumer Culture* 5 (2005): 315–37.

Hufford, David. "Cultural and Social Perspectives on Alternative Medicine." *Alternative Therapies* 1 (1995): 53–61.

Hutt, Peter Barton. "FDA Statutory Authority to Regulate the Safety of Dietary Supplements." *American Journal of Law and Medicine* 31 (2005): 155–76.

Jackson, Charles O. "Muckraking and Consumer Protection: The Case of the 1938 Food, Drug and Cosmetic Act." *Pharmacy in History* 13 (1971): 103–10.

Janssen, Wallace. "Outline of the History of U. S. Drug Regulation and Labeling." *Food, Drug, Cosmetic Law Journal* 36 (1981): 420–41.

Jarvis, William T. "Quackery: A National Scandal." *Clinical Chemistry* 38 (Aug. 1992): 1574–86.

McFadyen, Richard E. "Thalidomide in America: A Brush with Tragedy." *Clio Medica* 11 (1976): 79–93.

Marks, Harry M. "Revisiting The Origins of Compulsory Drug Prescriptions." *American Journal of Public Health* 85 (January 1995): 109–15.

Nahin, Richard L. and Stephen E. Straus. "Research into Complementary and Alternative Medicine: Problems and Potential." *British Medical Journal* 322 (Jan. 20, 2001): 161–63.

Nichols, John. "Medical Sectarianism." *JAMA* 60 (1913): 331–37.

Numbers, Ronald. "The History of American Medicine: A Field in Ferment." *Reviews in American History* 10 (1982): 245–63.

Parascandola, John. "Patent Medicines in Nineteenth-Century America." *Caduceus* 1 (1985): 1–39.

Perkins, Barbara Bridgman "Economic Organization of Medicine and the Committee on the Costs of Medical Care." *American Journal of Public Health* 88 (1998): 1721–26.

Pescosolido, Bernice A. and Jack K. Martin. "Cultural Authority and the Sovereignty of American Medicine: The Role of Networks, Class, and Community." *Journal of Health Politics, Policy and Law* 29 (Aug.–Oct. 2004): 735–56.

Pescosolido, Bernice A. "Beyond Rational Choice: The Social Dynamics of How People Seek Help." *American Journal of Sociology* 97 (1992): 1096–1138.

"Relations of Pharmacy to the Medical Profession." Parts I through VIII. *JAMA* 34 (April 21, 1900): 986–88; (April 28, 1900): 1049–51; (May 5, 1900) 1114–16; (May 12, 1900); 1178–79; (May 26, 1900) 1327–29; (June 2, 1900) 1405–07; *JAMA* 35 (July 7, 1900): 27–29; (July 14, 1900): 89–91.

Ross, Joseph S. "The Committee on the Costs of Medical Care and the History of Health Insurance in the United States." *Einstein Quarterly Journal of Biological Medicine* 19 (2002): 129–34

Sherman, Max and Steven Strauss. "Thalidomide: A Twenty-Five Year Perspective." *FDCLJ* 41 (1986): 458–66.

Shryock, Richard H. "Empiricism versus Rationalism in American Medicine, 1650–1950." *Proceedings of the American Antiquarian Society* (April 1969): 99–150.

Simmons, George H. "Proprietary Medicines: Some General Considerations." *JAMA* 44 (May 5, 1906): 1334–40.

Sollmann, Torald. "The Broader Aims of the Council on Pharmacy and Chemistry." *JAMA* 50 (April 4, 1908): 1134–38.

Sollmann, Torald. "Experimental Therapeutics." *JAMA* 58 (Jan. 27, 1912): 244–45.

Sollmann, Torald. "Therapeutic Research." *JAMA* 58 (May 4, 1912): 1390–92.

Sollmann, Torald. "Yesterday, Today and Tomorrow: The Activities of the Council on Pharmacy and Chemistry." *JAMA* 61 (July 12, 1912): 5–6.

Swann, John P. "FDA and the Practice of Pharmacy: The History of Prescription Drug Regulation Before the Durham-Humphrey Amendment of 1951." *Pharmacy in History* 36 (1994): 55–70.

Temin, Peter. "The Origin of Compulsory Drug Prescriptions." *Journal of Law and Economics* 22 (April 1979): 91–105.

Tomes, Nancy. "The Great American Medicine Show Revisited." *Bulletin of the History of Medicine* 79 (Winter 2005): 627–663.

Torbeson, Michael S. and Jonathan Erlen. "A Case Study of the Lash's Bitters Company: Advertising Changes after the Federal Food and Drugs Act of 1906 and the Sherley Amendment of 1912." *Pharmacy in History* 45 (2003): 139–49.

Wailoo, Keith. "Sovereignty and Science: Revisiting the Role of Science in the Construction and Erosion of Medical Dominance." *Journal of Health Politics, Policy and Law* 29 (Aug.–Oct. 2004): 643–59.

Waitzkin, Howard. "A Critical Theory of Medical Discourse: Ideology, Social Control, and the Processing of Social Context in Medical Encounters." *Journal of Health and Social Behavior* 30 (June 1989): 220–39.

Warner, John Harley. "The 'Nature-Trusting Heresy': American Physicians and the Concept of the Healing Power of Nature." *Perspectives in American History* 11 (1977–1978): 291–324.

Warner, John Harley. "Science in Medicine." *Osiris* 1 (1985): 37–58.

Warner, John Harley. "Ideals of Science and Their Discontents in Late Nineteenth-Century American Medicine." *Isis* 82 (1991): 454–78.

Warner, John Harley. "Grand Narrative and Its Discontents: Medical History and the Social Transformation of American Medicine." *Journal of Health Politics, Policy and Law* 29 (Aug.–Oct. 2004): 758–80.

Wynn, Frank B. "The Physician: Pathies, Isms and Cults in Medicine." *Journal of the Indiana State Medical Association* 14 (June 1921): 187–88.

INDEX

NDA. *See* New drug application
Neurosine poisoning, 55, 56
New and Non-Official Remedies (American Medical Association), 23, 25, 44, 54, 92; FDA and, 141, 142; Luminal (phenobarbital) in, 48; Pure Food and Drugs Act and, 36, 38; rules governing inclusion in, 26–27
New Deal reforms, 91, 102, 103. *See also* Federal Food, Drug and Cosmetics Act (1938)
New drug application (NDA), 113, 121, 143, 145, 149
New England Journal of Medicine, 171–72
Newspapers. *See* Press; *specific newspapers*
Newsweek (magazine), 170–71
New York Medical Journal, 29–30, 44
Nightingale, Stuart L., 166, 169
NIH. *See* National Institutes of Health
Nostrums. *See* Patent medicines; Secret nostrums
Nostrums and Quackery (Cramp), 65–67
Nutritional myths, 156
Nutting, J. H., 5–6, 11

OAM. *See* Office of Alternative Medicine
Office for the Study of Unconventional Medical Practices, 170
Office of Alternative Medicine (OAM) at the National Institutes of Health, xxi, 175
Office of Technology Assessment, 168, 169
100,000,000 Guinea Pigs (Schlink & Kallet), 98
Ornish, Dean, 170
Osler, William, 8–9, 11
Osteopaths, 87, 96

Palisade Manufacturing Company, 49
Patent medicines, 1–2, 4, 62; advertising of, 10–11, 12, 13, 18, 40–45, 105; Cramp on, 68–69; cures for epilepsy, 48–49; labeling of contents, 18–19, 99, 109, 112; muckrakers and, 98; press and,
40–45, 82; proprietary medicines compared, 23, 67–68; Pure Food and Drugs Act and, 34–38; scientific imagery used to promote, 10–11, 18, 49–50; self-care option and, 10, 17, 93. *See also* Drug (pharmaceutical) manufacturers; Secret nostrums
Pennsylvania Congress to Combat Health Quackery, 146
Pennsylvania Orthopaedic Institute and School of Mechano-Therapy, 57
Pennsylvania State Medical Society, 19–20
Pepper Committee (U.S. Congress), 151–52, 158, 166, 169
Petrolagar, 49
Pharmaceutical companies. *See* Drug (pharmaceutical) manufacturers
Pharmaceutical Manufacturers' Association, 144
Pharmacist (journal), 19
Pharmacists lobby, 115, 147
Phoenix *Republican* (newspaper), 41
Placebo effect, 160, 161, 169
Postal Service, U.S., 152, 162, 175
Post Office Department, U.S., 74, 76–77, 100; mail fraud and, 75, 77, 134–35, 158
Prescription medications, xix, 111, 112, 115, 161; chemotherapeutic revolution and, 118–19; over-the-counter drugs and, 116–17; sulfathiazole case and, 113–14
Press, 81, 105–6, 140, 141; freedom of, 6, 156; patent medicine advertising and, 40–45; thalidomide disaster and, 145. *See also* Muckraking journalists
Propaganda Department, American Medical Association, 60, 62–74, 77, 80, 88; cancer cures and, 85; chiropractic and, 86–87; correspondence network and, 78–81; educational efforts of, 63, 69, 70–74; establishment of, xviii; homeopathic remedies and, 84; "knocks and boosts" file, 81–83; self-medication and, 92. *See also* Bureau of Investigation,

About the Author

ERIC W. BOYLE earned his PhD in the History of Science, Technology, and Medicine from the University of California–Santa Barbara in 2007. He has taught courses in the history of medicine at the University of California-Santa Barbara, Cal Poly State University, and the University of Wisconsin–Madison. He is currently an archivist at the National Museum of Health and Medicine and lecturer for the University of Maryland.